Techniques in
GENERAL THORACIC SURGERY

Techniques in
GENERAL

THORACIC SURGERY

R. MAURICE HOOD, M.D.

Formerly Professor of Clinical Surgery,
Department of Surgery, New York University,
School of Medicine, New York, New York
Attending Surgeon, Bellevue Hospital,
Manhattan Veterans Administration Hospital,
New York, New York

With Contributions by:
    Homer S. Arnold, M.D.
    John H. Calhoon, M.D.

Second Edition

Illustrations by GRANT LASHBROOK

Lea & Febiger

PHILADELPHIA · BALTIMORE · HONG KONG
LONDON · MUNICH · SYDNEY · TOKYO

A WAVERLY COMPANY
1993

Lea & Febiger
Box 3024
200 Chester Field Parkway
Malvern, Pennsylvania 19355-9725
U.S.A.
(215) 251-2230

Executive Editor—Carroll C. Cann
Development Editor—Susan Hunsberger
Manuscript Editor—Jessica Howie Martin
Production Manager—Robert N. Spahr

Library of Congress Cataloging-in-Publication Data

Hood, R. Maurice (Raleigh Maurice), 1924–
    Techniques in general thoracic surgery / R. Maurice Hood;
illustrations by Grant Lashbrook.—2nd ed.
        p.   cm.
    Includes bibliographical references and index.
    ISBN 0-8121-1546-5
    1. Chest—Surgery. I. Title.
    [DNLM: 1. Thoracic Surgery—methods.   WF 980 H777t 1993]
    RD536.H654   1993
    617.5′4059—dc20
    DNLM/DLC   93-3486
    for Library of Congress   CIP

Reprints of chapters may be purchased from Lea & Febiger in quantities of 100 or more. Contact Sally
Grande in the Sales Department.

Print number: 5   4   3   2   1

Dedication

This volume is dedicated to Dr. Herbert Sloan. Dr. Sloan completed his surgical training at the Johns Hopkins Hospital in 1943 after a 3-year period of Army service in the Far East, during which time he became interested in thoracic surgery. He returned to the University of Michigan and completed an additional 3 years of training under John Alexander and Cameron Haight.

Dr. Sloan was appointed Assistant Professor of Surgery in 1950 and rose progressively through the academic ranks to become Professor of Surgery in 1962. He assumed the chairmanship of the section of Thoracic Surgery in 1970. At the time of this writing, he is retiring from the chairmanship of the section and assuming a new role as Chief of Clinical Affairs of the University Hospital. He received recognition by being elected president of both the American Association for Thoracic Surgery and the Society of Thoracic Surgery. He has received numerous awards and honors. Among his accomplishments have been positions of responsibility on the American Board of Thoracic Surgery and 19 medical societies.

Dr. Sloan served as the editor of the Annals of Thoracic Surgery from 1969 to 1984. He has written 143 papers and has co-authored 11 chapters in textbooks, including a text on chest trauma.

More than these tangibles, Dr. Sloan perpetuated the tradition of excellence of the thoracic surgical training program at Ann Arbor begun by John Alexander and continued by Cameron Haight. He has, more than anyone, maintained the professional interest in general thoracic surgery while creating a first-rate cardiac surgery program at the university.

I came under his influence in 1952 as a resident in thoracic surgery. He is an outstanding surgeon, teacher, and counselor, and ever a model of honesty and integrity. He has influenced the lives of more young surgeons than did his predecessors.

It is with profound respect and gratitude that this book is dedicated in the hope that it meets Herb's standard of excellence.

R. Maurice Hood

Preface

The 7 years since the first edition of this book was published have seen many changes in thoracic surgery and in surgery in general. The development of lung transplant as a viable, practical operation for chronic pulmonary disease has opened a new era in surgery scarcely dreamed of a generation ago. Lung transplantation is becoming an integral part of the specialty. Likewise, the technologic advances in fiberoptics and electronics have made surgical endoscopic procedures the fastest-growing area of all surgery including those involving the thorax.

The multidisciplinary approach to lung cancer and esophageal malignancies has modified the surgical approach to these diseases. Some of the developments have been real advances and some have been counterproductive.

New chapters have been added to cover these developing areas. Many new illustrations have been added, particularly in the section on esophageal surgery.

I have endeavored to write in a style that will be most helpful to residents in surgery, thoracic fellows, and general surgeons. The response of faculty and trainees to the first edition has been gratifying. I hope this edition will be a credit to my teachers and associates. Dr. Frank C. Spencer, who encouraged me to write the first volume, has continued to be an inspiration to me and to many others.

Austin, Texas

R. MAURICE HOOD

Contributors

Homer S. Arnold, M.D.
Captain, U.S. Navy Medical Corps, Retired
Attending Surgeon, Seton Medical Center
St. David's Community Hospital
Brackenridge Hospital
Austin, Texas

John H. Calhoon, M.D.
Assistant Professor
Co-Director Thoracic Transplantation
Department of Surgery
Division of Cardiothoracic Surgery
University of Texas Health Science Center
    at San Antonio
San Antonio, Texas

Contents

1

Preoperative Management

PREOPERATIVE EVALUATION AND CARE OF THE PULMONARY RESECTION PATIENT

Selection and evaluation of the patient for major pulmonary resection is a complex and demanding task. To simplify discussion of the problems involved, this chapter covers the following topics: (1) neoplasm, (2) suppurative disease, and (3) tuberculosis.

Before scheduling surgery, the patient's pulmonary function status should be evaluated. Evidence of significant coronary arterial or valvular disease should be fully evaluated, even to the point of catheterization and angiography. The patient who is in overt congestive heart failure is rarely a candidate for major resection.

Evaluation of Pulmonary Function

Prediction of the result of an operation with respect to the patient's ability to survive and function postoperatively is a highly desirable goal. Unfortunately, there is a considerable gap between the expectation and the actual results of pulmonary function testing. A basic understanding of normal cardiopulmonary physiology is necessary for the surgeon to make use of data from the pulmonary laboratory. An abstract interpretation of data by someone who has no clinical knowledge of the patient cannot be relied upon.

Figure 1–1 demonstrates a typical pulmonary laboratory report. Table 1–1 lists normal values for pulmonary function testing. Pulmonary function is made up of five basic components—volumes and capacities, pulmonary ventilation, distribution of inspired gas, pulmonary circulation and ventilation-perfusion ratios, and diffusion—and a disease process may alter one or more of these.

Volumes and Capacities. Space-occupying lesions, such as pneumothorax, hemothorax, pleural effusion, abdominal distention with air, fluid, or a mass, and parenchymal consolidation by inflammation or neoplasm, are common problems that may produce significant alterations. Pulmonary emphysema increases the total lung capacity and residual volume and reduces the inspiratory and vital capacities. Not only must abnormal values be identified but, in addition, the cause and nature of temporary or reversible changes, as opposed to fixed changes, must be identified.

Pulmonary Ventilation. This area of function is made up of respiratory rate, tidal volume, and evaluation of respiratory dead space. From these values, alveolar ventilation per minute can be estimated. It may also be measured by determining the amount of CO_2 in expired gas and percentage of CO_2 in alveolar gas as well as the expired volume. In normal people these values would be the same. Hypoventilation or hyperventilation can be thus identified. In addition, the causes of each can usually be identified.

These values must be interpreted in light of blood gas determinations.

```
                              MALE        AGE   43.
        HEIGHT   73.  WEIGHT   188.


          DETERMINATION        ACTUAL  PRED   %PRED

       VITAL CAPACITY,L (FVC)    5.73   5.16   111.
       FORCED EXP VOL,L(FEV1)    4.23   4.07   104.
       TIMED VC,%1SEC,(FEV1%)    74.    79.    94.
       MAX MID FLOW, L/SEC       3.25   4.30   76.     ARTERIAL BLOOD
       PEAK FLOW, L/MIN          580.   513.   113.
       MAX BR CAP,L/MIN (MVV)    218.7  171.9  127.    pH          7.44
                                                       PaO2        77
       RESPIRATORY RATE (F)      25.                   PaCO2       36
       VENTIL,L/MIN (VE)         14.44                 O2Sat       96%
       TIDAL VOL,ML (VT)         580.
       02 UPT.,ML/MIN (VO2)      265.
       VENT EQUIV L/100 ML       5.5    <2.5

       INSP CAPACITY,L (IC)      3.99
       EXP RESERVE,L (ERV)       1.36
       CALC VC, L                5.36   5.16   104.
       FUNC RES VOL,L (FRC)      3.52
       TOT LUNG CAP,L (TLC)      7.51   6.74   111.
       RESID VOL,L (RV)          2.15   1.62   133.
       (RV/TLC) X 100,%          29.    24.    121.
       HE MIX TIME,MIN           2.0    <3
```

Figure 1–1. A standard pulmonary function laboratory report. Initially, one should look at the static volumes to see whether they are normal, increased, or decreased. The residual volume and functional residual capacity are noted with respect to their fraction of the total lung capacity. Dynamic flow rates (FEV_1) indicate if there is obstruction or restriction. Arterial blood gas will detect whether there is hypoxemia. The P_{CO_2} of 36 mm Hg is probably based on hyperventilation prior to the needle stick. If marked abnormalities are noted on these initial studies, determinations of CO diffusing capacity, dead space ventilation, compliance, and airway resistance should be obtained.

Distribution of Inspired Gas. Partial or complete bronchial occlusion, retained secretions, and regional changes in elasticity can all produce significant inequality of air flow to the various areas of the lung. When alteration of air distribution is present, calculation of alveolar ventilation is inaccurate. Bronchospirometry may be of help in evaluating air distribution, although often disease processes are not unilateral but diffuse.

Pulmonary Circulation and Ventilation-Perfusion Ratios. The circulatory component of pulmonary function may be impaired by several disease processes (Fig. 1–2). Cardiac disease, whether ischemic, congenital, or valvular, may alter cardiac output. Severe myocardial disease may result in diminished ventricular output. Valvular obstruction on the left side produces left atrial hypertension, which is transmitted to the pulmonary vasculature. Congenital lesions with left-to-right shunts increase the flow through the pulmonary circulation and result in arterial wall changes with an increase in pulmonary vascular resistance. Pulmonary emphysema results in a loss of capillary vascular bed, which in turn results in pulmonary hypertension and also increases pulmonary artery resistance.

Emphysema and other diseases may occlude pulmonary vascular flow to aerated areas of the lung, causing shunting of blood to the venous system without contact with alveoli. The fraction of blood involved in shunting can be calculated. The ventilation-perfusion ratio can be ascertained with accuracy.

The ventilation-perfusion ratio can be increased by pulmonary artery obstruction by ligature, embolism, or thrombosis (such as in disseminated intravascular coagulation), by pulmonary hypertension, but principally by emphysema, in which both ventilation and circulation are impaired.

Table 1–1. Typical Values in Pulmonary Function Tests*

These are values for a healthy resting, recumbent young male (1.7 m² surface area) breathing air at sea level, unless other conditions are specified. They are presented merely to give approximate figures. These values may change with position, age, size, sex, and altitude; there is variability among members of a homogeneous group under standard conditions.

Lung Volumes

Inspiratory capacity, mL	3600
Expiratory reserve, volume, mL	1200
Vital capacity, mL	4800
Residual volume (RV), mL	1200
Functional residual capacity, mL	2400
Thoracic gas volume, mL	2400
Total lung capacity (TLC), mL	6000
RV/TLC × 100, %	20

Ventilation

Tidal volume, mL	500
Frequency, respirations/min	12
Minute volume, mL/min	6000
Respiratory dead space, mL	150
Alveolar ventilation, mL/min	4200

Distribution of Inspired Gas

Single-breath test (% increase N_2 for 500 mL expired alveolar gas), $\%N_2$	<1.5
Pulmonary nitrogen emptying rate (7 min test), $\%N_2$	<2.5
Helium closed-circuit (mixing efficiency related to perfect mixing), %	76

Diffusion and Gas Exchange

O_2 consumption (STPD), mL/min	240
CO_2 output (STPD), mL/min	192
Respiratory exchange ratio, R (CO_2 output/O_2 uptake)	0.8
Diffusing capacity, O_2 (STPD) resting, ml O_2/min/mm Hg	>15
Diffusing capacity, CO (steady state) (STPD) resting mL CO/min/mm Hg	17
Diffusing capacity, CO (single-breath) (STPD) resting, mL CO/min/mm Hg	25
Diffusing capacity, CO (rebreathing) (STPD) resting mL CO/min/mm Hg	25

Alveolar Ventilation/Pulmonary Capillary Blood Flow

Alveolar ventilation (L/min)/blood flow, L/min	0.8
Physiologic shunt/cardiac output × 100, %	<7
Physiologic dead space/tidal volume × 100, %	<30

Pulmonary Circulation

Pulmonary capillary blood flow, mL/min	5400
Pulmonary artery pressure, mm Hg	25/8
Pulmonary capillary blood volume, mL	75–100
Pulmonary "capillary" blood pressure (wedge), mm Hg	8

Alveolar Gas

Oxygen partial pressure, mm Hg	104
CO_2 partial pressure, mm Hg	40

Arterial Blood

O_2 saturation (% saturation of Hb with O_2), %	97.1
O_2 tension, mm Hg	100
CO_2 tension, mm Hg	40
Alveolar-arterial P_{O_2} difference (100% O_2), mm Hg	33
O_2 saturation (100% O_2), %	100
O_2 tension (100% O_2), mm Hg	640
pH	7.4

Mechanics of Breathing

Maximal voluntary ventilation, L/min	125–170
Forced expiratory volume, % in 1 sec	83
% in 3 sec	97
Maximal expiratory flow rate (for 1 L), L/min	400
Maximal inspiratory flow rate (for 1 L), L/min	300
Compliance of lungs and thoracic cage, L/cm H_2O	0.1
Compliance of lungs, L/cm H_2O	0.2
Airway resistance, cm H_2O/L/sec	1.6
Work of quiet breathing, kg-m/min	0.5
Maximal work of breathing, kg-m/breath	10
Maximal inspiratory and expiratory pressures, mm Hg	60–100

*From Comroe, J. H., Jr., et al.: The Lung. 2nd Ed. Copyright © 1962 by Year Book Medical Publishers, Inc., Chicago. Used by permission.

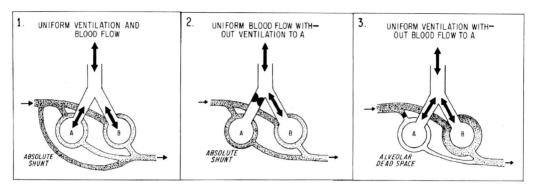

Figure 1–2. This figure illustrates the problem of uneven ventilation and blood flow. In Plate 1, there is uniform ventilation and blood flow, but an absolute shunt or an anatomic shunt is present. Plate 2 illustrates the problem seen with bronchial obstruction or atelectasis, whereby there continues to be uniform blood flow but absent ventilation, producing a shunt. Plate 3 illustrates uniform ventilation but pulmonary vascular occlusion, such as that seen with pulmonary emboli, in which dead space is increased. (Adapted from Comroe, J. H., Jr.: Physiology of Respiration. 2nd Ed. Copyright © 1974 by Year Book Medical Publishers, Inc., Chicago. Used by permission.)

Diffusion. The ultimate lung function is diffusion of oxygen and carbon dioxide across the alveolocapillary membrane. Diseases that produce interstitial or alveolar fibrosis impair diffusion. These include sarcoidosis, asbestosis, and interstitial hemorrhage. Emphysema is generally considered a problem of shunting and poor distribution of inspired air, but a loss of absolute surface area below the patient's requirements and an absolute loss of lung tissue by trauma or resection can reduce the diffusion area below the patient's needs.

Anemia and polycythemia may alter diffusion capacity.

The diagnosis of a diffusion defect may be made in the pulmonary laboratory, but its pathologic basis can be determined only by the pathologist.

Mechanics of Respiration. The ability of the patient to do the work of respiration is a vital part of pulmonary function evaluation. Fatigability, generalized weakness, neurologic dysfunction of intercostal muscles or diaphragm, hyperexpanded rib cage, and flattened diaphragm of chronic obstructive pulmonary disease all can interfere with the ability of the patient to breathe. The loss of compliance in emphysema makes the mechanical effort impossible. Airway resistance, whether from tracheobronchial mechanical obstruction, such as in neoplasm or stricture or from small airway obstruction seen in asthma, adds to the work of ventilation and perhaps at a level that results in hypoventilation.

Evaluation of this area of pulmonary function may be by determination of maximum ventilatory volume as an overall assessment. Measuring the maximal negative pressure the patient is able to produce is also helpful. Airway resistance can be determined. The forced expiratory volume (FEV_1) is the most useful study in this area and relates well to risk (Fig. 1–3).

Unrelated diseases such as angina pectoris, congestive heart failure, and weakness from illness may prevent or terminate testing in this field.

It should be noted that clinical evaluation is at least as important as the pulmonary laboratory data.

This brief summary is not intended to present a comprehensive view of evaluation of cardiopulmonary testing. Laboratory tests may be able to identify the specific defect and partially determine the impact on the patient's ability to tolerate a surgical procedure; to a lesser degree they may help predict the patient's postoperative pulmonary functional status.

The difficulties with pulmonary function studies are several.

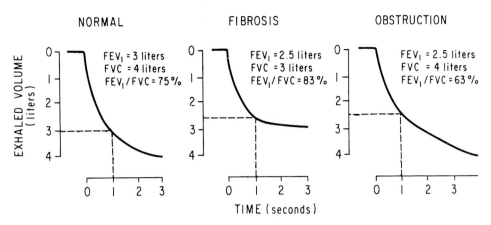

Figure 1–3. Graphs illustrating changes in the forced expiratory volume in the normal patient, in fibrosis or restrictive lung disease, and in obstruction. Because FEV_1 may at times be decreased in restrictive lung disease, it should be related to the total exhaled vital capacity. The ratio of FEV_1 to vital capacity may be decreased in the presence of bronchial obstruction but is normal in restrictive disease. (From Wolfe, W. G.: Preoperative assessment of pulmonary function: Quantitative evaluation of ventilation and blood-gas exchange. *In* Sabiston, D. C., Jr., and Spencer, F. C.: Gibbon's Surgery of the Chest. 4th Ed. Vol. 1. Philadelphia, W. B. Saunders Company, 1983, pp. 1–16. Used by permission.)

1. **They require a high level of patient understanding and cooperation.**
2. **They depend on the physical ability of the patient to exercise.**
3. **The function of the lung tissue to be resected cannot easily be physiologically separated from the remainder of the lung.**

There is also a ±25% chance of error inherent in the techniques. It can be assumed that there is no certain way of accurately predicting postoperative function or survival in some patients. The FEV_1 and the maximal voluntary ventilation (MVV) are more likely to accurately reflect operative risk than are any of the other commonly performed tests. Studies that show pulmonary function to be within normal limits are of little use because clinically the patient with such findings could easily be predicted to sustain a resection without difficulty. A patient whose pulmonary function studies indicate that no operative procedure is possible is not an operative candidate by ordinary observation. The patient in whom a clinical decision is equivocal shows indeterminate results on pulmonary function testing. Having the patient walk at a rapid pace for 100 yards or asking the patient to climb four flights of stairs and then observing the degree of resultant dyspnea and tachycardia are about as predictive as the pulmonary laboratory tests are for decisions on resection. Therefore, an accurate clinical appraisal and common sense are necessary in patient evaluation.

There simply are no laboratory values that relieve the surgeon of a clinical decision of operability based on all clinical data, laboratory values, and experience.

NEOPLASM

Bronchogenic carcinoma is the most common diagnosis requiring pulmonary resection today. Unfortunately, in many centers, staging of lung cancer, determination of operability, and selection of adjuvant therapy have passed to the oncologist or pulmonary internist, and the surgeon has become merely a technician. This approach has denied many patients an opportunity for survival and has resulted in excessive use of laboratory and diagnostic procedures that are irrelevant to either diagnosis or treatment. This test will proceed on the assumption that, except for small cell carcinoma, diagnosis and management are primarily surgical considerations. The surgeon should be familiar with the staging classification of Mountain, which will not be reprinted here.

Useful procedures in diagnosis and staging include bronchoscopy, scalene node biopsy, mediastinoscopy, computed tomographic (CT) scanning, conventional tomography, thoracentesis, liver biopsy, possibly thorascoscopy, and bone scanning. Not all of these are productive in every patient. For example, in the absence of pain, a bone scan usually does not yield diagnostic information. Liver metastases are not likely to be discovered if laboratory chemical data are normal. The surgeon must be wary of accepting a CT scan interpretation of positive mediastinal nodes if they are less than 1 cm in size and should also be wary of what appears to be chest wall or mediastinal invasion. Under these conditions, CT scans produce a fairly high incidence of false positive diagnoses.

A blind search for an extrapulmonary primary tumor when there is a single peripheral, circumscribed mass is a futile, expensive exercise. Solitary primary neoplasms are more than 100 times more frequent than solitary metastatic lesions if there is no known primary lesion.

A positive approach is necessary to manage the cancer patient; the surgeon should be seeking the indications for operation rather than searching for reasons not to operate. There are several findings, however, that should rule out any form of resection. These include the following:

1. **Recurrent laryngeal nerve paralysis.**
2. **Phrenic nerve paralysis (not invariably nonresectable).**
3. **Horner's syndrome.**
4. **Gross mediastinal invasion proved by biopsy.**
5. **Neoplastic cells identified in pleural fluid.**
6. **Proven distant metastases.**
7. **Extensive chest wall invasion (relative).**
8. **Bronchoscopic evidence of tracheal or carinal involvement.**

Many surgeons are tempted to perform "palliative" resections. These operations are hazardous and associated with excessive morbidity; moreover, they rarely, if ever, result in significant palliation.

Controversy over pneumonectomy versus lobectomy raged in the literature for many years, although a consensus was reached that lobectomy had a higher survival rate. No preplanned randomization study has ever been done, and because the operative mortality rate of pneumonectomy must be considered, the question of which procedure cures more patients has never been answered. The lesions that require pneumonectomy are more central and frequently larger, whereas those in which lobectomy can be done are more peripheral and smaller. Several reports indicate that local excision or segmental resection in the older or poor-risk patient has a survival rate comparable to that for the more extensive procedures; however, these lesions are smaller and more peripheral also.

Therefore, the extent, location, and size of the neoplasm, and the condition of the patient, determine which procedure is used. Several authors have reported on "extended" or "radical" pneumonectomy as a routine approach. Their mortality figures have failed to justify this approach. Routine preoperative irradiation to the hilum and mediastinum also results in an unacceptable rate of bronchial disruptions with a significant mortality increase that would appear to offset any theoretical advantage.

An ultraconservative approach may also be chosen. This approach excludes all patients from thoracotomy except those whose conditions can be managed easily without problem. Surgeons using this approach can demonstrate a better operative mortality rate and a higher resectability rate, and they have better 5-year survival figures. Although they appear to have a better set of statistics, it is at the expense of denying many patients their only chance of survival. The most desirable set of operative criteria is elusive but lies somewhere between the extreme of an overly aggressive attitude and the other extreme of accepting only the most favorable patients for operation; it demands a certain amount of common sense.

Routine preparation for operation should include cessation of smoking for at least 2 weeks, aggressive treatment of pulmonary infection and bronchitis, bringing the patient's cardiac status into an optimum state, and liberal use of pulmonary inhalation and physical therapy when chronic pulmonary disease is present. Preoperative instruction in coughing will help the patient in the postoperative period.

SUPPURATIVE DISEASE

Suppurative disease has become a relatively rare cause of pulmonary resection in the United States. Underdeveloped nations still must cope with high incidences of lung abscess and bronchiectasis, which are no longer seen in the United States. Recently, at the NYU Medical Center, a striking increase in the incidence of lung abscess related to intravenous drug abuse has been seen. Abscess from nosocomial infection has also increased in incidence.

The indications for resection of a primary (putrid, anaerobic, aspiration) lung abscess include failure to respond to antibiotic therapy, an abscess that has reached the chronic phase, one that ruptures into the pleural space, and one with massive hemoptysis. Bronchiectasis is relatively rare, but there are still patients who produce large amounts of purulent sputum, who have repetitive episodes of pneumonitis, or who have massive hemorrhage or multiple episodes of bleeding. Operation should be considered for these patients.

Preoperative mapping of the lesion by high-quality bronchograms and localization of a bleeding site by bronchoscopy are necessary. If the procedure is being done for symptoms other than bleeding, it is unwise to operate upon a patient with bronchiectasis unless all of the diseased tissue is resected. Also, as with tuberculosis, the state of the patient's pulmonary function and the impact of the planned operation must be considered. Many patients have inadvertently become respiratory cripples in the past because of an overly aggressive surgical approach.

The patient with either a lung abscess or bronchiectasis should be treated with appropriate antibiotics, postural drainage, repeated bronchoscopy, and other measures to ensure that the patient's condition is as good as possible at the time of surgery. Sputum should be minimal if proper preparation has been made. Copious purulent bronchial secretions at the time of surgery almost guarantee a difficult postoperative period.

TUBERCULOSIS

Fifty years ago, **tuberculosis** was one of the most common diagnoses for which pulmonary resection was performed. Today, in developed nations, tuberculosis is an uncommon, if not a rare, reason for resection. The underdeveloped nations must still cope with the disease as it was in the United States before effective antibiotics were available. In fact, in New York and other metropolitan areas where there are large populations of people who have immigrated recently and where alcohol and drug abuse are rampant, there has been a striking increase in the incidence of tuberculosis and in surgical problems related thereto. Further, the need for surgical resection in atypical disease is much higher than in patients with infections caused by typical organisms, and the incidence of atypical infection appears to be increasing.

General principles developed years ago still apply despite the changed disease pattern. It is preferable to postpone any thought of surgery until the maximal effect of antibiotic therapy has been obtained, which usually means not less than 4 months of therapy. There are, however, certain pathologic states for which resectional therapy is considered:

1. **Massive hemoptysis not otherwise controllable.**
2. **Destroyed lobe or lung.**
3. **Persistent cavitary disease with positive sputum.**
4. **Bronchial stenosis secondary to tuberculous bronchitis.**
5. **Extensive atypical disease not responding to therapy.**
6. **Tuberculous bronchiectasis with recurrent bleeding.**
7. **A peripheral "tuberculoma" when a diagnosis of carcinoma cannot be excluded.**
8. **Drug-resistant, progressive disease**

Evaluation of radiographic studies, which should include standard chest x-rays, CT scans, and tomography, must be accurate. It is not physically possible to resect all diseased tissue, but the surgeon must be able to resect the damaged tissue that neither the patient's defenses nor the therapy are able to cope with. It should be determined which lobes and segments are involved and the resection preplanned, based not only on the extent of the disease but also on (1) whether the remaining lung will fill the pleural space or a thoracoplasty will be required, and (2) whether the proposed resection is compatible with the patient's pulmonary function.

PREOPERATIVE MANAGEMENT OF PATIENTS HAVING ESOPHAGEAL RESECTION FOR CARCINOMA

Surgical treatment of carcinoma of the esophagus is in poor favor in many areas because of the low postoperative survival figures and high operative mortality and morbidity rates. The experience in China and Japan clearly shows that good survival rates will be seen only when it becomes possible to make a diagnosis much earlier than is usually done in the United States. The mortality and morbidity rates can be acceptable if there is proper patient selection for surgery, adequate preparation for operation, a well-performed operation, and good postoperative management.

Many times there is poor selection for operation. Patients manifesting mediastinal invasion or evidence of distant metastatic disease should be excluded from considerations of surgery. Findings that should preclude attempts at resection include the following:

1. **Pleural effusion with neoplastic cells in the fluid.**
2. **Evidence of liver metastases by CT scan or liver scan.**
3. **Visible cervical lymph node involvement.**
4. **Recurrent laryngeal or phrenic nerve paralysis.**
5. **Bone metastases or vertebral invasion.**
6. **Pulmonary metastases.**
7. **Tracheoesophageal fistula or visible neoplasm in the bronchus at bronchoscopy.**
8. **Other evidence of distant metastases.**

Some of these patients may have a bypass procedure for relief of dysphagia and to prevent aspiration pneumonia, but attempts at resection are usually futile and hazardous.

There is some evidence at this time to suggest that preoperative radiation or chemotherapy can convert a nonresectable tumor into a resectable lesion. Should there be good evidence of extensive mediastinal involvement, my preference is for cervical esophagogastrectomy with the primary lesion treated with radiation and chemotherapy.

The postoperative management of the patient who has had an esophagectomy requires a careful and preplanned approach, both preoperatively and intraoperatively. Although many factors influence the postoperative course and complication rate, the preoperative status and therapy of the patient are most important. In this regard, certain aspects should be considered and evaluated:

1. The nutritional status is most critical. Individuals who have lost extensive amounts of weight are likely to be anergic and obviously in negative nitrogen balance. These

patients are subject to poor wound healing and vulnerable to infection. A 3- or 4-week period of hyperalimentation will at least partially correct this aspect. They may also require transfusion.

2. The cardiopulmonary status of the patient must be evaluated and cardiac disease identified. Chronic pulmonary obstructive disease is also common. The patient's condition should be as optimal as possible.

3. The operative procedure performed influences the postoperative course greatly. Gastric replacement has proved to be the safest method in most centers. Colon replacement in resections for carcinoma in the older patient has consistently had a much higher mortality rate (seldom lower than 15%). Jejunal transplant has fared no better. The newer approach of free jejunal transplant with a microvascular anastomosis holds much promise for the future. Transhiatal esophagectomy, although widely accepted, is not the ideal procedure in my opinion.

4. Preoperative irradiation and chemotherapy adversely affect the patient's course. There is as yet insufficient data to determine whether the increased risk is warranted by an increase in resectability or in long-term survival. It would seem unwise to perform an anastomosis in an irradiated area of esophagus, and if the thoracic esophagus has been given a significant amount of radiation, cervical esophagogastrostomy is preferable, preceded by total thoracic esophagectomy.

Should preoperative therapy result in severe leukopenia, anemia, platelet depression, or anergy, the operative procedure must be delayed; perhaps complete re-evaluation as to suitability for operation may be necessary.

Preoperative alimentation, transfusion, antibiotic therapy, and other supportive measures all may help in avoiding disastrous postoperative problems.

It has been my routine practice to use a bowel preparation preoperatively, including neomycin solution if the patient is unable to swallow tablets.

At the termination of the operative procedure, the surgeon should evaluate the procedure objectively with respect to its technical result. Any deficiencies or unsatisfactory anastomosis or poor vascularity must be taken into consideration as the postoperative period is entered.

THE DAY BEFORE OPERATION

The current epidemic of malpractice litigation has resulted in many proposals to reduce risks. The patient's postoperative course and final result depend, to a considerable degree, not only on the technical operative procedure but also on the attitude and cooperation of the patient throughout the hospital course. The patient's expectation of the final result may not agree with that of the surgeon.

Many of the surgeon's problems originate in failure to accept the role of physician with the patient. A large number of surgeons wish to be only technicians and leave the patient's general and specialized care to the referring physician, the anesthesiologist, the cardiologist, the pulmonary internist, the oncologist, or the radiotherapist, or all of the above. When this occurs, responsibility is so diffused that no individual really takes responsibility. The result is chaotic care and a multiplicity of unnecessary complications. The patient is quick to sense the fact that no one is in charge and that the surgeon is uncaring or unconcerned.

The degree of rapport or lack of it which the surgeon establishes determines more than any other factor whether the patient's appraisal of the total care or result is good or bad. Rapport means accepting the role of physician. It means taking the time to become knowledgeable about the patient, the spouse, children, occupation, and economic status. It means just sitting and talking. The surgeon should not give the impression of being hurried at daily visits. Always sit down, touch the patient, and be truly concerned, not merely try to appear concerned. A patient or family member who expresses concern, apprehension, or uncertainty requires time for explanation, encouragement, or just emotional support.

Sometimes the surgeon fails to appreciate the impact that a diagnosis of cancer or the prospect of a dangerous operative procedure has on the individual. It may take time and repetitive explanation, kindness, and patience during a most difficult time for the patient. This is one reason why an impersonal approach to surgery is to be condemned. It robs the patient of his or her identity, and frequently of dignity as well, and leads to a situation fraught with fear and uncertainty. If the surgeon fails to supply answers and explanations, to give reassurance, or to show kindness, the patient receives only minimal support, physical or emotional.

Some physicians excuse their lack of involvement with the patient as necessary for them to remain objective. This is a lame excuse for failing to be concerned enough to take care of a sick person. Objectivity is necessary but does not justify what has just been described.

I believe that the day or evening before operation is an especially important period. The surgeon should sit down with the patient and family and give a lucid, detailed explanation of the disease, the operative procedure (using drawings or illustrations), and the result expected. A review of possible complications and poor results must be presented in a way designed to inform and not terrify the patient. A discussion of the procedures to be expected in the immediate postoperative period, including monitoring, laboratory work, intratracheal suctioning, bronchoscopy, and ventilating machines should be detailed and reasons for use made clear. The chart should reflect this discussion in detail.

This visit should include signing of the operative permit, which I believe should be filled out personally by the surgeon, with explanations made by the surgeon in the presence of legally required witnesses.

For reasons that should be obvious from the foregoing discussion, the current practice of same-day admissions has many disadvantages, is adverse to the patient's welfare, and makes a good doctor-patient relationship more difficult to establish.

It is highly desirable that an intensive care nurse visit the patient also and acquaint him or her with purpose and facilities of the intensive care unit (ICU), explaining its procedures. It is also productive to have the patient visit the ICU preoperatively for a brief orientation.

These activities require time, coordination, and a genuine concern for the patient. They will be rewarded by a smoother postoperative course, a good doctor-patient relationship, and minimal resort to legal action.

ANESTHESIA CONSIDERATION AND INTRAOPERATIVE MONITORING

There are considerable controversy and dialogue today regarding the respective responsibilities of the anesthesiologist and surgeon during and following a major operative procedure. One group would have the anesthesiologist assume full control of all aspects of the patient's care intraoperatively and postoperatively except the technical conduct of the operative procedure. In fact, this is being done at many centers. At the opposite end of the spectrum, another group would have the surgeon or surgical house staff be responsible for at all times every facet of care, including respiratory management.

These opposing and irreconcilable views are responsible for many acrimonious confrontations and endless personality conflicts, at the same time reducing the quality of care the patient receives. I will not try to diminish or defuse this controversy here, but it would seem apparent that, in this age of high technology and extraordinary volume of knowledge, no individual can be all things at all times. Anesthesia, cardiology, pulmonary medicine, and thoracic surgery, although all dealing with similar problems, are separate disciplines, and each works from a different core knowledge and data base. It would seem that a cooperative effort based on mutual respect and common courtesy will produce a better care situation. It is not possible for the surgeon to have infinite knowledge regarding anesthesia techniques, cardiac physiology, or complex ventilatory problems.

Similarly, the anesthesiologist is at a greater disadvantage when faced with decisions that may involve reoperation or a radical change in management. Certainly, it is necessary for one individual to coordinate, consult, evaluate, and at some point make decisions with which others may disagree. This person should be the surgeon, but he or she must use to a maximum the expertise of others.

It is beyond the scope of this book to discuss various anesthetic techniques. The advantages and disadvantages of various agents can be found in other publications. The techniques, agents, type of induction, type of endotracheal tube, ventilating techniques, intraoperative monitoring, fluid administration, and immediate postoperative care are all critical to patient management and should be agreed upon in advance by surgeon and anesthesiologist.

The decision to ventilate for longer than the recovery period is best made by surgeon and anesthesiologist before operation. The preoperative drugs to be given, as well as those used during operation, can be selected or modified based on this decision. The seeming trend toward ventilating most patients for 24 hours or longer is probably unwise. Of course, a preoperative decision not to ventilate may be changed because of the condition of the patient and the result and duration of the operative procedure.

The monitoring or determination of various biochemical data during operation varies widely from one institution to another. A teaching institution is likely to engage in more extensive electronic and biochemical determinations than a private nonteaching institution. When there is little or no cost consciousness or necessity of cost containment, this area is severely abused. What level of monitoring is necessary or minimally required for the safety of the patient? There is no simple answer. The patient's age, disease, and immediate condition will indicate what parameters must be determined or monitored.

For discussion, assume that a pneumonectomy is to be performed in a 65-year-old male patient with pre-existing coronary artery disease. Arterial pressure recording, a central venous pressure (CVP) recording, electrocardiogram, urinary output, and periodic blood gas and pH determinations seem necessary. A more critical cardiac status may require a Swan-Ganz catheter for pulmonary artery and wedge pressure recording.

The number of major and fatal mishaps from CVP and Swan-Ganz catheters reported in the last 10 years should prohibit their use when not indicated. A carefully observed protocol and training period must be a part of the catheterization procedure if major problems are to be avoided.

Determinations of electrolyte values in noncardiac procedures are rarely necessary intraoperatively if preoperative values were normal unless inappropriate fluid volumes or composition are given. Cardiac enzyme determination is similarly not indicated unless there is immediate evidence of myocardial injury. Hematocrit levels are useful but often misleading because of the delay in hemodilution and because of fluid therapy. A careful assessment of blood loss by measurement and sponge weighing is probably more accurate. A good knowledge of the expected physiologic impact of a pneumonectomy in this type of patient will be invaluable in interpreting various data and determining which values are needed. A measure of common sense is also desirable. The urinary output is often used as a measure of need for volume infusion. In the absence of preoperative dehydration or hypovolemia, it is not necessary to insist on a fixed urinary output of over 25 mL/hour, assuming that blood loss is being replaced and that there is no preoperative renal dysfunction. Many factors other than fluid intake modify urine flow. It is a serious error to terminate a procedure of 3 hours' duration after having administered 4 to 6 liters of crystalloid in excess of blood and urine loss. This fluid surplus is not always tolerated.

Determination of cardiac output may be of value when there is known cardiac disease, or may assist in diagnosis when there is persistent hypotension or otherwise unexplained abnormal pulmonary artery pressure values.

The use of the central venous catheter and the Swan-Ganz catheter has become commonplace in trauma patients and in many elective thoracic surgical patients. In fact,

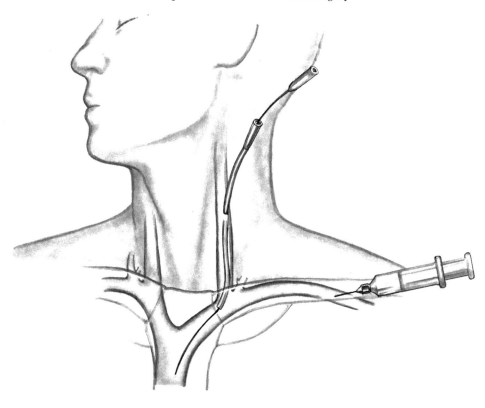

Figure 1–4. The correct technique of inserting either a central venous pressure (CVP) monitoring catheter or a Swan-Ganz catheter. Injury to the pleural and arterial structures can usually be avoided. (From Hood, R. M., Boyd, A. D., and Culliford, A. T.: Thoracic Trauma. Philadelphia, W. B. Saunders Company, 1989, p. 396. Used by permission.)

in many university centers their use has become routine in all patients, presumably as a teaching exercise.

The use of these catheters has resulted in a number of serious and fatal complications. These mishaps are all preventable and do not seem to be abating as experience accumulates (Fig. 1–4). The insertion of the central venous catheter and its use have resulted in tension pneumothorax, hydrothorax and hemothorax, injury to the subclavian artery, air embolism, and embolism of sheared-off catheters.

The Swan-Ganz catheter has had a similar list of mishaps, and, in addition, rupture of a pulmonary artery. If a rupture occurs in a heparinized patient, a fatality usually results. Rupture in the nonheparinized patient results in hemoptysis of varying degree, intrapulmonary hematoma, and hemothorax.

The guidelines in Tables 1–2 and 1–3 are those in use in the New York University Medical Center and, if used, should prevent this series of injuries.

Table 1–2. Guidelines for Intra-Clavicular Subclavian Catheterization*

I. Introduction
  A. Indications
    1. Hyperalimentation.
    2. Monitoring central venous pressure (when no other route is available).
  B. Contraindications
    1. A struggling uncooperative patient.
    2. Severe pulmonary disease with gross distortion of the chest wall.
    3. Bleeding diathesis or patients on anticoagulants.
    4. S/p radical mastectomy (affected side).
    5. S/p clavicular fracture with deformity.

II. Some Anatomic Considerations
    1. The axillary vein becomes the subclavian vein behind the junction of the medial and middle thirds of the clavicle. The subclavian vein joins the internal jugular vein to form the innominate vein just behind the sternoclavicular joint. The innominate veins from either side join behind the manubrium to form the superior vena cava.
    2. The subclavian vein is bordered by the clavicle anteriorly, the anterior scalene muscle posteriorly and the first rib inferiorly.
    3. The subclavian artery and brachial plexus lie posterior to the anterior scalene muscle. This provides a 10 to 15 mm distance between the subclavian vein and these structures.
    4. The pleura is in contact with the posteroinferior aspect of the subclavian vein.

III. Technique
    1. The patient's need for a central line is reviewed and the relative safety of the subclavian route is assessed with regard to (a) coagulation disorders, (b) degree of patient cooperation, (c) presence of any known anomalies, and (d) proper nursing supervision after insertion.
    2. All the needed equipment is obtained and checked for completeness.
    3. The right side is preferred to avoid injury to the thoracic duct.
    4. The patient is placed on his back and in Trendelenburg position. The head should be turned away from the puncture side for three reasons: (a) this tenses the scalenus anticus muscle and helps engorge the vein; (b) it makes the landmark more prominent; and (c) it helps to prevent contamination of equipment. Pillows and sheets should be removed from beneath the head and neck, since these will disturb the anatomy. In the awake patient, some reassurance at this point will help prevent any voluntary change in position (such as inwardly rotating the shoulder).
    5. A large-bore 20-cm long Bardick Intercath is disassembled and the needle is placed on a 10-cc syringe. The needle and syringe are held parallel to the ground at all times.
    6. The needle (bevel down) enters the skin over the clavicle 1 to 2 cm medial to the midpoint of the clavicle. When the periosteum is struck, it is "walked" under the clavicle always hugging its inferior surface.
    7. The index finger of the left hand is firmly held in the suprasternal notch and the tip of the needle is directed toward it. While the needle is being slowly moved, constant mild negative pressure is being maintained on the syringe.
    8. When blood is obtained, the needle is advanced another 1 to 2 mm so that the entire beveled end of the needle lies within the vein.
    9. The needle is stabilized with the left thumb and index finger or a clamp and the syringe is removed. After the syringe is removed, the needle must be quickly covered with a gloved finger to prevent air embolization.
    10. The catheter is then introduced and threaded in for its entire length. The needle position should be carefully maintained during this transfer. The guidewire should be removed if any difficulty is encountered in positioning the catheter.

*From Hood, R. M., Boyd, A. D., and Culliford, A. T.: Thoracic Trauma. Philadelphia, W. B. Saunders Company, 1989, p. 392. Used by permission.

Table 1–2.   Guidelines for Intra-Clavicular Subclavian Catheterization* (Continued)

11. The catheter must never be pulled out from the needle alone, since the needle point may shear off a piece of the catheter.
12. Before attaching to the skin, the free aspiration of blood from the catheter should be demonstrated.
13. The needle guard is then attached to the needle and the catheter attached to an anesthesia extension set. Three-point fixation with a 3-0 silk or nylon should be achieved.
14. The patient should be returned to a comfortable position and the chest auscultated.
15. The procedure should never be regarded as complete until the post-subclavian puncture chest x-ray is seen. This should be obtained as soon as possible.

IV. Special Consideration for Subclavian Puncture Prior to Open Heart Procedures
1. These should not be attempted until the patient is fully asleep, intubated and relaxed. This will allow for a full Trendelenburg position, which is essential in the fluid-restricted, diuretic-treated patient.
2. All pillows and sheets should be removed from beneath the head and shoulders.
3. No more than two sticks should be attempted on the same side.
4. If arterial blood is obtained, attempts on that side should be stopped, and following sternotomy the area visualized and any injury repaired. This is to be done prior to heparinization for bypass.
5. The subclavian route for central pressure monitoring should be used after peripheral lines for the antecubital fossa and external jugular lines have been unsuccessful.
6. Only rarely should it be necessary to use bilateral subclavian catheters.

V. Complications
A. Pneumothorax
   1. *Cause:* Laceration of the pleura or lung parenchyma with the needle.
   2. *Signs and Symptoms:* Dyspnea, cyanosis, diminished breath sounds, hyper-resonance, sudden withdrawal of large amounts of air during insertion of the needle.
   3. *Prevention:* Never change the axis of the needle once it is through the skin. If you want to change the direction of the needle, remove it completely and reinsert.
   4. *Treatment:* A chest tube is usually required.
B. Hemothorax
   1. *Cause:* Laceration of the subclavian vein, artery or other vessel with associated puncture of the pleural space, or laceration of the lung parenchyma producing a hemo-pneumothorax.
   2. *Signs and Symptoms:* Dyspnea, cyanosis, diminished breath sounds, hypo-resonance.
   3. *Prevention:* Same as for pneumothorax.
   4. *Treatment:* Frequent chest x-rays and hematocrit determinations, chest tube or thoracentesis.
C. Hydrothorax
   1. *Cause:* Intrapleural placement of catheter.
   2. *Signs and Symptoms:* Dyspnea (especially several hours after insertion), hypo-resonance.
   3. *Prevention:* Be sure that venous blood is aspirated from the catheter before starting the IV infusion.
   4. *Treatment:* Removal of the catheter and thoracentesis.

---

*From Hood, R. M., Boyd, A. D., and Culliford, A. T.: Thoracic Trauma. Philadelphia, W. B. Saunders Company, 1989, p. 393. Used by permission.

Table 1–2. Guidelines for Intra-Clavicular Subclavian Catheterization* (Continued)

D. Catheter Embolism
   1. *Cause:* Shearing off of part of the catheter as it is withdrawn through the needle.
   2. *Signs and Symptoms:* A piece of catheter is missing on withdrawal.
   3. *Prevention:* Never withdraw the catheter through the needle; withdraw as a unit.
   4. *Treatment:* Angiography and snaring are required.
E. Air Embolism
   1. *Cause:* Entrance of air via the catheter into the great veins. This can occur during insertion or by accidental disconnection. The hypovolemic patient is especially prone to this complication.
   2. *Signs and Symptoms:* Dyspnea, cyanosis, cardiac arrest.
   3. *Prevention:* Trendelenburg position, guarding of the hub from air during insertion and maintenance of tight connections.
   4. *Treatment:* Cover the needle or catheter hub. Place the patient in Trendelenburg in the left lateral decubitus position. If the patient cannot be resuscitated, open the left chest and aspirate the right ventricle. The potential for systemic air embolization in this situation exists, therefore the left ventricle should also be aspirated prior to defibrillation. In addition the aorta should be vented for the first few minutes after defibrillation.
F. Hemomediastinum
   1. *Cause:* Laceration of a great vessel during insertion.
   2. *Signs and Symptoms:* Dyspnea, SVC syndrome.
   3. *Prevention:* Care in insertion.
   4. *Treatment:* Observation, frequent CXR and Hcts. Median sternotomy may be required.
G. Arterial Puncture
   1. *Cause:* Improper technique.
   2. *Signs and Symptoms:* Return of arterial blood through the needle, large hematoma on needle withdrawal.
   3. *Prevention:* Proper anatomic technique.
   4. *Treatment:* Observation. Rarely tracheostomy will be required for extrinsic airway compression.

*From Hood, R. M., Boyd, A. D., and Culliford, A. T.: Thoracic Trauma. Philadelphia, W. B. Saunders Company, 1989, p. 394. Used by permission.

Table 1–3.   Guidelines for Swan-Ganz Catheterization*

I. Indications for Use

1. Acute heart failure—cardiogenic shock.
2. Cardiac tamponade.
3. Severe hypovolemia with suspected LV failure.
4. Medical emergencies, i.e., gram-negative sepsis, acute renal failure, hemorrhagic pancreatitis, etc.
5. Intra- and postoperative management of high-risk patients, i.e., history of pulmonary or cardiac disease, fluid shifts, extensive intra-abdominal operations.
6. Cardiac output determinations.
7. Monitoring during anesthetic induction in open heart surgery.

II. Contraindications to Use

1. There are no absolute contraindications to flow directed balloon-tipped catheter use. Some relative contraindications are the same as for any venous catheterization and include:
   a. Recurrent sepsis.
   b. Hypercoagulable states as well as patients on extensive anti-coagulants.
   c. Arrhythmias such as complete LBBB, WPW syndrome, and Ebstein's malformation.
   d. Severe long-standing pulmonary hypertension.

III. Technique

1. Assemble and check all equipment, including the monitoring system. Inflate the balloon of the Swan-Ganz catheter, check for leaks and there should be no asymmetry to balloon when fully inflated.
2. Insert catheter into vein either by percutaneous method or cutdown. Sterile techniques and procedures as previously outlined for internal jugular, subclavian, and brachial vein cutdown should be followed. With the use of introducer and percutaneous venipuncture in internal jugular, subclavian veins, the advantage of immediate partial inflation of balloon can be used to facilitate passage of catheter. The disadvantages are those of any subclavian or jugular percutaneous venipuncture. The advantage of the antecubital fossa cutdown is the safety of the procedure; however, passage of catheter may be difficult due to venous anatomy and/or venospasm, which will make manipulation of the catheter difficult.
3. With the balloon half inflated, the catheter is advanced into the SVC and right atrium (RA), continuously monitoring the venous pressure which will indicate when the RA is reached. When catheter tip is in the RA, the catheter has been inserted about 40 cm from the right and 50 cm from the left antecubital fossa in adults of average size.
4. Now inflate the balloon maximally.
5. While continuously monitoring the venous pressure and ECG, advance catheter, and note after passing the tricuspid valve, the right ventricle (RV) pressure curve.
6. Further advance the catheter with balloon still maximally inflated across the pulmonary valve into the pulmonary artery. If pulmonary artery (PA) pressure trace is not obtained, deflate the balloon and withdraw catheter until RA pressure curve noted on monitor. Then, re-inflate balloon maximally and advance catheter as before.
7. Once PA pressure curve is noted, further advance catheter with balloon maximally inflated until the curve is dampened and a pulmonary capillary wedge pressure is noted on monitor. At this point, deflate balloon completely.

*From Hood, R. M., Boyd, A. D., and Culliford, A. T.: Thoracic Trauma. Philadelphia, W. B. Saunders Company, 1989, p. 395. Used by permission.

Table 1–3. Guidelines for Swan-Ganz Catheterization* (Continued)

8. The catheter may be advanced 1 to 2 cm after deflation, as it tends to recoil when deflated toward the pulmonary valve and redundant catheter in right ventricle may cause arrhythmias. Redundant catheter in RV may lead to migration of catheter tip into the periphery of the pulmonary vascular bed. Therefore, reinflate balloon slowly, watching pressure monitor until wedge is noted. If volume needed is maximum balloon capacity, the catheter may be advanced a centimeter or two with balloon deflated. If volume in balloon to obtain wedge is less than half of maximum balloon volume, then deflate balloon and withdraw catheter to a position at which nearly full balloon volume is required to obtain wedge.

9. The balloon should always be inflated slowly; continuously watch the PA pressure and watch for wedge pressure. Stop inflating the balloon when wedge pressure noted. In patients with long-standing pulmonary hypertension, the pulmonary vessels are thin-walled and can be easily ruptured by overdistention by the balloon.

10. Always monitor the PA pressure with the balloon down continuously; this will facilitate quick recognition if the catheter tip should migrate to a wedge position. Also a constant infusion through the catheter lumen of a heparinized infusion solution should be maintained at all times. This further prevents catheter migration and, if so, the continual rise in wedge pressure will be quickly noticed on the monitor. This also aids in preventing embolization from the catheter tip.

11. Once catheter has been properly positioned, it should be sutured to the skin to secure its position. Immediate supine chest x-ray should be taken to check catheter tip location. Properly placed catheters may advance peripherally due to lung volume changes, postural changes of patient, positive pressure ventilation, etc. Therefore, a supine chest film should be taken daily to verify catheter tip location.

12. Dressing changes should be made with strict aseptic technique. At no time should catheter be advanced after initial positioning. If catheter dislodges from PA, then it should be removed entirely and a new catheter placed.

IV. Complications and Considerations

1. *Pulmonary infarction:* This usually occurs when the catheter tip has migrated into the periphery and wedge, therefore excluding that segment of lung from blood supply. This may also occur if the balloon is left inflated. This complication can be avoided by:
   a. Continually monitoring the PA pressure curve.
   b. Never allowing redundancy of catheter in the right ventricle.
   c. Never leaving syringe in balloon inflate position.
   d. Daily chest x-rays.

2. *Hemoptysis:* This usually occurs when the balloon is inflated rapidly while in the periphery of the pulmonary vasculature. It usually occurs in people with severe pulmonary hypertension and on anticoagulant therapy. This can be avoided by:
   a. Never allowing the catheter tip to get in peripheral position.
   b. Always inflating the balloon slowly watching the PA pressure curve and stop inflating the moment the PA trace occurs. If such a complication occurs, and massive hemoptysis is evident, the balloon can be fully inflated and withdrawn slightly to hopefully tamponade the ruptured pulmonary vessel.

3. It is important to understand the different *pressure values and curves* that one will see on the monitor to understand location of the catheter tip. Normally the RA pressure runs between 0 to 5 mm Hg, the RV is normally 25/0 and the PA normally 25/10. The pulmonary wedge pressure usually simulates the PA diastolic and runs between 8 to 12 mm Hg.

*From Hood, R. M., Boyd, A. D., and Culliford, A. T.: Thoracic Trauma. Philadelphia, W. B. Saunders Company, 1989, p. 396. Used by permission.

Table 1–3.   Guidelines for Swan-Ganz Catheterization* (Continued)

4. Common *arrhythmias* encountered in complete LBBB is an increased risk of complete heart block by RV stimulation by catheter tip. In the case of WPW and Ebstein's malformation, there is an increased risk of tachyarrhythmias. The catheter should be withdrawn with the balloon deflated immediately if any arrhythmia is encountered.
5. *Eccentric inflation of the balloon* can lead to problems. It can result in the inability to obtain a good wedge, as the balloon inflating eccentrically will force the catheter tip up against the wall of the vessel. Also, the eccentric inflation can result in rupture of the pulmonary artery.
6. It must be kept in mind that the ideal position of a Swan-Ganz catheter is in a large PA from which it can advance into the wedge position on inflation of the balloon and slip back to the previous location on deflation.
7. *Pulmonary hypertension* increases:
    a. Inability to obtain proper wedge.
    b. Chance of PA rupture, either by an eccentric balloon, repeated overinflation, or peripherally located balloon.
    c. The chance of peripheral location of catheter tip. The peripheral vessels are larger in pulmonary hypertension, and therefore wedge curve may be found more toward periphery.
8. *Pulmonary embolism* from venous thrombosis developing around the catheter can occur in cases in which there is a hypercoagulable state or congestive heart failure, etc. This results in a pulmonary infarction. In cases such as these, anticoagulation may be instituted to help prevent this complication.
9. *Occult catheter sepsis* is a complication presumably encountered when catheter is left in place much longer than 7 to 10 days. It is recommended that catheters be changed after 7 days.
10. Complication of the attempted percutaneous insertion of catheter into subclavian and/or internal jugular veins consists of neck hematomas, pneumothorax, hemo-pneumothorax, etc. as described in the procedures for subclavian and internal jugular venipuncture.

Abbreviations: LV = Left ventricular; LBBB = left bundle branch block; WPW = Wolf-Parkinson-White syndrome; SVC = subclavian vein catheter; ECG = electrocardiogram.
    *From Hood, R. M., Boyd, A. D., and Culliford, A. T.: Thoracic Trauma. Philadelphia, W. B. Saunders Company, 1989, p. 396. Used by permission.

2
Postoperative Care

The demands of postoperative care are more exacting in thoracic surgery than in any other field of surgery. The survival of the cardiac patient is totally dependent on the quality of care supplied. Following pulmonary resection the patient requires care that is just as exacting as the care given to the cardiac surgical patient. For the general thoracic surgical patient, not only survival but the extent of recovery and rehabilitation depend on intelligent, conscientious care. It must be emphasized that cardiac surgery and pulmonary surgery, although they have some similarities, are entirely different disciplines requiring a different body of knowledge relating to physiology, disease process, and technique. A different set of complications may follow, and much more active participation is required in the care of the pulmonary patient. Care must not be delegated; the surgeon must remain personally and actively involved, with the assistance of the anesthesiologist, the nurse, and other members of the pulmonary care team.

Eternal vigilance is the key idea in postoperative care. Much thoracic surgery today is performed by general surgeons and by cardiac surgeons as a side issue. Without a basic knowledge of pulmonary physiology, pulmonary disease, pathologic physiology accompanying disease, x-ray interpretation, and the necessary procedures, techniques, and methods from which to choose the best approach to a problem, these surgeons cannot intelligently serve a thoracic surgical patient. The surgeon who attempts thoracic surgery without the background knowledge is at best a technician rather than a surgeon. Much personal time is required by each patient. In no other field of surgery does the statement of Halsted, "The surgeon should be a physician who operates," apply more accurately.

The following discussion is based on the premise that the surgeon, personally, is responsible for the patient's detailed care.

POSTOPERATIVE VENTILATORY STATUS

Most pulmonary resection patients should not require postoperative ventilation. Patients with severe chronic pulmonary disease are exceptions, and a preoperative decision can usually be made that ventilation may or will not be necessary.

This area must involve good communication and cooperation with the anesthesiologist. As already noted, the decision to ventilate or not to ventilate should be made preoperatively. The preoperative medication and the intraoperative agents and relaxants must be given with the idea of extubating immediately postoperatively. An oversedated or narcotized patient has an impaired respiratory drive, prohibiting an early attempt at extubation.

Everything else being equal, the pulmonary resection patient will do better and have fewer pulmonary complications if prolonged ventilation is not necessary.

19

Before and after extubation, estimating the tidal volume by observation or by use of a Wright spirometer will help in making decisions, and the values of blood gases will determine the immediate course. Postoperative sedation must be minimal if adequate ventilation is to be maintained.

A decision to ventilate is a major one and should not be taken lightly. Certainly it should not be substituted for high-level professional attention, with the resident staff member assuming that if the patient is on a ventilator, everything is simplified and the effort being expended can be reduced.

The patient with emphysema should not be ventilated unless it is imperative; if it is, positive end expiratory pressure (PEEP) or continuous positive airway pressure (CPAP) should not be used unless necessary, and insufflation pressure should not be allowed to exceed 30 to 35 cm H_2O.

Weaning from the Ventilator

A patient who has been ventilated for some time and whose laboratory values and clinical findings suggest that the ventilatory support can be terminated may be weaned. This can be easily accomplished or may present difficulties.

Usually, the $F_{I_{O_2}}$ is reduced gradually to 20%; then the tidal volume is adjusted at a physiologic level. The IMV rate should be diminished, and once a rate of 2 to 4/minute is reached and blood gas values are satisfactory, the endotracheal tube may be removed.

The patient with chronic respiratory disease whose blood gas values are abnormal preoperatively cannot be simply or rapidly weaned with safety.

Attempts at rapid weaning when the patient has normal gas values are usually not successful for two principal reasons. First, preoperatively the patient will have been expending considerable physical effort to breathe. Postoperatively, the patient's respiratory center, after a period of ventilation, will have "forgotten" how much physical effort is required. If support is withdrawn rapidly, the patient's body does not rise to the demand, and instead decompensates. Pain and weakness may also make the mechanical effort of ventilation difficult to accomplish.

The second factor to be considered in weaning the chronic respiratory patient is the fact that the patient may have become chronically used to a P_{CO_2} greater than 40 mm Hg and a pH less than 7.35 and has been able to function at P_{O_2} levels around 60 mm Hg. In fact, the lowered P_{O_2} level may represent the patient's principal respiratory drive. Therefore, preoperative values must again be established before he or she can become independent of breathing support.

I have usually been successful through following this protocol. First, discontinue PEEP or CPAP gradually. Second, slowly—day by day—reduce the $F_{I_{O_2}}$ to room air level (i.e., 20%), without altering other parameters. Then, slowly reduce the tidal volume, day by day, until a value is reached that is within the patient's range and which should have been measured preoperatively. Following the patient's clinical status and the arterial blood gas (ABG) levels closely, diminish the IMV rate very slowly until it is apparent that the ABG levels are stable and the patient is comfortable.

Convert the tube to a T-piece for 30 to 45 minutes, then extubate if an endotracheal tube is being used. A tracheostomy may be left for an additional period.

This process may require a week to 10 days or may be accomplished much sooner in patients who are less ill. The pitfall, to repeat, is to try to wean the patient from the respirator when normal values are present.

FLUID BALANCE AND ADMINISTRATION

Intraoperative and postoperative fluid administration is complicated by conflicting views and aims. Resolution of differences and an agreed-upon plan of fluid administration should be accomplished before operation if possible.

Removal of approximately 50% of the pulmonary vascular bed renders the pneumonectomy patient vulnerable to fluid overload. Blood replacement should not be empirical but must be based on an accurate estimate of loss during the procedure. Unless there is unusual loss from vascular adhesions or a surgical mishap, transfusion is rarely needed. Crystalloid infusion should be based on a projected requirement with the object of keeping the patient somewhat on the dry side. Often, giving 1500 mL during the intraoperative period and the first 4 hours postoperatively is sufficient unless the patient was dehydrated or hypovolemic preoperatively.

Assuming a state of normal fluid balance preoperatively, only maintenance fluids and fluid volume are required to counteract the relative vasodilatation hypovolemia that occurs during induction with virtually all anesthetic agents. Rarely would more than 500 mL/hour be necessary during the operation.

Likewise, disturbances of composition and of acid-base balance will not need correction unless they were present preoperatively or induced by inappropriate fluid therapy.

Before postoperative fluid orders are written, the intraoperative fluids should be added up carefully and considered in the total. Because ileus is an unusual complication, oral administration is possible shortly after operation and use of intravenous fluids can be minimized. Intravenous administration should not exceed 50 to 75 mL/hour under the circumstances described. The common procedure of trying to regulate fluids by a central venous line reading and urinary output determination during operation is an invitation to disaster. Excess fluid administration, if diagnosed, should be managed by rapid diuresis. Respiratory distress from this cause is ominous in the pneumonectomy patient. Other than diuresis, intubation, and ventilation using PEEP at 10 to 15 cm H_2O may be life-saving.

Patients who have known cardiac disease, those whose fluid balance is in disarray, or those in whom considerable blood loss has occurred or is anticipated would be better served by placing a Swan-Ganz catheter preoperatively so that fluid administration may be more accurately accomplished.

To summarize, most thoracic surgical patients have normal fluid volume and composition status preoperatively. Nausea, vomiting, and ileus are not common, and oral intake can usually be resumed soon after surgery. Therefore, unless there is unwise use of fluid and blood intraoperatively and postoperatively, fluid volume deficit or overload and electrolyte disturbances should not occur.

I have a firm commitment to the principle of replacing blood loss with whole blood rather than with packed cells plus crystalloid, plasma protein fraction (Plasmanate), heta starch, or albumin. All of these agents have their advocates and regardless of the virtues of whole blood, blood bank policies make the use of whole blood nearly impossible.

PAIN RELIEF AND SEDATION

The patient with a posterolateral incision generally has more pain than one with the median sternotomy and also has greater need to cough and breathe deeply. Therefore, pain relief is important. The intubated patient may be sedated to a comfortable level, but the spontaneously breathing patient must not be narcotized to a point of manifesting respiratory depression, although at the same time he or she should be receiving enough analgesia to permit effective coughing and restful sleep. Therefore, a compromise is always necessary.

I prefer morphine given often in 1 to 3 mg increments intravenously. It may be given as often as every 30 to 45 min, but preferably less frequently. This dosage produces some analgesia with no significant depression. After the first 36 hours, codeine (30 to 60 mg orally in the form of Empirin with codeine) or acetaminophen (Tylenol with codeine, No. 3 or No. 4) is usually adequate.

Doses of meperidine hydrochloride (Demerol, 50 to 100 mg) and morphine (6 to 12 mg) are to be condemned.

The use of diazepam (Valium), at least in my experience, is of no value and may be dangerous.

Patients must be permitted time to sleep and, unless specific orders are written to let them sleep undisturbed, they may be kept awake unnecessarily during the night hours.

A recent phenomenon in intensive nursing care units has been development of agitation in a patient who begins to hallucinate and develops striking paranoia. Much has been written on this subject, and there is considerable disagreement as to its cause. Sleeplessness is probably a primary causative factor, however. The elderly patient is much more susceptible, and it has been observed that patients who are excessively fearful and apprehensive preoperatively are more likely to become disoriented. Those who use alcohol or tranquilizers are very susceptible to toxic psychosis unless these drugs are maintained at their preoperative levels.

Prevention of disorientation involves several factors.

1. Allow the patient to sleep undisturbed for intervals of at least 3 hours and see that a total of 6 to 8 hours of sleep is obtained in each 24 hours.

2. Relieve pain but do not produce mental confusion with narcotics or tranquilizers.

3. Keep the patient oriented to night and day by means of windows, clocks, lighting, conversation, and, if possible, keeping the same nurses with the patient each day.

When the patient begins to show early signs of disturbance, such as picking at bedclothes or inappropriate responses, becomes agitated, or becomes unable to sleep, treatment should begin and should consist of the following measures:

1. Discontinue all narcotics and sedation.

2. Remove all sources of pain and discomfort and keep them as far away as possible (i.e., chest tubes, blood pressure cuff, respiratory therapy apparatus).

3. Sedate the patient with paraldehyde (6 mL orally), followed by 4 mL intramuscularly or by stomach tube every 30 minutes until the patient is sound asleep and cannot be aroused. This may require a total dosage of 20 to 30 mL. Paraldehyde produces a deep, dreamless sleep, which usually terminates the toxic psychosis. This drug has the widest margin of safety of any currently used sedative. It does not produce respiratory depression at levels employed clinically.

Once asleep, the patient should be left alone for 8 to 12 hours without being disturbed.

Some older patients do not become reoriented until they return to a familiar environment among members of their families.

Diazepam, chlorpropamide, and similar drugs are contraindicated for this syndrome and almost invariably make the patient worse.

MANAGEMENT OF BRONCHIAL SECRETIONS

There is no other single aspect of postoperative care that is as critically important as keeping the bronchial tree free of obstructing and infected bronchial secretions. At the same time, no area is generally so poorly managed. This responsibility cannot be delegated to the nursing staff or to the inhalation therapist. It cannot be managed from home or some other part of the hospital. Ordering chest physical therapy is not a substitute for proper care. Nor can this problem be managed by writing orders or doing laboratory work.

There is no substitute for the surgeon at the bedside. Atelectasis, which is the most common complication of thoracic surgery, can be prevented; it can be anticipated, and the early process can be managed. Atelectasis should never be an unpleasant surprise to a resident house staff; its presence is sufficient evidence that the postoperative or postinjury care has been deficient, and the responsible person is always the operating surgeon.

The treatment begins in the preoperative period by bringing the patient to optimal condition, minimizing infection, and forbidding smoking. The patient should be taught how to cough preoperatively, and the techniques of nasotracheal suctioning and bronchoscopy should be explained to the patient. The patient should not be surprised and frightened by these procedures. He or she should understand the importance of clearing secretions.

The cause of atelectasis depends on several factors: (1) the presence of pre-existing pulmonary and bronchial disease; (2) following general anesthesia, the occurrence of a purulent bronchitis within hours, with a marked increase in volume of secretions, attenuated ciliary action, and abnormal surfactant activity; (3) splinting of the chest wall from pain, weakness, narcotics, and sedatives.

Postoperatively, it must be assumed that retention of bronchial secretions will occur and the surgeon must see that they are cleared and also continually be aware of the patient's status hour by hour.

The chest x-ray shows little sign until complete atelectasis is fully developed, and may appear normal when the bronchus has been occluded for 8 to 12 hours.

Assisted coughing by the trained, motivated patient is the most effective method of preventing atelectasis. Much emphasis has been placed on chest physical therapy in recent years. There is a growing body of evidence that all measures included in this area, such as intermittent positive pressure breathing (IPPB), percussion, and the incentive spirometer, are either of no value or are distinctly counterproductive. To put it bluntly, secretions must either be coughed up by the patient or removed by suction. There are no other useful measures.

Physical examination of the patient who is retaining secretions and progressing to atelectasis will alert the observant surgeon to the problem. First noted is an ineffective cough in a patient who is splinting excessively or is just not making the effort. As secretions accumulate, the cough becomes "wet," with audible rhonchi. Auscultation will reveal rales, rhonchi, and wheezing. Intervention at this point with nasotracheal suction will probably suffice.

Dyspnea is also an early finding. Flaring of the nares is a pertinent observation. Some patients become somnolent, and therefore the patient's mental status must continually be evaluated, keeping in mind the amount of narcotics used.

The disappearance of breath sounds over an area of lung where they were present previously and should be heard is a clear danger signal. Tachycardia is almost invariably present, and the rate is usually disproportionately rapid.

All these findings antedate x-ray changes by many hours. The x-ray film first shows patchy consolidation and diminished volume before complete opacification and collapse of the lobe or lung occurs. These findings are frequently misdiagnosed as pneumonitis, and treatment may be limited to antibiotic therapy.

Fever at levels of 39° to 40° C (102° to 104° F) also heralds atelectasis hours ahead of x-ray findings. As hypoxemia and hypercapnea increase, the patient may become apprehensive, agitated, and even disoriented or combative. These symptoms may lead to ordering additional sedation, which may prove to be a fatal mistake.

Management of secretions consists of three approaches. First, preoperative education and postoperative encouragement and assistance will result in effective coughing up of secretions. The surgeon and the nurse who continuously assist the patient with coughing will be able to prevent most postoperative problems associated with secretions. Assistance is best provided by having the patient sit up with the doctor or nurse standing on the opposite side from the area operated on and reaching with both arms around the patient, locking the fingers over the midportion of the chest, and pulling firmly, with the patient being held firmly against the assistant's chest, splinting while the patient coughs. Occasionally, excessive pain that is preventing coughing may be relieved by intercostal block to a point that a patient may completely clear the secretions. This is more applicable in the trauma patient with rib fractures than following thoracotomy.

Second, the method of nasotracheal suction proposed by Haight in 1947 (Fig. 2–1) is the method of choice for most patients. It requires a minimum of equipment, is easily mastered, and is relatively atraumatic to the patient. Unfortunately, much of the effort expended only serves to upset the patient and irritate the surgeon. The usual suction catheters provided are difficult to introduce and too small to do effective suctioning. Most

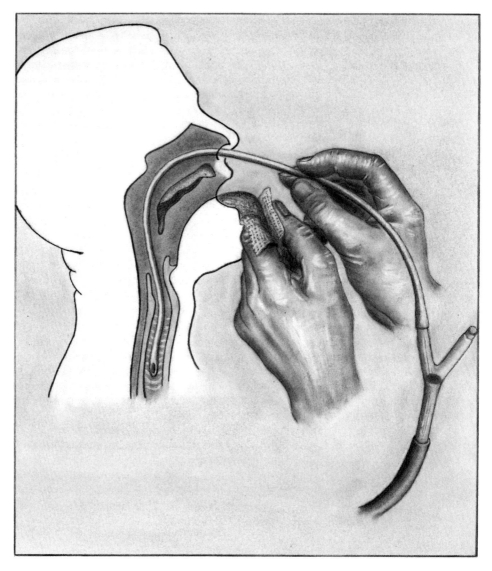

Figure 2–1. Diagrammatic representation of Haight's technique of intratracheal suction for removal of secretions.

often an attempt to introduce a catheter is made with the patient in the supine or head-elevated position, which makes tracheal intubation difficult.

I find it best to obtain a quantity of No. 16 or No. 18 French red rubber Robinson catheters, insert one end into the other, and have them sterilized. This gives the catheter sufficient curve to make intubation easy. A glass or plastic Y-tube is connected to the catheter and the suction tubing for suction control.

The patient should be sitting and an assistant should grasp the tongue with a 4 × 8 piece of gauze or a washcloth; while the tongue is held extended, the well-lubricated catheter is introduced through whichever nostril will accept it freely. Then the patient is asked to breathe deeply and slowly, and with a quick jabbing motion the catheter is introduced past the vocal cords. The patient should have already been informed that breathing will be possible and that the catheter will be in for only a short time. Suctioning is then carried out, turning the patient's head from side to side so that both main bronchi are intubated. The suction is interrupted every 2 to 3 seconds to avoid collapse of bronchi and to prevent hypoxia. If a large quantity of secretions is present, the catheter may have to be withdrawn into the trachea with the finger removed from the Y-tube; the patient is instructed to breathe and stop coughing. If oxygenation is poor, momentarily connect an oxygen source to the free arm of the Y-tube. After 20 to 30 seconds, suctioning may be resumed. Saline may be introduced for irrigation. A bronchoscopic suction trap may be placed in the circuit for collection of secretions for culture.

Effectively done, this technique — used one to three times daily — should prevent and treat most episodes of atelectasis and make bronchoscopy unnecessary.

Bronchoscopy by means of the fiberoptic bronchoscope can be used for secretion removal. It is best performed when the patient is still intubated or has a tracheostomy. The suction port is small, and if the secretions are thick, considerable time and irrigation may be required, or the procedure may be ineffective altogether.

Bedside bronchoscopy with a rigid bronchoscope is most effective, but should be reserved for the patient who has a completely collapsed lung or lobe and in whom catheter suctioning and fiberoptic bronchoscopy have been ineffective.

This technique consists of removing the headboard of the ICU bed and elevating the head to about 30 degrees. Topical anesthesia is produced by spraying the pharynx with an atomizer containing 0.5% tetracaine hydrochloride (Pontocaine) solution. The tonsillary fossae can be further anesthetized with a cotton sponge on a Jackson laryngeal forceps, and with each application the posterior one third of the tongue is also coated with Pontocaine. About 5 minutes are required before the gag reflex is abolished. No attempt is made to anesthetize the trachea as coughing is desirable. A 7 mm × 40 cm rigid bronchoscope is introduced and each orifice of the bronchial tree is cleared of secretions. Irrigation with saline is also helpful. It is best to spend 10 to 15 minutes with the bronchoscope in place to recover secretions that continually run into the larger bronchi from smaller, inaccessible ones. Oxygen may be introduced through the ventilating arm. Before the bronchoscope is removed, listen to the chest with a stethoscope to check for return of breath sounds.

Vigorous supported coughing during the first hour postbronchoscopy will produce a larger quantity of secretions than were removed by suctioning. A chest x-ray should show immediate clearing, and if it does not, another useful tool is to intubate the patient and, with the assistance of the anesthesiologist, attach an Ambu bag, applying up to 45 to 50 cm H_2O of inspiratory pressure for 15 to 30 minutes in an effort to expand the lung.

Secretion control requires effort, but the prompt, uncomplicated recovery of the thoracic surgical patient is a satisfying reward.

THE POSTOPERATIVE CHEST X-RAY

Postoperative x-ray films are an invaluable tool in the daily evaluation of the patient. To be of any value, the film must be of good quality. The surgeon should insist that, when at all possible, the patient be in an upright position, with the x-ray tube 6 feet away and the beam horizontal. Films are usually made with the patient in a semirecumbent position on the x-ray tube at an oblique angle 3 to 4 feet away. This produces a wide variety of interesting but uninterpretable films.

A patient who cannot sit up should have the film made in the supine position with the tube vertically over the patient and as high as possible. Do not accept underexposed or overexposed films, and do not try to read films in which the patient is in a rotated position or is otherwise malpositioned. This may cause considerable irritation for the radiologists and ICU nursing staff, but the patient's welfare is heavily dependent upon the interpretation of the postoperative film; therefore, film quality must not be compromised. Certainly, the surgeon must not be pushed into operative procedures or deterred from them on the basis of films of poor technical quality.

It is worthwhile each day to compare the current film with all preceding films rather than to trust imperfect memories.

The interpretation of the postoperative chest x-ray requires experience, and fellows and residents should spend much time reviewing the films with an experienced surgeon.

Findings that should be noted include mediastinal position, mediastinal widening, pneumothorax, estimate of the amount of pleural fluid and loculations of pleural fluid, position of chest tubes, air in the mediastinum or chest wall, consolidation or atelectasis of the lung, position of each leaf of the diaphragm, and changes in the shape or size of the cardiac silhouette.

All findings must be interpreted in light of the known pathologic processes and surgical defects rather than merely deviation from normal. This knowledge enables the thoracic surgeon to render a more accurate appraisal of the postoperative chest film than the radiologist. For this and other reasons, the surgeon must not develop the habit of accepting the radiologist's opinion instead of developing the skill to interpret postoperative films.

ANTIBIOTIC ADMINISTRATION AND WOUND INFECTION

There is no uniformity of opinion regarding preoperative, intraoperative, and postoperative antibiotic usage.

Excluding cardiovascular procedures from discussion, it is unclear whether a lesser incidence of postoperative wound infections results when prophylactic antibiotics are used. Wound infection of thoracotomy incisions, with the exception of the median sternotomy, are rare, and when they occur usually represent an extension of empyema of bronchial or esophageal origin. Most empyemas complicating pulmonary or esophageal procedures that did not reflect preoperative infection are traceable to technical error, errors in judgment, or poor postoperative care. Therefore, in Lindskog's words, antibiotic therapy becomes a kind of bib in attempting to prevent infections produced by poor surgical technique.

The control of surgical infection is a complex problem involving many professionals and departments and cannot be approached simplistically. Design of operating rooms; control and quality of air flow; isolation of known infections; an ongoing program of education in sterile procedure; adequate cleaning and maintenance techniques; a continuous program of surveillance of infections; screening of personnel and epidemiologic study; and high standards of operating techniques and perioperative care are all features that determine the incidence and seriousness of surgical infections.

Pre-existing pulmonary, mediastinal, or pleural infection should be treated with appropriate antibiotic therapy and the timing of operation coordinated with optimal response.

A pulmonary resection when there is no pre-existing infection probably requires no antibiotic therapy. Postoperatively, the majority of surgeons will probably use brief broad-spectrum antibiotic coverage.

The patient undergoing esophageal resection should, in my opinion, receive a preoperative bowel preparation including neomycin. Intraoperatively, 1 gram of a cephalosporin is given prior to surgery, and the dose is repeated 4 hours later. Postoperatively, cephalosporin and gentamicin are given for 36 hours. Unless there is evidence of clinical infection, no further therapy is required.

The practice of using the newest, most potent drugs, such as clindamycin, cefoxitin, or amikacin for prophylaxis is to be condemned.

The patient who, for any reason, is immunocompromised represents a significant risk. Institutions such as city hospitals or Veterans Administration hospitals have patient populations in which alcohol abuse, drug addiction, and poor nutrition—all unrelated to the surgical disease—are common. Tuberculosis is much more common than one would suppose. Cirrhosis and chronic renal disease are also frequent. Anergy in some patients with carcinoma of the esophagus and lung is well documented.

The patient in an immunocompromised state, regardless of its cause, should be identified. Those who have carcinoma are usually in a catabolic state, with malnutrition playing a major role. A period of 3 to 4 weeks of hyperalimentation may reverse this process in some patients when malnutrition is obvious.

Often, however, the higher risk must be accepted; certainly judicious antibiotic therapy may be of help, but it will not eliminate the risk of infection, particularly nosocomial infections.

PRINCIPLES OF PROPHYLACTIC ANTIBIOTIC ADMINISTRATION

1. There are no prophylactic doses as opposed to therapeutic doses. The drugs must be given in such quantity as to produce an effective concentration in the blood.

2. There is no single drug that will serve as an all-purpose prophylactic or therapeutic agent.

3. Duration of therapy should be short to prevent complications caused by various agents and to prevent emergence of or colonization by resistant organisms.

As suggested by Altemeir and colleagues, a 24-hour dose of the agent to be used is given, one third immediately preoperatively and one third every 4 hours two more times. Special situations or prolonged procedures may require a longer period of therapy.

Many combinations of agents are useful. Examples include the following:

1. **Penicillin G (or ampicillin) plus streptomycin or gentamycin.**
2. **A cephalosporin plus an aminoglycoside.**
3. **Erythromycin plus an aminoglycoside.**
4. **Cephamandol.**
5. **Clindamycin.**
6. **Vancomycin.**

In addition, other combinations are possible. An agent with significant toxic properties should not be selected for prophylactic use.

3
Postoperative Care: Special Problems

PNEUMONECTOMY

The pneumonectomy patient is at considerable risk, more so than most thoracic surgical patients, and requires careful attention and monitoring.

Immediate Postoperative State

A chest x-ray must be made as soon as the patient is turned to the supine position to determine the volume of air in the pleural space and the mediastinal position. Do not allow the scrub nurse to break scrub, and keep surgical instruments sterile until the patient leaves the room. After the x-ray is available, it can be determined whether the volume of air is sufficient, too little, or excessive. Thoracentesis with removal or addition of air may be required. A repeat film is then obtained before the patient is moved.

An alternative method is to use a U-shaped water manometer and adjust the volume until the pleural pressure is minus 6 to 8 cm of H_2O.

The pneumonectomy patient should lie on his or her back or on the operated side and never turn onto the unoperated side; the shift of mediastinum and chest wall splinting may result in hypoventilation if the remaining lung is dependent.

The patient should be extubated as soon as possible unless respiratory insufficiency is anticipated. Prior discussion with the anesthesiologist should prevent use of long-acting premedications or intraoperative use of agents whose actions cannot be reversed. Early ambulation, particularly in those over 75 years old, should be initiated. These patients are best gotten out of bed into a chair within 3 to 4 hours and made to stand and walk within 4 to 5 hours.

Some surgeons prefer to drain the pleural space so that mediastinal position can be easily controlled. The tube may remain clamped or connected to a water-seal drainage system without suction.

Postoperative Bleeding

Because a chest tube is not usually used, bleeding into the pleural space will not be observed easily. Evidence of hypovolemia as manifested by hypotension, tachycardia, diminished urine output, and lowered filling pressures may be identified. The hematocrit change may lag hours behind and not be useful in the early stage. A chest x-ray should be made immediately with the patient in the upright position to estimate the amount of pleural fluid accumulation since the last film. Any sudden increase should be a cause for concern. A massive hemorrhage signifies a pulmonary artery or vein ligature or a suture line disruption. This situation justifies rapid opening of the incision immediately and control of the bleeding site with the hand. The Ambu bag will be necessary for ventilation

28

while the patient is being transported to the operating room or sufficient equipment is being brought to the scene. There is not enough time to wait until the patient can be gotten to the operating room, or even to wait for a chest x-ray. Probably a time period of less than 1 to 2 minutes is the limit for establishing control.

Respiratory Insufficiency

Some patients requiring pneumonectomy display either respiratory insufficiency or acute cor pulmonale postoperatively.

This may represent an error in preoperative evaluation of pulmonary ventilatory and circulatory function. It may be the result of pneumonectomy that is required because of technical problems in a patient known to have diminished pulmonary function, when lobectomy had been planned. The patient may require prolonged ventilatory support and may or may not survive.

Before a fatalistic attitude is adopted, the surgeon should eliminate several factors that are mostly iatrogenic and are readily correctable.

1. **Excessive blood or crystalloid infusion. The total fluids should be added up and categorized. Diuresis using furosemide (Lasix) or ethacrynic acid (Edecrin) may be resorted to; even venisection may be performed. The best method of preventing fluid overload is to limit intravenous intake to replacement of measured blood loss and crystalloid infusion to about 1500 mL for the operative period and the first 4 to 6 hours. A Swan-Ganz catheter may be inserted if there is doubt, and the filling pressure determined.**
2. **Check the mediastinal position to be certain that acute mediastinal shift has not occurred and that the remaining lung has adequate expansion room.**
3. **Exclude pneumothorax on the nonoperated side.**
4. **Exclude unreversed muscle relaxant.**
5. **Be certain that excessive sedating drugs or narcotics have not been administered.**
6. **An intercostal block may be performed for pain relief to ascertain that hypoventilation is not due to pain.**

When all correctable factors have been excluded or corrected, continue ventilatory support, probably digitalize, and keep patient relatively dry. Often the patient will adjust to his limitations and recover, even though dyspnea may be permanent.

Postoperative Bronchopleural Fistula

Disruption of a bronchial suture or staple line represents one of the major complications in pulmonary surgery and requires prompt diagnosis and management if the patient is to survive.

A bronchial fistula rarely appears before the seventh day unless produced by endotracheal instrumentation; therefore, the patient is usually out of the critical care area or even at home. The disruption is heralded by a sudden onset of coughing, which produces a serosanguineous fluid. The pleural cavity is usually at least half full of fluid by this time. The danger is that the pleural fluid may enter the tracheobronchial tree faster than it can be coughed up, and the patient literally drowns. This can be fatal in minutes if not managed. There is no time for an x-ray to be made or for laboratory procedures to be carried out. Once it is established that a thin serosanguineous fluid is being coughed up, the pleural space must be drained immediately. A small incision (1 to 2 cm) is made in the midaxillary line in the fifth or sixth interspacing using whatever instruments are available. If a chest tube is not available, merely use a hemostat to make an opening into the pleura and drain the fluid into the bed. A chest tube may be inserted properly later. If there must be even a brief delay, have the patient lie on the operated side and instruct him or her to try not to cough or breathe deeply.

After the fluid has been drained, a chest tube is inserted or open drainage should be established on the most dependent site. A bronchial leak occurring within the first week warrants an attempt at surgical closure. The chest is opened and the bronchial stump identified. The stump is then resutured with 4-0 Prolene, Tev-Dek, or No. 32 stainless steel wire. The sutured stump should be covered with a vascularized muscle graft from an intercostal space or another source. If the pleural space is infected, however, closure will probably not be successful.

Empyema

Rarely, an empyema will develop in the absence of bronchopleural fistula. Diagnosis is confirmed by thoracentesis and culture. Drainage should be established. Then one of several protocols can be utilized in an attempt to sterilize the pleural space. The original article by Claggett should be consulted. After bacterial cultures are negative, the chest tube is removed and the tract excised and closed. The probability of control of infection without recurrence is about 50%.

Cardiac Problems

From 30 to 50% of pneumonectomy patients develop rapid atrial fibrillation or atrial flutter in the immediate postoperative period. The cause of this phenomenon is poorly understood. The pneumonectomy patient does not tolerate this arrhythmia well and usually manifests hypotension or rapid onset of congestive failure in the form of pulmonary edema or both. Early diagnosis and termination of the arrhythmia is necessary. Continuous electrocardiographic monitoring is a necessary part of care for the first week. Atrial fibrillation usually responds within a few hours to digitalization. Lantoside-C or digoxin may be used. Give half of the digitalizing dose intravenously, followed by one quarter of the total dose after 4 hours and the remaining one quarter after another 4 hours. Usually conversion occurs in the first 3 to 4 hours. Should the patient show evidence of heart failure and early conversion does not occur, cardioversion may be necessary. Some physicians prefer to slow the heart rate with propranolol and depend on digitalization.

Evidence of cor pulmonale should be managed with digitalization and diuretics, but usually the patient does not respond well and the prognosis is usually poor.

One more word about mediastinal position postoperatively. Occasionally, pleural fluid may be secreted faster than air is absorbed, or occasionally the reverse may occur. Should marked shift take place, it should be corrected by removing or adding additional air to achieve a stable state. Also, a poor chest wall closure may result in expelling the pleural air with the positive pressure of the respirator or with coughing. Again, this may require replacement by thoracentesis.

LOBECTOMY, SEGMENTECTOMY, AND LOCAL EXCISION

These procedures differ from pneumonectomy in several respects. First, respiratory insufficiency is not usually a problem unless a patient with severe chronic pulmonary disease has undergone surgery. Second, retention of bronchial secretions represents a greater problem and therefore atelectasis is a greater threat. Third, air leakage from lung parenchyma is almost universal and produces problems that require management.

Intraoperatively, the surgeon must continuously take care not to damage lung that is not to be resected and must meticulously close inadvertently produced leaks, particularly those that are larger or will not come into contact with the chest wall.

Inflammatory pleural disease that restricts motion of the remaining lung requires decortication, which must be performed meticulously.

Preoperative assessment of remaining lung volume and the amount of lung to be removed may require pre-section thoracoplasty or the combining of thoracoplasty with pulmonary resection. It is pointless to leave a volume of lung that cannot fill the thorax. Experience, more than anything else, will enable the surgeon to judge the disparity of lung volume with the volume of the pleural space after mediastinal shift and diaphragmatic elevation have occurred.

Other complications are managed similarly to those described for pneumonectomy.

Hemorrhage is a threat, but it has different manifestations. The chest tubes, if open, will result in lost blood appearing in the drainage system. It is normal for a thoracotomy wound to drain 500 to 800 mL of serosanguineous fluid in the first 24 hours. Occasionally this may mask real hemorrhage. To resolve doubt, obtain hematocrit readings on the drainage fluid to determine the blood content and measure loss every 10 min. Should loss exceed 100 mL/hour for more than 4 hours, reoperation should be considered. Any sudden increase of several hundred milliliters requires urgent reoperation, even in the ICU, depending on the volume of loss and the patient's condition.

MANAGEMENT OF THE POSTOPERATIVE BRONCHOPLEURAL FISTULA

Postoperative air leak is the most common sequela of pulmonary resection. It is a constant source of concern and frustration. The surgeon faces daily doubt and indecision as to how to proceed and whether or not to intervene surgically. Each surgeon tends to formulate a plan based on experience that generally deals well with the problem.

This section is designed, not for the purpose of educating the experienced surgeon, but to give some guidelines to the inexperienced one. Opposing views may be offered or other methods found that may be equally effective.

The first and foremost technique of coping with the persistent air leak is to prevent it. Be certain that the bronchial staple or suture line is secure and airtight before closure. Even a tiny bubble of air is not acceptable; the closure must be perfectly secure.

Second, during dissection in lysis of adhesions, the surgeon should not be hurried or use crude techniques and must, so far as is possible, prevent injury to the lung. Each incision into the parenchyma produces a leak that must either close spontaneously or be closed surgically.

Separating interlobar fissures requires patience and skill to remain in the interlobar plane. Separation of the incomplete fissure by the stapling instrument prevents many parenchymal leaks, but at the cost of compressing some lung tissue and distortion of the lung. This sacrifice is preferable in view of the risk that bronchopleural fistula and empyema may develop otherwise.

The patient with pulmonary emphysema represents a special problem. The peripheral air spaces are large and tend to leak more. The parenchyma is fragile and does not hold sutures well. The lung is avascular and, because of this, healing of the air leak may be slow or not occur at all. Therefore, these patients deserve the greatest of care and gentleness of tissue handling in order to minimize postoperative morbidity.

The surgeon must be certain that the amount of lung remaining following pulmonary resection is adequate to fill the pleural space. This should involve preoperative planning and knowledge of pulmonary function. It is usually possible to predict that there will be a space problem, and a preliminary or concomitant thoracoplasty may be done. Do not launch a resection plan that guarantees a postoperative problem. An example is a patient requiring an upper lobectomy and partial or complete resection of the superior segment. Without thoracoplasty or other measures, complete expansion is not likely to occur.

Segmental resection using the classic technique of Overholt always leaves a raw intersegmental plane from which air leakage is unavoidable. The stapling device may be used to remove the segment and minimize air leakage at the expense of distortion of the remaining lung. Otherwise the surgeon must accept a persistent fistula requiring prolonged or secondary drainage in about 15% of cases.

Because tuberculosis and bronchiectasis are now uncommon reasons for surgical intervention, the surgeon should exercise considerable discretion before performing segmental resection unless the stapling technique is applied.

Air leaks of any size produced by surgical trauma should be closed if possible. At least two methods are useful. The first is to grasp the area of the fistula gently with an Alyce forceps and carefully ligate the tissue. This avoids needle holes, which in turn will leak. The second is to oversew the area of fistula with 5-0 or 6-0 Prolene or similar suture material using a very small vascular needle. A small fragment of skeletal muscle may be excised and sutured over the air leak. A point of diminishing return is reached, after which the surgeon accepts a certain amount of air leakage. The volume of the sum of all air leaks cannot always be appreciated with the thorax open, but once the chest is closed, the volume of air leakage is fully apparent.

Occasionally, it is immediately obvious that the volume of leakage is excessive. Reopening the incision and making further efforts at control is preferable to a futile wait-and-see approach.

Once the postoperative period has been entered, how should the surgeon manage air leakage? This cannot be answered simply, but the following protocol is offered. Lung expansion must be maintained, and keeping the lung fully expanded is the best way of being certain that a peripheral leak will close. A negative pressure of -25 cm is suggested. If the lung cannot be kept expanded with this pressure, it may be increased to as much as -35 to -40 cm; however, the volume of leakage may be so great as to interfere with ventilation. In this case reoperation may be required.

A conservative course is in order if full expansion is being maintained. Rarely does a fistula fail to close under these circumstances, although it may persist for some time. Chest x-rays must be made often to be certain that expansion is being fully maintained.

Should a partial pneumothorax persist or appear after several days, the first approach is to ascertain that the chest tubes are patent and properly placed, correcting any defect that is present. The surgeon may then be tempted to reduce or remove suction in order to try to minimize the amount of air leakage on the theory that the fistula is being kept open by the suction. This is usually unwise, but it may be attempted if complete lung expansion has been maintained for several days. A chest film should be made 1 or 2 hours after reducing or removing suction. If a partial pneumothorax appears, immediately resume suction. **Never** attempt this maneuver in the presence of **incomplete** expansion.

Pneumoperitoneum (Fig. 3–1) is a procedure that dates back several years and may be useful when lung expansion appears to be insufficient for the pleural space. To be of value, it should be instituted early. The technique consists of inserting a No. 19 or No. 20 gauge needle into the peritoneal cavity at about the edge of the rectus sheath in either lower quadrant. After making certain that the needle is not in a vessel or vascular structure, 100 to 200 mL of air is instilled initially. After 3 or 4 minutes, the air volume is increased to 1000 mL. This produces considerable discomfort, including shoulder pain, a sense of fullness, and occasionally dyspnea. After an hour or so, most of the discomfort subsides. Then an abdominal binder is applied to increase intra-abdominal pressure. An upright chest film is made after 24 hours to assess the position of the diaphragm. Additional increments of air are instilled daily to produce an elevation of the diaphragm of about 5 cm. Temporary phrenic nerve paralysis was utilized frequently in the past to augment elevation of the diaphragm, but this maneuver is rarely used today.

Thoracoplasty may be needed if all measures fail, but when chest tubes are traversing the chest wall, there is risk of subscapular space infection. This is a complication of considerable magnitude not easily managed. It is far better to discern the need for thoracoplasty preoperatively or intraoperatively.

A small apical or localized space may be acceptable and may not require drainage unless obviously infected. Many of these spaces prove to be innocuous.

A major air leak appearing after the first 5 to 7 days may represent bronchial stump disruption. This may be considered a surgical problem. Reoperation and its risks must be assessed in view of the patient's general condition, the time interval since surgery, and the

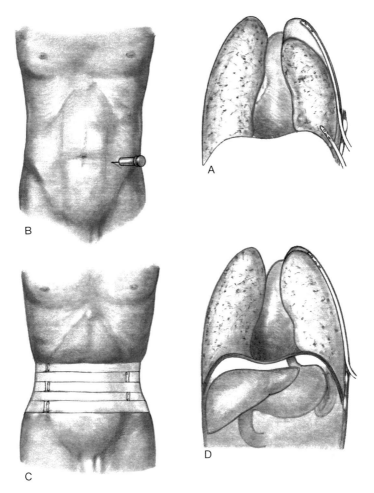

Figure 3–1. Use of pneumoperitoneum to assist in expansion of the lung after resection and closure of bronchopleural fistula. *A,* diagram of the postoperative situation with incomplete lung expansion. *B,* A needle is inserted into the left lower quadrant lateral to the pectal sheath and 500 cc of air is installed, to be followed later by an additional 1000 cc of air. *C,* An abdominal binder may be used to increase intra-abdominal pressure and increase diaphragmatic elevation. *D,* Diagram illustrating the elevated diaphragm that permits the lung to fill the pleural space. (From Hood, R. M., et al.: Surgical Diseases of the Pleura and Chest Wall. Philadelphia, W. B. Saunders Company, 1986, p. 154. Used by permission.)

surgeon's knowledge of the operative field. Long-term drainage may be chosen rather than an attempt at secondary closure. However, if reoperation is to be done, it must be done as early as possible.

Closure of a persistent bronchopleural fistula may be advisable. A major air leak appearing in the first week should be considered as originating from the bronchial stump. If the procedure has been a lobectomy or segmental resection, the inability to maintain expansion should probably be an indication for reoperation and secondary bronchial closure or reamputation and closure.

An early leak from the bronchial stump should also be considered for reoperation and resuture. The use of biologic glue to occlude a small bronchial fistula has been proposed. This may or may not prove effective.

A persistent bronchopleural fistula following a pneumonectomy poses a major therapeutic problem. Considerable attention has been focused in the past 7 years on

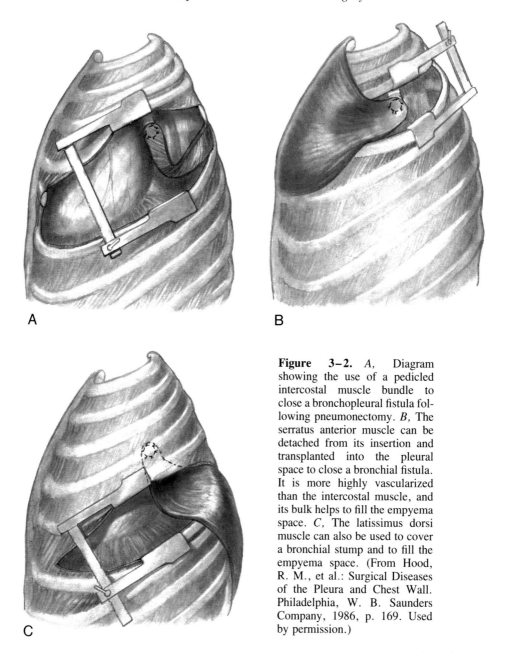

Figure 3–2. *A,* Diagram showing the use of a pedicled intercostal muscle bundle to close a bronchopleural fistula following pneumonectomy. *B,* The serratus anterior muscle can be detached from its insertion and transplanted into the pleural space to close a bronchial fistula. It is more highly vascularized than the intercostal muscle, and its bulk helps to fill the empyema space. *C,* The latissimus dorsi muscle can also be used to cover a bronchial stump and to fill the empyema space. (From Hood, R. M., et al.: Surgical Diseases of the Pleura and Chest Wall. Philadelphia, W. B. Saunders Company, 1986, p. 169. Used by permission.)

pedicled muscle grafts to suture over the fistula and also to obliterate the pleural space to avoid thoracoplasty. The various muscles that may be used include intercostal muscle, pectoralis major, latissimus dorsi, serratus anterior, and rectus abdominus. (Fig. 3–2 *A–C*). The greater omentum can also be used for this purpose (see Chap. 11).

It is a serious error to try to close the pleural space by this method too early. The pleural space in the first 3 months is simply too large. There is progressive shrinking of the space produced by mediastinal shift, elevation of the diaphragm and constriction of the chest wall. By the end of the sixth month, the space remaining will be less than one-third to one-fourth the volume it was during the first few weeks. The amount of muscle required to fill the space or the extent of thoracoplasty required can be minimized by waiting.

One point is worth mentioning at the risk of appearing snide. The cosmetic defect of thoracoplasty is undesirable, but disability is not severe. If all of the muscle grafts are used as recommended by some authors, the disability of arm and shoulder motion will exceed that of thoracoplasty.

In summary, bronchopleural fistula is a common problem. It should be prevented if at all possible. Once it is established, a watchful, nonsurgical approach is usually adequate. Surgical intervention is occasionally useful.

Patients who have undergone partial resection have more difficulty with retention of secretions and subsequent atelectasis than pneumonectomy patients or thoracotomy patients who have not had pulmonary resection. The extent and severity of pulmonary and tracheobronchial infections parallel the patient's difficulty with secretions. Therefore, the surgical procedure should be done after maximal efforts at control of infection and reduction of the volume of secretions have been made (see earlier discussions on this subject).

Local excision and wedge resections are simple to do, and the surgeon may be tempted not to use a chest tube. This will usually prove to be bad judgment. With rare exceptions, any time the chest is opened, a chest tube should be used, and if any pulmonary resection is done, two tubes are preferable.

ESOPHAGEAL RESECTION

If the operative approach was a posterior thoracotomy, a portable chest film must be made immediately, as soon as closure is completed, to determine the presence of contralateral pneumothorax or hemothorax and the need for chest tube insertion. The position of the nasogastric tube should be noted and adjusted if necessary.

Retention of bronchial secretions is common, and atelectasis is a major problem that must be prevented. Nasotracheal suction after extubation may be hazardous if there is a cervical or a high intrathoracic anastomosis. The suctioning must not be delegated to someone who is unskilled or unaware of the danger of injuring the anastomotic suture line. Bronchoscopy poses similar risks and must be done with care. Tracheostomy may be necessary occasionally; however, in the presence of a cervical anastomosis, it may result in infection in the area. It should be done above the thyroid isthmus at the level of the second cartilage if it is required.

Cardiac arrhythmias are common, particularly atrial fibrillation, which occurs in from 30 to 50% of patients. Early diagnosis is necessary. Management usually requires only digitalization, but propranolol may be useful in slowing the heart rate. Cardioversion can be used if the arrhythmia is refractory.

Many surgeons prefer to use digitalization preoperatively rather than wait for a specific indication. In the absence of evidence of congestive heart failure or preoperative rhythm disturbances, I do not perform digitalization preoperatively.

There is always a question of when to remove the nasogastric tube postoperatively. Its presence is probably detrimental to the esophagogastric anastomosis. If it is removed too soon, however, the intestinal ileus or poor gastric emptying persist, and reintroduction of the tube is hazardous.

I prefer to wait until there is active peristalsis, a minimum of gastric drainage, and the passage of flatus before removing the tube. The integrity of the anastomosis should be verified by contrast study before feeding begins. The patient is given clear liquids, progressing to a bland diet over 1 week.

Early dilatation with a Hurst-Maloney dilator is helpful in preventing stricture formation. A size 36 dilator is passed on the ninth or tenth postoperative day and repeated weekly, increasing to a size 44. This is terminated after 4 to 6 weeks.

Although it is common practice to leave chest tubes in longer than usual because of the risk of anastomotic leak, this is probably unwise. The chest tube will become walled off early, and in the event of a leak, the tube will probably not communicate with the area of leakage. In addition, the longer a tube remains in place, the more likely it is that it will serve as an entry route for infection. Therefore, the tube should be removed, as in any other thoracotomy.

Postoperative bleeding is unlikely unless there has been invasion of neoplasm into the paraesophageal tissues, necessitating extensive dissection and the leaving of a large, raw wound area. This is made worse if bacterial infection has been present in the area of the neoplasm. Careful hemostasis intraoperatively is necessary if reoperation is to be avoided.

Anastomotic leak is the most feared complication in esophagectomy. Intrathoracic leak probably occurs in about 5% of patients. Cervical anastomotic leaks have been variously reported in from 5 to 30% of patients. An intrathoracic leak will produce a life-endangering mediastinitis and empyema unless promptly diagnosed and drained. The character of the chest tube drainage must be noted daily. Any evidence of purulent material or bile requires an immediate contrast study. Once the chest tube has been removed, the surgeon must rely on the appearance of the chest x-ray and the clinical findings. Any evidence of otherwise unexplained sepsis, air or fluid in either pleural space, mediastinum, or the cervical wound, and pain or swelling of the neck must be sought and the diagnosis established by contrast study.

Occasionally, the vascularity and viability of the transplanted stomach or colon may be questionable at the time of surgery, and the survival of the organ may not be certain. Re-exploration of the cervical incision, that is, a "second look," 24 to 36 hours postoperatively will establish the fact so that a necrosing stomach or colon can be removed before perforation and infection have occurred.

Management of an anastomotic leak once the diagnosis is established requires immediate intervention. The cervical leak should be exposed by reopening the incision and placing a Penrose or Jackson-Pratt drain in the area. Occasionally, if this is done early, an attempt may be made to repair the area of disruption. Generally, there is too much induration for sutures to hold. A cervical skeletal muscle may be detached and sewn into the leak. The wound must be left open. Most cervical fistulas close, although frequently with stricture formation. Dilatation of the anastomosis may be accomplished even though the salivary fistula is present.

The surgeon must remember that the cervical anastomosis area usually communicates with the right pleural space, and because of this fact, early drainage may not prevent empyema. Empyema may occur regardless of the timing or method of drainage and make drainage of the pleural space necessary.

Disruption of an intrathoracic anastomotic leak is a much more serious matter. Diagnosis is frequently delayed, and the reluctance to reoperate is also a cause of delay. A simple chest tube should not be considered effective drainage. It is preferable to reopen the thoracotomy incision and free the lung, exposing the anastomosis and placing drains about the area of disruption.

These drains should be Jackson-Pratt drains. A chest tube should also be sutured in place, close, but not in contact with, the stomach or esophagus. The mediastinum should be opened widely enough to be certain that no area of infection is left undrained. Occasionally, drainage of the contralateral pleural space is also necessary.

The patient's clinical course should be followed carefully and should be one of rapid improvement. A failure to improve, a rising white blood cell count, and persistent fever should be warnings that drainage has not been adequate or that mediastinitis or empyema is progressing in spite of the drainage procedure.

A decision must be made early whether to attempt additional drainage or to reoperate and take out the transplanted organ entirely. The procedure must be accompanied by cervical esophagostomy and closure of the wound in the fundus of the stomach. It may be necessary to resect a part of the stomach, and on occasion the stomach may be replaced in the peritoneal cavity and gastrostomy or jejunostomy established for feeding.

Usually drainage is adequate, and the leak will close or can be closed later with a pedicled muscle graft. Stricture formation is almost inevitable. However, if the patient continues to show evidence of sepsis, it is preferable to sacrifice the esophagogastrectomy rather than have a fatality from infection.

A second reconstructive procedure will have to follow at a later date.

4

Operations for Trauma

The procedures described in this chapter are those related to thoracic trauma. Some, like thoracentesis and chest tube insertion, are widely used for other purposes as well. This is not intended to be a comprehensive guide to trauma management but rather a description of operative procedures that are useful in trauma patients. The lesser procedures are described in considerable detail because these are more likely to be employed by those with least experience and because of the frequency of major technical mishaps related to these operations.

PROCEDURES FOR TRAUMA AND CONDITIONS REQUIRING SURGERY

1. **Thoracentesis.**
2. **Chest tube insertion—chest suction apparatus.**
3. **Cricothyroidotomy.**
4. **Tracheostomy.**
5. **Flail chest.**
6. **Decortication.**
7. **Repair of ruptured bronchus.**
8. **Repair of ruptured diaphragm.**
9. **Cardiac tamponade.**
10. **Repair of atrial or aortic injury.**
11. **Repair of ventricular injury.**
12. **Repair of cervical esophageal injury.**
13. **Repair of thoracic esophageal injury.**
14. **Management of penetrating injuries to the base of the neck.**
15. **Intercostal block.**

THORACENTESIS

Thoracentesis is one of the most commonly performed procedures, yet despite its frequent use and simplicity, the number of major mishaps associated with it is very high. Thoracentesis is included here to help prevent these largely unnecessary complications.

First, examine x-rays to evaluate the pleural effusion. The effusion may be localized; if so, its position must be accurately determined. A large generalized or unilocular effusion should pose few problems. The surgeon must remember that the position of the diaphragm at the time of the procedure will be 3 to 5 cm higher than that seen on the typical, full inspiration film. When pleural disease is present, it is not unusual for the diaphragm to be elevated above its normal position. Cardiac size is also important. Gross enlargement of the heart, which may be observed by pleural effusion, has resulted in cardiac injury during attempts at thoracentesis.

Procedure (Fig. 4-1)

Have the patient assume a sitting position with the arms resting on an overbed table or supported by a nurse. The patient should be comfortable. Prepare the skin with povidone-iodine (Betadine) or other agent. Drape only below the area of thoracentesis.

Anesthesia.   1% lidocaine (Xylocaine). A large skin wheal is produced by intradermal injection, followed by subcutaneous infiltration. As the rib area is entered, try, by touching the rib and feeling your way, to enter the intercostal space just above the rib below and infiltrate 5 mL of lidocaine in this area (Fig. 4-2). Do not try to find the intercostal nerve. Then wait 2 to 3 minutes before proceeding. Thoracentesis should not be painful.

Site of Puncture.   A localized pleural effusion demands careful localization before attempting thoracentesis. The sixth or seventh interspace just below the tip of the scapula

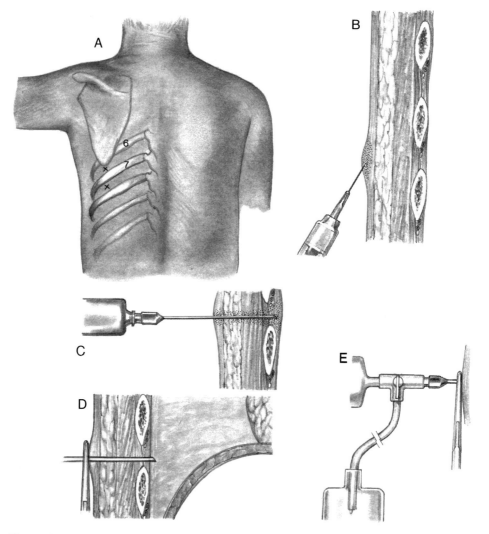

Figure 4-1.   Thoracentesis. Basic technique. *A,* The usual site of thoracentesis, the sixth or seventh inner space. *B, C,* Lower aspiration points than those illustrated should be avoided. *D,* A method of controlling the length of a needle inserted into the pleural space to minimize injury to the lung and avoid causing secondary pneumothorax as a complication. *E,* The procedure should be a closed one to minimize the aspiration of air into the pleural space with emptying of the syringe.

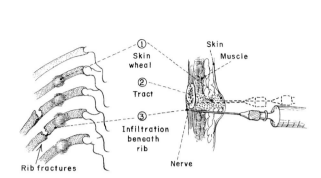

Figure 4–2. The technique of intercostal nerve block as described in the text. Note that the infiltrating needle is "walked" under the lower rib margin, unlike the technique of thoracentesis. (From Zuidema GD, Rutherford RB, Ballinger WF: The Management of Trauma, 4th ed. Philadelphia, WB Saunders Co, 1985, p 402.) Reprinted in Hood, R. M., Boyd, A. D., and Culliford, A. T.: Thoracic Trauma. Philadelphia, W. B. Saunders Company, 1989, p. 105. Used by permission.)

should be used for a generalized effusion. **Do not use a lower interspace.** A plastic cannula with a removable needle is desirable to avoid lung injury. Otherwise a 14 gauge needle is preferable.

Place the needle to be used on a 10 mL syringe with a three-way stopcock. Clamp a hemostat on the needle at the estimated length to be used. Make a 2 mm incision with a No. 11 blade. Introduce the needle slowly, again noting the top edge of the rib, and enter the pleural space very carefully. As soon as free fluid is obtained, readjust the hemostat so that the depth of the needle is fixed. Exchange the 10 mL syringe for a 50 mL syringe and attach tubing from the stopcock to the receptacle to be used.

Withdraw fluid at a steady rate. The procedure should be terminated if the patient complains of dyspnea, vertigo, or pain or begins to cough. The maximum amount of fluid removed at any one time should be 1000 mL. As soon as the lung is felt to touch the needle, stopping the fluid flow, discontinue the effort rather than persist and produce a pneumothorax.

An alternative method is to introduce a plastic catheter through the needle and thereby minimize the risk of lung injury, although fluid removal is slower.

Resist the temptation to attach the needle to a suction system to speed up fluid removal; also, if the patient becomes agitated or dyspneic, do not persist.

Observe the patient for several minutes to be certain that hypotension does not occur. Syncope is frequent.

Should the patient not be able to sit, move him or her to the edge of the bed and have someone support the arm and tap as far posteriorly as possible, but again not below the seventh interspace in the posterior axillary line.

A portable chest film should be obtained immediately to be certain whether pneumothorax is or is not present.

INTERCOSTAL NERVE BLOCK

Procedure (Figs. 4–3 and 4–4)

The patient is placed in the lateral or sitting position.

Anesthesia

Lidocaine 1%. A 5 mL syringe armed with a No. 25 or No. 26 gauge ½ inch needle is used to make an intradermal welt over each rib that is to be blocked at the posterior rib angle. A 10 mL syringe with a No. 20 1½ inch (3 cm) needle is then employed. The needle is inserted through the area of skin anesthesia and used to palpate the rib. The

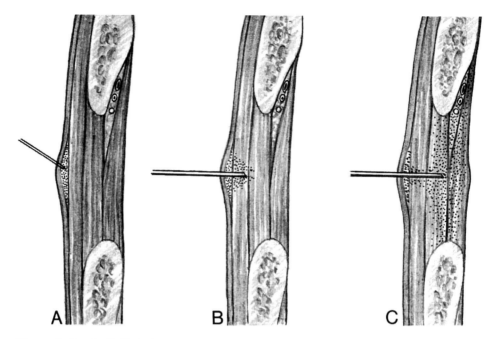

Figure 4–3. *A–C,* Techniques of local anesthesia to the chest wall prior to needle biopsy or thoracentesis. Adequate anesthesia should be produced and the procedure should be painless.

needle is "walked" off the edge of the rib and then advanced about 0.5 cm. After one is certain that the needle is extravascular, 5 cc of anesthetic solution is injected into the intracostal space with no attempt being made to touch the intercostal nerve. Attempting to inject in or near the nerve is painful, may injure the intercostal artery, and is not necessary. One must avoid entering the pleural space, and attempts at injection posterior to the rib angle are more likely to result in intradural injection, arterial injury, and in entering the pleura. The dural sheath extends laterally up to 1″ from the foramen. There is no internal intercostal muscle in this area, and the vessels and nerve lie directly on the pleura in the middle of the intercostal space. The number of intercostal spaces to be blocked depends on the extent and number of ribs fractured.

CHEST TUBE INSERTION

Indications

1. **Any traumatic pneumothorax and selected cases of spontaneous pneumothorax.**
2. **Significant hemothorax.**
3. **Penetrating thoracoabdominal injury.**
4. **Prophylactically in patients with rib fractures or penetrating wounds without evidence of pneumothorax, who (a) are going to surgery for other reasons or (b) are going to be intubated and placed on a respirator.**
5. **Two tubes are often necessary.**

Procedure: Pneumothorax (Fig. 4–4)

A 2 cm incision is made over the fourth interspace in the anterior axillary line. The chest wall is penetrated with a hemostat, which is spread until a finger can be introduced.

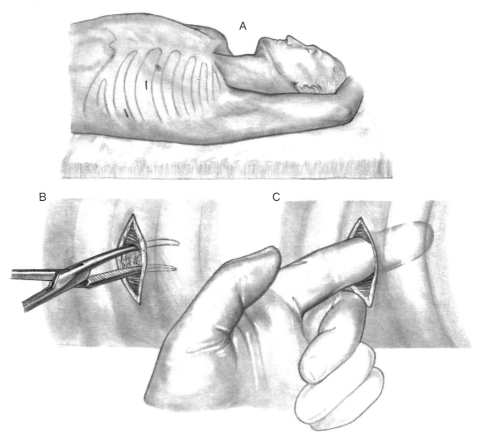

Figure 4–4. Chest tube insertion.

A, Two sites for chest tube insertion. The upper site is in the anterior axillary line in the fourth interspace and is the site preferred for pneumothorax. The lower site is the fifth or sixth interspace in the posterior axillary line. A tube for drainage of hemothorax or a pleural effusion would use this site.

B, A skin incision has been made and a sharp hemostat (tonsil or Crile) is used to enlarge the wound, penetrate the musculature, and enter the pleural space.

C, A finger is introduced to explore and further widen the wound.

Illustration continued on following page

The presence of a free pleural space is ascertained. A No. 28 chest tube is usually used. A No. 20 or No. 24 tube is adequate for spontaneous pneumothorax. The length of tube to be inserted is determined and marked with a ligature around the tube, or a hemostat may be clamped across the tube. Four to six inches of tube should be inserted into the pleural space.

Insert the tube with the aid of a large hemostat, directing and guiding it with a finger superiorly and anteriorly. Do not tunnel the tube tract. A tube containing a rigid trochar may be used (Fig. 4–4*F*). This will make a smaller incision possible, and the metal trochar may be bent at an angle of about 35 degrees to facilitate placement of the tube anteriorly or laterally. The trochar must not be used with force as an introducer or serious injury to the lung or other structures may result. It should be used as a guide for placement.

Sutures (size 0 or 2-0) are placed at either side of the tube, closing the wound, and are tied around the tube. A horizontal mattress suture is placed in the center of the wound and

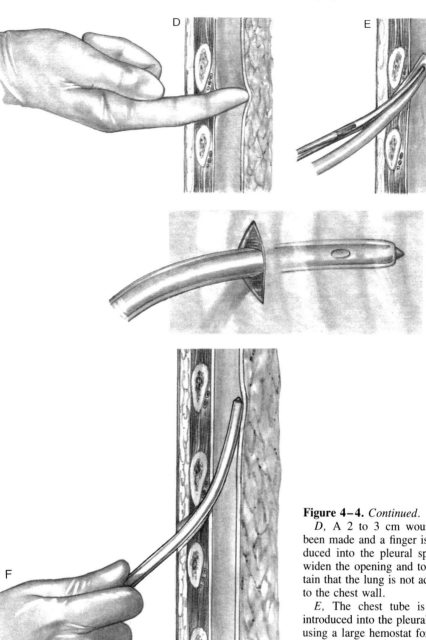

Figure 4–4. *Continued.*

D, A 2 to 3 cm wound has been made and a finger is introduced into the pleural space to widen the opening and to ascertain that the lung is not adherent to the chest wall.

E, The chest tube is being introduced into the pleural space using a large hemostat for guidance.

F, The trochar chest tube has been bent to an angle of about 30 degrees and is being gently introduced and guided into position.

Illustration continued on opposite page

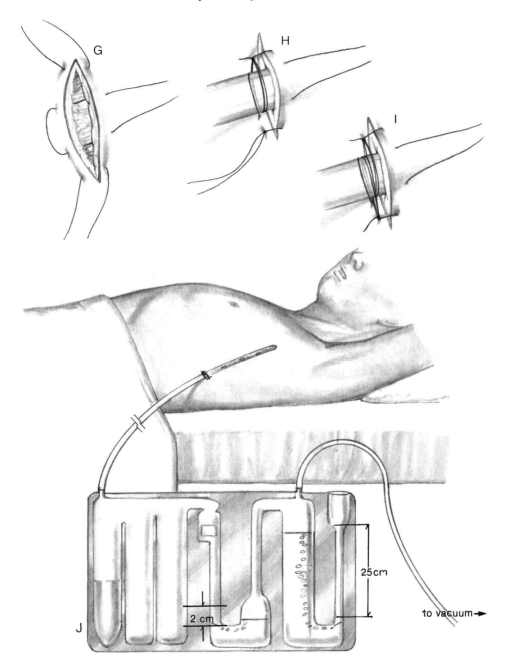

Figure 4–4. *Continued.*

G–I, A technique of suturing the chest tube to the skin and leaving a suture to tie when the tube is removed.

J, The chest tube has been inserted, sutured in place, and connected to one of the available drainage systems. These drainage systems consist of a collection area, a waterseal apparatus, and a suction-regulating system (on the right).

left untied to use for wound closure at the time of tube removal (Fig. 4–4G, H, and I).

Connect the chest tube to waterseal apparatus. The amount of negative pressure to be used should be individualized but is usually in the range of 20 to 25 cm H_2O (Fig. 4–4J).

Rapid re-expansion of the lung may produce pain, dyspnea, and violent coughing. Therefore, the waterseal system alone is used initially, and after lung expansion is well advanced, suction may be added.

The common, older method of introducing a mushroom or Foley catheter through the anterior second interspace should be abandoned. It is unnecessarily painful. When the lung expands, it covers and occludes the catheter, leaving an apical pneumothorax. The lung seals about the tube, rendering it useless. A tube in this site is ineffective in removing pleural fluid or blood.

CRICOTHYROIDOTOMY

Cricothyroidotomy is particularly useful in emergency situations when tracheal intubation from above cannot be carried out. It is also of value in patients who have had recent median sternotomy incisions. Cricothyroidotomy is contraindicated in patients with significant laryngeal inflammation because of the risk of subglottic stenosis. I consider any patient having an endotracheal tube in place for 5 days or longer to have significant laryngeal inflammation.

Procedure (Fig. 4–5)

Cricothyroidotomy is a rapid, technically simple, and precise procedure. It is carried out under sterile conditions with the neck in moderate extension. The neck is carefully palpated and the cricothyroid space identified at the lower end of the thyroid cartilage. Care must be exercised in identifying the cricothyroid space because the thyrohyoid space can be mistaken for the lower cricothyroid space. A transverse incision is then made over the cricothyroid space. Veins encountered in this area are clamped and tied with absorbable suture except in emergency situations, when this may be omitted. The cricothyroid membrane is then pierced with a No. 15 blade, taking care not to injure the posterior trachea. A Trousseau dilator or fine clamp is inserted into this stab wound and gently spread, separating the thyroid and cricoid cartilages. Heavy scissors are then inserted in the opening and spread transversely, paralleling the cricoid cartilage until the cricoid membrane is opened sufficiently so that a tracheostomy tube can be inserted. A Lanz, Shiley, or American high-volume, low-pressure cuff tracheostomy tube is then inserted. Usually an 8 mm tube is used.

TRACHEOSTOMY

Tracheostomy is a standard tool in management of the thoracic surgical patient. Unfortunately, in most centers a retrospective review of this operative procedure will show: (1) that a significant number of patients did not require tracheostomy, and (2) that the morbidity and mortality rates were excessive, particularly in view of the usual belief that a tracheostomy is a relatively simple operation and should not be associated with major complications or death.

Observation over many years has conclusively demonstrated that many house officers do not have a clear understanding of the indications for tracheostomy and have an even less clear understanding of the contraindications. Many avoidable technical errors, a number of them fatal, occur far too often, and poor postoperative management has resulted in additional complications and death.

This section assumes that the reader has no previous knowledge of tracheostomy techniques.

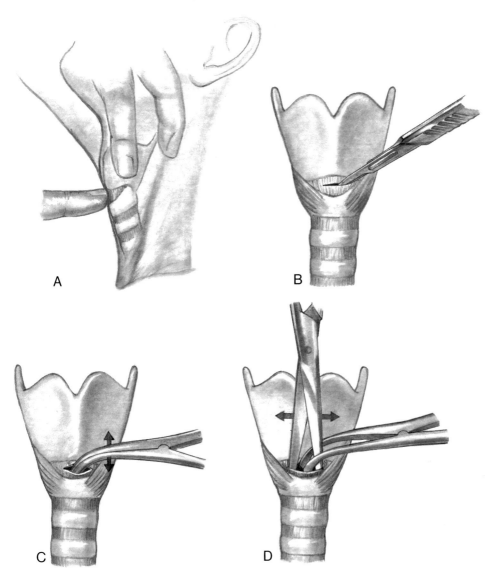

Figure 4–5. Cricothyroidotomy. *A,* With the patient in position with the neck extended, the thyroid cartilage is held with one hand and the forefinger is used to palpate the space between the thyroid and cricoid cartilages. *B,* The skin is incised over the thyrocricoid membrane. The membrane is incised and the lumen entered. *C,* A tracheal spreader is introduced. *D,* The opening is enlarged to the point that a tracheostomy tube can be introduced.

Indications

1. When access is required for suctioning of secretions not otherwise manageable.
2. When laryngeal or subglottic obstruction is present.
3. When oral or nasal intubation is not technically possible and intubation is mandatory.
4. When extensive head, facial, or oral injuries are present and there is need to provide an airway and to prevent aspiration of blood and secretions.
5. When a patient requires endotracheal intubation for a longer period than 72 to 96 hours.

6. **When suctioning via endotracheal tube is inadequate to control secretions and prevent atelectasis or infection.**
7. **When it is necessary to decrease airway dead space volume.**

Contraindications

1. **Do not use for establishment of airway if orotracheal or nasotracheal intubation is possible.**
2. **Tracheobronchitis.**
3. **Recent aortic or cardiac surgery (relative).**
4. **Infants under 6 months (relative).**
5. **Asthma.**
6. **When safe operation is not possible.**
7. **Lack of positive indication.**

Requirements for Operation

1. **Surgical lighting.**
2. **Adequate instruments.**
3. **Assistant.**
4. **Suction.**
5. **Prior endotracheal intubation makes procedure safer.**

Note: Tracheostomy is usually relegated to the individual with the least surgical experience. The most experienced surgeon available should be at least a participant.

Procedure (Fig. 4–6)

The patient should be placed in the supine position with a folded or rolled sheet, approximately 3 inches in height, placed beneath the shoulders, allowing the head to be hyperextended slightly. One individual should hold the head in the vertical position to prevent the patient from moving the head during the procedure.

Local anesthesia is produced by intradermal and subcutaneous injection of 1% lidocaine. A transverse incision, 5 cm in length, is made approximately 1 inch above the suprasternal notch. The incision is carried through the platysma muscle with sharp dissection. From this point, it is best to use only blunt dissection, and certainly the operator should not cut blindly in an area where the structures cannot be perfectly identified. The anterior cervical musculature is separated in the midline by blunt dissection, opening the pretracheal fascia and entering the visceral compartment of the neck. The trachea will be found to be covered with adipose mediastinal tissue. This tissue should be dissected bluntly from the anterior tracheal wall until the trachea can be seen clearly. The trachea is then grasped with a tracheal hook or tenaculum and elevated into the wound. The first hook should preferably be placed to the right of the midline. A second hook is then placed in the same position on the opposite side, further elevating it into the wound and immobilizing it. The hooks should be directed from inferiorly to superiorly.

A vertical incision is made in the second or third tracheal ring using a No. 15 blade; it is preferable not to incise the fourth or fifth ring for fear of letting the tracheostomy tube come into contact with, or injuring, the innominate artery or vein. The artery should be palpated before making the tracheostomy incision. It may be necessary to place the incision above the thyroid isthmus to avoid an excessively low tracheostomy stoma.

A tracheal spreader is then introduced through the incision and the incision is opened widely. The surgeon should hold the tracheal spreader with the right hand while the assistant takes the tracheostomy tube (previously assembled and with the balloon tested), and insert it into the trachea and the obturator removed. The hooks and tracheal spreader should be removed from the wound and the patient connected to the ventilator. The

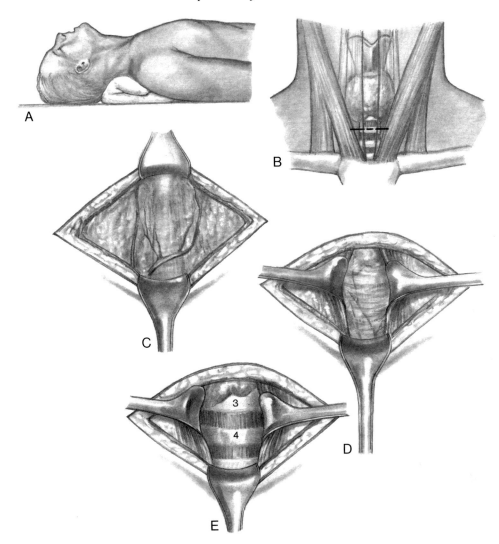

Figure 4–6. Tracheostomy. The basic steps in tracheostomy (see text for more detail).

Illustration continued on following page

tracheal balloon should be inflated slowly until there is just a minimal leak of air. Then the tracheostomy tube is tied in place to prevent its being extruded from the trachea.

At this point, a careful search is made for bleeding points, which are secured by cautery or ligature.

Technical Notes. It is my preference to use a No. 6 or No. 7 tracheostomy tube routinely. The fiberoptic bronchoscope will pass through the No. 7 tube. Using a No. 8 or No. 9 tube or an even larger one will merely result in an inordinate amount of injury to the anterior tracheal wall.

It is wisest to use a 6-inch flexible silastic tube between the respirator tubing and the tracheostomy tube to avoid undue torque being placed on the tube by the rigidity of the ventilator tubing.

Lessons from Experience. Technical errors include injury to the anterior cervical veins, left innominate vein, innominate artery, internal jugular vein, and carotid arteries; pneumothorax, particularly in children; placement of the stoma too low; and injury at the stoma site to a degree that will result in a stricture formation. All of these are preventable

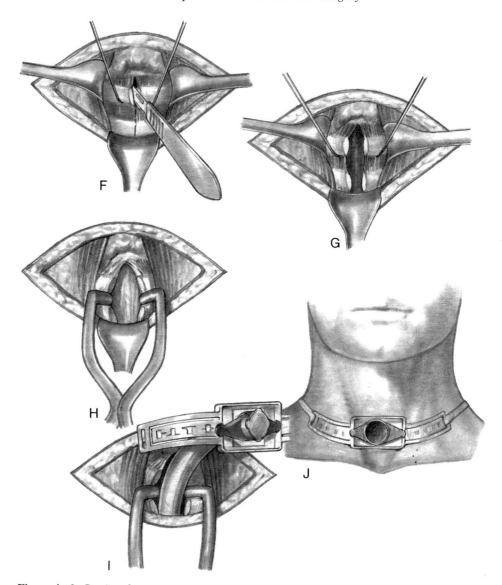

Figure 4–6. *Continued.*

if the surgeon has adequate light and assistance, and knows how to do the procedure. When possible, and particularly in children, tracheostomies should be performed with an endotracheal tube in place.

Tracheostomy Care

Each day the wound should be dressed, preferably twice daily. One should never allow the weight of the ventilator tubing to pull on the tracheostomy tube. The ventilator tubing should be secured by external fixation near the patient. Balloon inflation should never exceed the volume necessary to maintain a slight leak, and one should not inflate the balloon before the ventilator is connected. The tracheostomy should be suctioned using sterile gloves and catheters. The catheters should always have at least two terminal ports or holes. Extreme gentleness should be used in suctioning to avoid damage to tracheal mucosa. Added humidification is usually a significant component of all types of ventilator systems, but the surgeon should be certain that humidification of an adequate degree is available. It is hazardous to attempt oral feeding in the tracheostomy patient because aspiration will almost surely occur. The patient who requires a tracheostomy tube for many months may learn to eat without risk of aspiration, but it would be preferable if oral feeding were not attempted. Finally, the tracheostomy tube should be removed as soon as possible and not left in place any longer than is absolutely necessary.

Management of Complications

Injury or Erosion of an Innominate Artery.   This is a catastrophic complication of tracheostomy, which more often than not is fatal. The first requirement is to control hemorrhage. This is best done by using the tracheostomy tube to compress the innominate artery or by removing the tracheostomy tube and using the finger to compress the artery against the posterior surface of the sternum. As soon as this has been accomplished, the patient should be orally intubated and the trachea cleared as rapidly as possible of aspirated blood. Once this has been done, the patient's ability to survive is at least established. The patient is then taken to the operating room and anesthetized. While one person continues to tamponade the innominate artery, an assistant opens the sternum through a median sternotomy, retracting the sternum widely. As soon as the innominate artery can be visualized, it can be clamped proximally with a vascular clamp, and both the subclavian and carotid arteries should also be clamped. After both ends have been secured, the injured area is excised and the ends oversewn with 4-0 monofilament nonabsorbable suture. Never make an attempt to repair the injured artery at this time because this is an infected field, and any such attempt will prove disastrous when secondary hemorrhage occurs several days later. Should revascularization be required, an extra-anatomic graft outside the primary surgical field should be utilized. This graft may be from the left carotid artery, but probably is best taken from the axillary or subclavian artery on the left side to the axillary artery on the right side. To reiterate, primary repair should not be attempted.

Pneumothorax.   This is a complication that occurs most often in children under 5 years because the pleura approaches the midline in a small child. If the dissection is kept in the midline, pneumothorax is not likely to occur. When a tracheostomy is being done in a small child, postoperative chest films made immediately afterward are desirable to detect pneumothorax before it becomes a critical problem. In the small child, bilateral pneumothorax is common and immediately life-endangering.

Late Tracheal Stricture.   Stricture may result from excessive surgical trauma at the stoma site, but more often occurs at the balloon site and may be produced by overinflation, poor care, or merely the length of time that an inflated tracheostomy balloon is required. The routine use of a low-pressure cuff, properly inflated, is an important preventive measure. See Chapter 7 for the procedure for resection of tracheal stricture.

Intraoperative Bleeding.   Bleeding may be venous or arterial, and if it should occur, it should be controlled temporarily by digital pressure or pack. Then, if the patient is outside the operating room, the patient should be transported to the operating room, where adequate assistance and proper instruments are available. Blind efforts to clamp an unknown bleeding vessel can be disastrous. Usually, however, bleeding is from veins lying anterior to the trachea.

Wound Infection.   This is an unusual complication which is best prevented by leaving the wound open rather than suturing it closed, as well as by good surgical technique.

Marked Subcutaneous and Mediastinal Emphysema.   Rapidly advancing subcutaneous emphysema is most often caused by the tracheostomy tube lying in the anterior mediastinum instead of in the trachea. With each effort by the respirator, air is insufflated into the mediastinum. Air may also appear if there is a significant leak around the inflated cuff and if the wound has been tightly secured. If the tracheostomy tube is not in the trachea, respiratory distress will occur simultaneously, with the appearance of subcutaneous emphysema. Immediate wound inspection and determination of the cause are necessary.

Dislodgment of the Tracheostomy Tube. This mishap may occur at any time. It is more likely to happen in an obese patient with a short, thick neck or in a patient who is agitated and struggling. Tying the tube firmly in place and being certain that the tube is long enough and properly placed are important. Immediate recognition of displacement is critical. Replacement is simple if the tube has been in place for 3 days or longer. Should the tube be displaced in the first 24 hours, there will be no established tract, and replacement may be difficult. Attempting to reinsert the tube blindly is usually unsuccessful, and if the patient is respirator-dependent, or if proximal obstruction is present, the time available for replacement is very short. It is best to obtain a tracheostomy set, assistance, and good lighting and to re-establish surgical exposure so that the stoma may be visualized and the tube replaced. An endotracheal tube may be used if the tracheostomy tube is too short, rather than risk dislodgment.

MANAGEMENT OF UNSTABLE CHEST WALL (FLAIL CHEST) (FIG. 4–7)

A steering wheel injury and lateral chest trauma result in multiple rib fractures in which a variable area of the chest wall becomes unstable. If this area is large enough and mobile enough, the patient's ability to carry out the mechanical work of respiration is impaired.

The injuring force is not limited to the chest wall; major intrathoracic trauma is usually incurred and may include any number of entities. However, pulmonary contusion, pneumothorax, and hemothorax predominate. More often than not, management of the parenchymal tissues is more important than the injury to the rib cage.

The management, therefore, is determined by many factors, not just visible paradoxic motion. The patient must not be overloaded with fluid. Arterial gases must be monitored continually; hourly assessment is necessary to determine management. The procedures described assume that there is major destabilization of the chest wall and that assistance is required for this problem, regardless of coexisting pulmonary contusion.

Four approaches are possible. The simplest, which may be of temporary value if adequate ventilation is not possible and intubation cannot be performed right away, is a compression dressing taped in place (Fig. 4–7B). A sandbag or other weight may be similarly used. This will stabilize the thoracic wall in a collapsed position, which will improve ventilation but will limit expansion and favor retention of secretions.

The great majority of patients with flail chest can be managed by careful tracheal toilet, avoiding fluid overload, and utilization of intercostal block. The patient requires continuous observation, serial blood gas studies, and repeated measurement of the tidal volume. Fatigue and oversedation are also negative factors. In view of the high incidence of nosocomial infections related to prolonged ventilation, intubation should be avoided if possible. Nonventilatory management requires much more attentive care than the alternative.

Skeletal traction (Fig. 4–7A) applied to the unstable area by towel clips or wires can be very effective. This produces stability in an expanded position while permitting some mobility; it also allows the patient to cough.

Tracheostomy (Fig. 4–7C) can be performed and may serve two purposes. First, it removes the physiologic obstruction of the larynx and at the same time reduces airway dead space by about 150 mL in the adult, thereby improving ventilation efficiency significantly. The tracheostomy also provides access for control of pulmonary secretions, which is a critical aspect of management. Endotracheal intubation without a ventilator is not a comparable substitute.

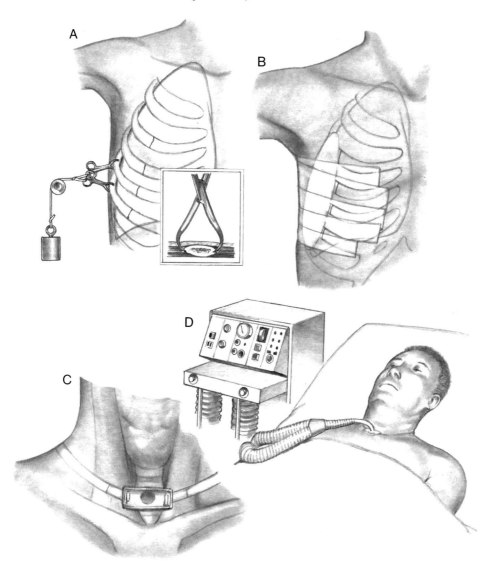

Figure 4–7.   Flail chest. Techniques available for stabilizing the unstable wall following multiple rib fractures.

A, External traction is exerted through towel clips attached to ribs in flail segment area. An alternative method is to use stainless steel wire passed around one or two ribs.

B, The chest wall is stabilized by gauze packing and tape. This can be used as a temporary expediency only since the chest wall is maintained in a collapsed position.

C, Tracheostomy may be of help by removing the obstruction of the laryngeal lumen, therefore requiring less inspiratory pressure; by giving access to secretions and by reducing dead space by about 150 mL, thereby increasing alveolar ventilation.

D, Support by a ventilator may be necessary if other measures are inadequate and hypoventilation of unacceptable degree as measured by blood gas determination is present.

Currently, if respiratory insufficiency is present (Fig. 4–7*D*), intubation and ventilatory support are generally used. If ventilation is required for more than 3 to 4 days, tracheostomy should be performed. Although much opinion to the contrary has been presented, I prefer to use hyperinflation with increased dead space and controlled ventilation. The intermittent mandatory ventilation approach does not stabilize the chest wall and requires excessive patient effort, with resultant fatigue. The addition of positive end-expiratory pressure or continuous positive airway pressure should not be routine but selected on the basis of blood gas determinations.

Chest wall stability is seldom acquired before 7 to 10 days.

STABILIZATION OF RIB FRACTURES (FIG. 4–8)

Indication

Stabilization of individual rib fractures is usually unnecessary even when fractures are multiple. However, displacement or overlapping may be extreme, so that union in an uncorrected position will produce an unsatisfactory result. In this situation, reduction and fixation may be indicated.

Position

Supine or lateral.

Procedure

An incision is made over the fracture. It may be transverse if a single rib is to be repaired. If fractures are multiple, a vertical incision may be chosen. Multiple incisions can be used. Hemostasis is produced by electrocautery. Injured intercostal vessels should be identified and ligated.

The fractured rib is exposed. Periosteum is left as intact as possible to preserve blood supply. Any of the techniques diagrammed in Figure 4–8 may be used, varying from simple suture with a steel wire to the more complex procedures. Other techniques not shown can also be used.

On completion of the bone work, the incision or incisions are closed. Excessive metallic materials, if used, will probably require removal at a later time.

PLEURAL DECORTICATION

Decortication is based on earlier observations that in organized hemothorax and empyema there is deposition of fibrinous material on the visceral and parietal pleural surfaces, which undergoes progressive fibrosis and hyalinization, slowly becoming thicker and more dense. The underlying pleural surfaces are generally normal, and once this ''peel'' is removed, the lung can be expanded and resume normal function.

A clotted hemothorax is best managed by early evacuation and immediate re-expansion. After a period of at least 10 days and until about 4 weeks have elapsed, removal of the ''immature peel'' will be difficult and unsatisfactory. Therefore, if a hemothorax is not managed well immediately, the surgeon should wait until decortication can be done effectively. A necessary requirement for satisfactory decortication is that the lung be sufficiently normal that complete expansion is possible. The patient with underlying disease, such as abscess, tuberculosis, fibrosis, or any of several processes that prevent expansion, should not be subjected to attempts at decortication. Occasionally resection and decortication may be combined.

Procedure (Fig. 4–9)

A posterolateral incision is made. A rib resection may be chosen if the process is old and ribs are contracted. This provides a wider area for beginning pleural dissection. One of two techniques may be chosen. An empyema space or hemothorax that is months old may sometimes be removed intact without entering the cavity. Dissection is begun in the

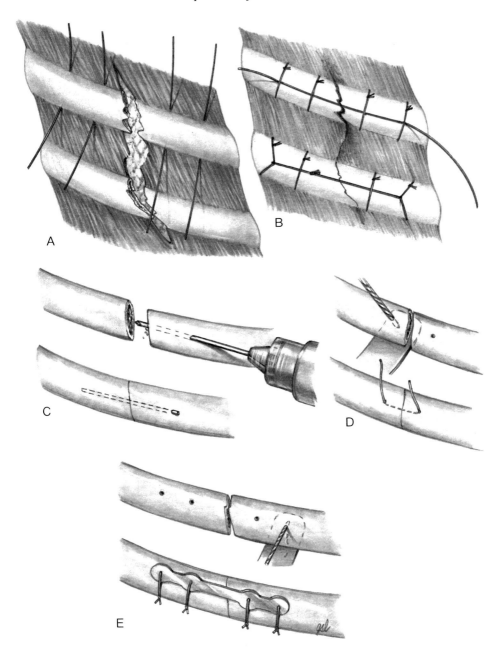

Figure 4–8. *A* and *B*, A method of fracture stabilization using only wire to impact the fragments under tension. *C*, A Kirschner wire or Keith needle may be utilized to stabilize a fracture site. The excess wire or needle is cut as close to the rib as possible. *D*, The easiest method of fracture stabilization utilizing a single wire to approximate the fragments. *E*, A bone plate with multiple points of fixation may serve to immobilize a fracture. (From Hood, R. M., et al.: Surgical Diseases of the Pleura and Chest Wall. Philadelphia, W. B. Saunders Company, 1986, p. 214. Used by permission.)

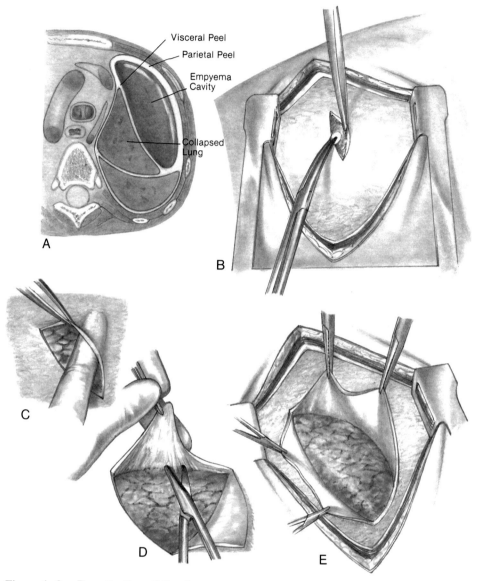

Figure 4–9. Decortication of the pleura.

A, A cross-sectional diagram of the thorax demonstrating the relationship of the empyema cavity and its walls to the chest wall pleura, lung, and mediastinal structures.

B, The chest has been opened and the empyema space entered. The thick parietal peel has only been incised and retracted. An incision in the visceral peel has been made and dissection of the peel from the lung has been begun with a "peanut" dissector.

C, Sometimes the peel can be detached by gentle finger dissection.

D, Sharp dissection may be occasionally or entirely necessary.

E, A large area of lung has been decorticated and is expanding from its semi-collapsed state.

wound area, freeing the peel from the chest wall. As the margin of the space is reached where the parietal peel is reflected onto the lung to become the visceral peel, this area becomes critical. The peel is thickest at this spot. Be careful to "turn the corner" and not carry the dissection plane retroaortic or retroesophageal, with disastrous results. The peel is then carefully removed from the lung surface.

The other technique involves entering the empyema or hemothorax cavity and beginning the visceral peel removal first. An incision is made carefully at a point not near a fissure, and as soon as the pleura is seen, the cut edges are grasped with a hemostat or an Alyce clamp, and the peel is lifted. The peel may be freed from the pleural surface using Metzenbaum scissors, "peanut" dissectors, Freer elevators, or any other instrument the surgeon may find useful. A combination of blunt and sharp dissection is required. As infolding of the lung is encountered, the lung is carefully mobilized. The fissures may pose a significant problem as the peel often dips deep into them, and the dissection plane may become obscure or lost. Every effort should be made to minimize injury to the lung. The procedure is time-consuming, and efforts to hurry will be rewarded by multiple entries into the lung.

The parietal peel can then be removed, again taking care at the reflection area. The diaphragm should also be decorticated carefully to mobilize it completely.

The procedure is best done with the lung partially expanded rather than completely collapsed. Occasionally, if the pleural process extends into the pleural apex, it may be wise to leave a portion attached to the chest wall rather than risk vascular or nerve injury.

After the procedure is complete, air leaks must be found and closed if possible, and assiduous efforts with electrocautery are made to produce complete hemostasis.

Drainage tubes are placed carefully; occasionally in an active empyema three tubes may be used.

The wound is then closed.

Notes

1. **Should excessive air leakage be present postoperatively and expansion is not complete, reoperation may be indicated.**
2. **The first postoperative chest film usually reflects complete expansion with minimal pleural opacification. However, subsequent films usually show progressive pleural reaction, and by the fourth or fifth postoperative day, the film may appear similar to the preoperative x-ray. This is temporary and should not result in any operative efforts.**

REPAIR OF TRAUMATIC BRONCHIAL RUPTURE

Traumatic bronchial rupture is one of the critical traumatic lesions that may present either as a life-endangering emergency or as a relatively asymptomatic condition that is diagnosed later, after complete healing and atelectasis have occurred. If the mediastinal pleura is torn or ruptured, a complete or tension pneumothorax will appear. Insertion of a chest tube results in uncontrollable air leak. Diagnosis, once suspected, is confirmed by bronchoscopy.

Procedure (Acute Rupture) (Fig. 4–10)

Unless the injury is shown to be on the left and is more than 2 cm distal to the carina, the lesion is approached through a right posterolateral thoracotomy. Initially, a long endotracheal tube is inserted to the tracheal level. The chest tube, if present, must not be clamped, but may be left unconnected once intubation is accomplished. The respiratory status of the patient may be extremely critical, and it may be necessary to make the chest incision with great speed. If the mediastinal pleura is already open, temporarily control the leak with the finger to improve ventilation. When exposure is fully obtained, the mediastinal pleura over the lower trachea and main bronchus is rapidly opened and the injury quickly assessed. An endobronchial catheter is guided into the uninjured bronchus and the cuff is inflated. This should provide adequate ventilation during the repair.

The area of injury is excised completely, and the edges of the torn bronchus are debrided. Significant resection of the bronchial wall is rarely necessary. Coincidental vascular injury, except for bronchial vessels, is rare. Suture material may be stainless steel

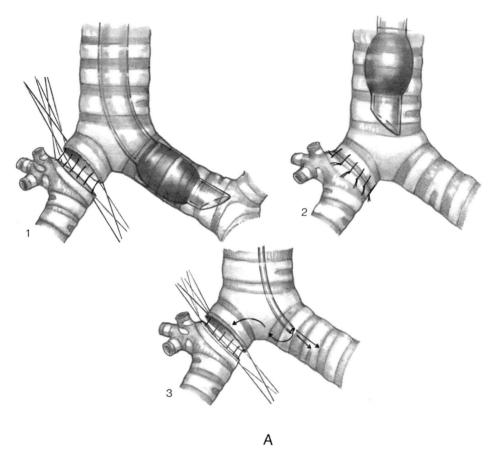

A

Figure 4–10. *A,* **Repair of traumatic rupture of the bronchus.**

1, An endobronchial tube has been introduced into the left main bronchus so that the area of injury is isolated and can be opened.

2, The suture-anastomosis has been completed and the endobronchial tube is withdrawn into the trachea so that the right lung may be reexpanded and the integrity of the suture line assured.

3, An alternative ventilation technique using high frequency jet ventilation with an open airway system.

Illustration continued on opposite page

wire (No. 34), 4-0 Prolene, 4-0 coated Dexon or Vicryl, or PDS (monofilament absorbable suture). The latter is probably better because it will not act as a foreign body, producing granulation or requiring endoscopic removal at a later time. Some prefer to keep the suture material submucosal, but this probably is not really possible. Sutures should be about 2 to 3 mm apart and include about 3 mm of bronchial wall. Interrupted sutures are used, and the knots are placed externally. It is better to place the posterior row of sutures before any are tied so that each may be accurately placed. Care and gentleness are necessary when suturing the membranous portion of the wall so that needle holes are not torn or enlarged. Sutures must be tied carefully to avoid cutting through bronchial cartilages. The anastomosis is submerged in saline after completion to be certain that the closure is complete. The endobronchial tube is retracted into the trachea and pressure is elevated to 30 to 40 cm H_2O. The advisability of covering the suture line with pleura or muscle is conjectural at best. Two chest tubes are placed, and the wound is closed.

Modification of Procedure (Late Repair). Dissection of the proximal and distal bronchial ends after a long period of time is time-consuming and difficult. Adhesions to

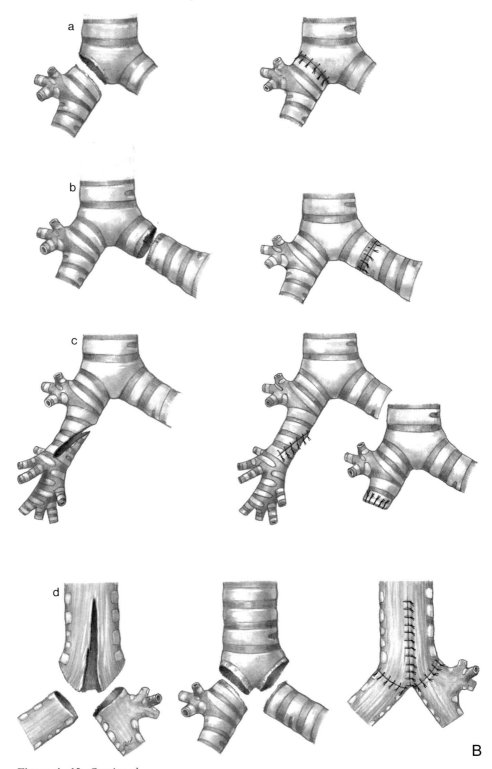

B

Figure 4–10. *Continued.*

B, a through *d,* **Four types of tracheal or bronchial injuries** that have been operated on and the suture techniques employed. The injury shown in *d* was repaired utilizing complete cardiopulmonary bypass.

the pulmonary artery and veins may be very firm. Proximal arterial control may be desirable if this dissection is too difficult. Once the two bronchial ends are freed, each end is excised. The distal bronchial tree will be filled with a gray-green mucus, which should be aspirated meticulously and irrigated. The two bronchial stumps are debrided back to normal tissue, and repair is carried out as described previously.

NOTES

1. **Anesthesia and ventilation may be done by high frequency jet technique using a small catheter and leaving the bronchus open. The absence of the cuffed tube in the area makes the technical procedure easier, and the ventilation may be better.**
2. **Bronchoscopy should be done immediately postoperatively and at least every other day for the first week to inspect the suture line and keep it free of secretions.**
3. **Proximal tracheostomy may be advantageous to permit suctioning and to prevent tussive force applied to the suture line, but at present the trend is away from elective tracheostomy.**

REPAIR OF INJURY TO THE CERVICAL TRACHEA

Etiology

1. **Direct blow (steering wheel, karate blow).**
2. **Penetrating (stab or gunshot wound).**
3. **"Clothesline" injury.**

Pathology

1. **Crushing of larynx or trachea with loss of airway.**
2. **Complete division with airway impairment.**
3. **Perforation by penetrating weapon or missile.**

Immediate Management (Fig. 4–11)

The immediate problem is to establish an airway. An attempt should be made to intubate orally. This will be successful most of the time unless the larynx is structurally collapsed. The direct-blow injury demands an urgent tracheostomy if intubation is not successful. Cricothyroidotomy is not likely to be helpful, because it would involve the injured area.

The penetrating injury does not usually produce a structural airway problem, but coincident vascular injury may result in fatal airway occlusion through aspiration of blood. Oral intubation should protect against aspiration and allow time for vascular control. Unless either an enlarging hematoma or exsanguination demands immediate operation, it is probably wise to delay operation long enough to obtain arteriograms and a contrast study of the esophagus. Esophagoscopy may also be warranted as a preoperative study. Arteriography, to be of significant value, must be immediately available, and surgical exploration should not be delayed if a long waiting period is involved.

An enlarging hematoma and continuous or massive hemorrhage demand immediate surgical intervention. If the wound is low in the cervical area, proximal control via sternotomy or left anterior thoracotomy may be necessary (see discussion on penetrating injuries of the base of the neck later in this chapter).

Rapidly advancing mediastinal and subcutaneous emphysema may be alarming. Once the tracheostomy or endotracheal tube balloon is inflated distal to the site of injury, this phenomenon should be controlled.

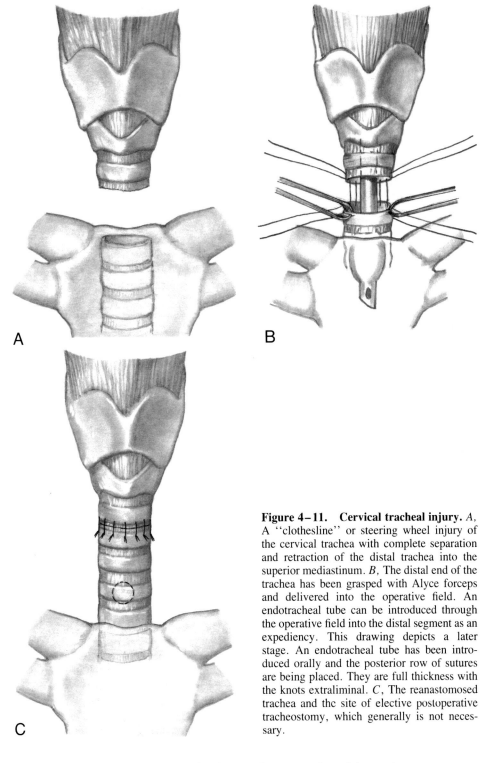

Figure 4–11. Cervical tracheal injury. *A*, A "clothesline" or steering wheel injury of the cervical trachea with complete separation and retraction of the distal trachea into the superior mediastinum. *B*, The distal end of the trachea has been grasped with Alyce forceps and delivered into the operative field. An endotracheal tube can be introduced through the operative field into the distal segment as an expediency. This drawing depicts a later stage. An endotracheal tube has been introduced orally and the posterior row of sutures are being placed. They are full thickness with the knots extraliminal. *C*, The reanastomosed trachea and the site of elective postoperative tracheostomy, which generally is not necessary.

The "clothesline" injury, resulting in complete separation of the trachea, may present without an immediate airway problem, but usually there is hoarseness and hemoptysis. Respiratory obstruction usually develops minutes to hours later. Oral intubation is occasionally possible even though the distal trachea usually retracts into the superior mediastinum. However, the unsuccessful intubation may lead to the correct diagnosis.

The only approach to airway establishment in patients with complete separation is to make a transverse cervical incision rapidly. As soon as the pretracheal fascia is incised, the trachea is seen to be missing. Retraction and good lighting will demonstrate the lower segment of the trachea in the retrosternal area. It can be grasped with an Alyce clamp and delivered into the wound. An endotracheal tube may be inserted into the open trachea or a tracheostomy tube may be inserted. At this point, the emergency has been terminated and definitive management begun.

Definitive Management

Crushing Injuries. The trachea so injured may be resected and an end-to-end anastomosis done. Frequently, there is accompanying severe structural damage to the larynx, which demands a distal tracheostomy. An otolaryngologist should become involved in the reconstruction. Management must be individualized since a wide variety of injuries may be present. A careful search for both recurrent laryngeal nerves must precede repair. The nerves should be carefully anastomosed if divided.

Penetrating Injuries. In the absence of vascular, esophageal, or nerve injury, penetrating injuries should simply be closed. A tracheostomy may or may not be indicated. A tracheostomy in the presence of an arterial anastomosis or graft will almost certainly be followed by secondary hemorrhage. Extra-anatomic arterial bypass grafting may be necessary if there is a major tracheal suture line or tracheostomy in the field.

A coexistent esophageal injury should be repaired and a pedicled vascularized muscle should be used to separate the trachea and esophagus.

Complete Tracheal Separation (Fig. 4–11). The most common site of separation is between the cricoid and second tracheal ring. Unless there are other injuries or the larynx is involved, repair should be by end-to-end anastomosis. Diagnosis must be accurate and intervention prompt. This should be preceded by oral intubation into the distal segment of trachea after removal of the previously placed airway tube. This repair is also preceded by a search for the recurrent laryngeal nerves so that they may be either protected or repaired. Distal tracheostomy is often done after repair; however, I prefer to not establish tracheostomy unless there is laryngeal injury or repair is tenuous. Steel wire, Prolene, Dexon, Vicryl, and PDS are all satisfactory suture materials.

If the surgeon is not experienced in tracheal repair, it would be better to leave the endotracheal tube or tracheostomy tube in place and refer the patient to another facility. This should also be done if the injury is extensive and complex.

Notes

1. **Establishment of an airway in a struggling, hypoxic patient may be extremely difficult. Time is critical and decision-making must not be wrong or occupy excessive time.**
2. **The temptation to stop the struggling of the patient with a muscle relaxant to facilitate intubation must be resisted because this is usually a fatal decision.**

REPAIR OF TRAUMATIC RUPTURE OF DIAPHRAGM

Traumatic rupture of the diaphragm is one of the critical thoracic injuries requiring early diagnosis and management. This description relates to rupture from blunt trauma rather than diaphragmatic injury from penetrating trauma. The injury may be approached either transthoracically or by laparotomy. Certainly if laparotomy is required for other reasons, it becomes the obvious approach. Thoracoabdominal penetrating injuries should be approached by laparotomy. However, in blunt trauma, if there is no evidence of injured abdominal viscera or if there is evidence of other intrathoracic injury, thoracotomy is preferable. The most common related injury is splenic rupture, which can actually be more easily managed via thoracotomy. Technically, the repair can be better accomplished through the thorax. Surgical repair being done within weeks or months postinjury must be approached through the thorax because of adhesions between abdominal viscera and intrathoracic structures.

Procedure (Fig. 4–12)

The patient is placed in the full lateral position and a left posterolateral thoracotomy is made overlying the seventh intercostal space. The pleura is opened and blood is cleared from the pleural space. The herniated viscera are inspected for evidence of injury. If none is found, the stomach and other structures are replaced in the peritoneal cavity. The surgeon should not hesitate to enlarge the traumatic laceration if necessary to simplify reduction of a hernia and to gain sufficient exposure for exploration of the upper abdomen.

The torn edges of the diaphragm are inspected for bleeding or for several branches of the phrenic artery, which are controlled by suture ligature. The wound edges are debrided to normal uninjured muscle. The upper abdomen is then explored, with particular attention to the spleen and liver, and the appropriate procedures are accomplished. The thoracic viscera are also carefully inspected.

Repair of the diaphragm is carried out by a two-layer overlapping technique similar to the Mayo umbilical hernia fascial repair, using interrupted, nonabsorbable sutures. The first layer is mattressed on one side and simple sutures are used on the opposing side. After these have been placed and tied, a second row is placed, securing the free edge with approximately a 2 cm overlap. Placing the end sutures first and using them for traction will be helpful in placing and spacing sutures quickly and accurately. A single drainage tube is placed posteriorly, and the chest incision is closed. Drainage of the subphrenic space is not done unless there has been injury to the liver, kidney, or a hollow viscus.

Notes

1. **Rapid opening of the chest may be critically necessary if the stomach has become massively dilated and the patient is in severe distress.**
2. **Either laparotomy or thoracotomy may be converted to a thoracoabdominal incision if exposure is inadequate.**

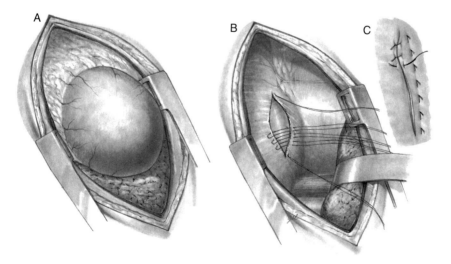

Figure 4–12.   Repair of traumatic diaphragmatic hernia—left side. *A*, The view usually seen when the chest is opened. The greater curvature of the stomach is uppermost, with a large amount of omentum, and usually the transverse colon is also seen. *B*, The herniated viscera have been reduced and the lacerations in the posterolateral aspect of the diaphragm are being closed with an imbricating two-layered closure using nonabsorbable sutures. *C*, Details of a diaphragmatic closure.

3. **A large rent in the diaphragm usually denervates the muscle distal to the tear; therefore, diaphragmatic motion is impaired in the postoperative period. Control of secretions may be more difficult because of the patient's inability to cough effectively.**

GENERAL MANAGEMENT OF EMERGENCY THORACOTOMY

Emergency thoracotomy has become a controversial procedure and has been overused in some centers. When it is used prematurely or when there is ample time to transfer the patient to the operating room, the patient's welfare is jeopardized, and fatal outcome may be the result.

This procedure should be reserved for patients in cardiac arrest that has occurred less than 5 minutes before admission, in those with massive hemorrhage in whom death is imminent, and when it is impossible to effect immediate transfer.

Adequate lighting, instrumentation, ventilation equipment and assistants are prerequisites. Emergency thoracotomy by inexperienced personnel is not likely to be successful.

The incision may be a left submammary thoracotomy, median sternotomy, or bilateral anterior thoracotomy.

Figure 4–13 demonstrates a method of controlling bleeding from hilar pulmonary vessels or the lung. The subsequent section demonstrates other techniques of the management of intrathoracic bleeding.

MANAGEMENT OF PENETRATING INJURIES OF THE HEART, AORTA, AND PULMONARY ARTERY

Cardiac Tamponade

Cardiac tamponade may be the result of injury to any cardiac chamber or the intrapericardial aorta and pulmonary artery. Diagnosis must involve a high degree of awareness and aggressiveness. Most patients with tamponade survive long enough to reach the operating room; therefore, Emergency Room thoracotomy is not advisable unless the patient is in an agonal state or in circulatory arrest upon arrival. Figure 4–14 demonstrates the techniques of pericardiocentesis and subxiphoid pericardiotomy, which may be used as a means of diagnosis and for temporary relief.

The technique of aspiration should be done with a plastic-covered needle (Fig. 4–14A). The needle is inserted in the subxiphoid area at a 45-degree angle, directed superiorly and at a 45-degree angle laterally to the left. As soon as fluid or blood is obtained, the metal portion is removed, leaving the plastic cannula in the pericardial sac. Aspiration may serve to confirm the diagnosis and provide temporary relief of tamponade. However, the

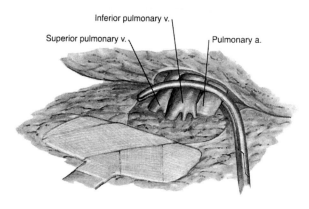

Inferior pulmonary v.

Superior pulmonary v.   Pulmonary a.

Figure 4–13. Technique of clamping the hilar vessels and branches "en masse" for emergency control of hemorrhage from vascular injury near the hilus of one or more strictures. (From Hood, R. M., Boyd, A. D., and Culliford, A. T.: Thoracic Trauma. Philadelphia, W. B. Saunders Company, 1989, p. 65. Used by permission.)

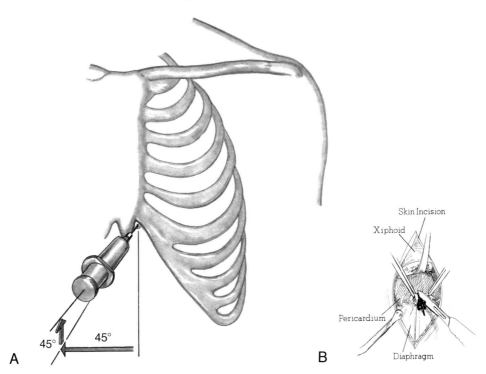

Skin Incision
Xiphoid
Pericardium
Diaphragm

A   B

Figure 4–14. *A*, Technique of pericardiocentesis. The degree of the inclination of the needle is important. The approach to the pericardium should be slow and with a gentle touch so that the operator can feel the puncture of the pericardium and the ventricular pulsation. (From Hood, R. M., Boyd, A. D., and Culliford, A. T.: Thoracic Trauma. Philadelphia, W. B. Saunders Company, 1989, p. 185. Used by permission.) *B*, Diagram of a limited pericardial exploration for diagnosis and temporary relief of hemopericardium with tamponade. (From Hood, R. M.: Trauma to the chest. *In* Sabiston, D. C., Jr., and Spencer, F. C.: Gibbon's Surgery of the Chest. 4th Ed. Philadelphia, W. B. Saunders Co., 1983, pp. 291–317.)

failure to retrieve blood in the presence of tamponade is not uncommon and does not exclude the diagnosis.

Subxiphoid pericardiotomy (Fig. 4–14*B*) may be an adequate means of proving the presence of blood in the pericardium and may relieve tamponading pressure altogether. A major tear into a cardiac chamber may be present, and the subxiphoid vent may convert tamponade to a situation where exsanguination is a threat. Therefore, this procedure is best done in the operating room, where full preparation for thoracotomy has been made.

Anterior or submammary thoracotomy is frequently chosen and is adequate unless there is aortic injury or injury to the right side of the heart. This incision may be converted to a transverse anterior thoracotomy by transecting the sternum and extending it into the opposite fourth or fifth interspace.

Median sternotomy is a better choice, however, if there has been time for full operating room preparation.

Atrial Injury. As soon as the incision has been made and is adequately retracted, the pericardium is rapidly and widely opened. Blood and clots are evacuated rapidly and the injury is visualized. Digital control of the perforation is usually effective. An injury to the atrium may be grasped with a curved vascular clamp (Fig. 4–15) and then oversewn.

Injury to the left atrium is less common and may require improvisation to effect repair and avoid air embolism. The use of complete cardiopulmonary bypass may be of value if it is immediately available.

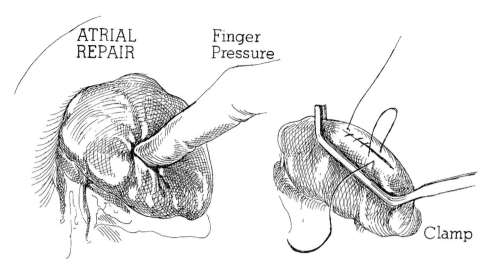

Figure 4–15. Control of hemorrhage from an injury to the right atrium using digital pressure followed by application of a curved vascular clamp to permit suturing of the isolated area. (From Hood, R. M.: Trauma to the chest. *In* Sabiston, D. C., Jr., and Spencer, F. C.: Gibbon's Surgery of the Chest. 4th Ed. Philadelphia, W. B. Saunders Co., 1983, pp. 291–317.)

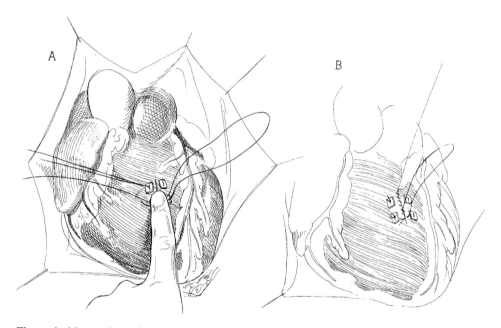

Figure 4–16. *A, B,* An injury through the ventricular wall is controlled by digital pressure, while pledgeted sutures in horizontal mattress form are used to control bleeding. A more superficial continuous suture is used to complete the closure. (From Hood, R. M.: Trauma to the chest. *In* Sabiston, D. C., Jr., and Spencer, F. C.: Gibbon's Surgery of the Chest. 4th Ed. Philadelphia, W. B. Saunders Co., 1983, pp. 291–317.)

Ventricular Injury. Laceration of the right ventricle is the most common injury. Application of the technique shown in Figure 4–16 is generally effective. Sutures should be 2-0 in size and the needle used must be large enough to pass beneath the tamponading finger. The left ventricle poses a more difficult problem because of the pressure of the left side of the heart. Control of bleeding may be more difficult. Hypovolemia is more likely to be present, and ventricular fibrillation is also more likely during repair efforts. If digital pressure is not effective, a Foley catheter and balloon may be useful in establishing control. Pledgeted sutures are advisable. Lacerations near major coronary vessels should be managed by horizontal mattress sutures passed beneath the vessel, excluding it from any occlusive suture. An injury to a major coronary vessel, such as the left anterior descending artery, calls for immediate bypass vein graft as soon as cardiopulmonary bypass is available. A wait-and-watch policy is not advisable.

Many patients are hypovolemic or become so during efforts to control and achieve fibrillation or arrest while repair is being done. It is wise to complete the repair rapidly while someone times the period of arrest. Then, when cardiac chambers are intact, effective massage and restoration of volume can be accomplished. Attempts at massage with an open wound are usually ineffective and may also result in air embolism.

Pulmonary Artery. Pulmonary artery injury can usually be controlled with digital pressure followed by application of a partial occlusion clamp and simple continuous sutures.

Aorta. Aortic injuries are most difficult. A single injury may be managed as diagrammed in Figure 4–17, but major blood loss will be the rule. Through-and-through injuries of the aorta are extremely difficult to control. Complete cardiopulmonary bypass may be helpful if enough time is available. More often, loss of volume requires a more direct approach. Inflow occlusion of both vena cavae gives the surgeon 1 to 2 minutes of time to gain control or to close the wound, and requires no special equipment.

Lessons from Experience

1. **A well-planned protocol approach is desirable.**
2. **Emergency Room thoracotomy, although occasionally successful, is usually an error in judgment unless full operating room capabilities are present.**
3. **Should fibrillation occur before the injury is sutured, complete suture closure rapidly before attempting to massage or defibrillate.**
4. **Do not waste valuable time in the Emergency Room trying to resuscitate the patient. Transfer to the Operating Room and begin operating as soon as possible.**
5. **Should personnel and preparations be inadequate, relieve tamponade, control bleeding digitally, and await adequate help and equipment.**

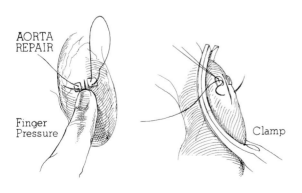

AORTA
REPAIR

Finger
Pressure

Clamp

Figure 4–17. Principle of temporary control of bleeding from a penetrating injury to the aorta followed by application of a partial occlusion clamp. Buttressed sutures are used to close the defect. (From Hood, R. M.: Trauma to the chest. *In* Sabiston, D. C., Jr., and Spencer, F. C.: Gibbon's Surgery of the Chest. 4th Ed. Philadelphia, W. B. Saunders Co., 1983, pp. 291–317.)

SURGICAL MANAGEMENT OF CERVICAL ESOPHAGEAL PERFORATION

Cervical esophageal injury is produced most often by endoscopic trauma and by dilatation procedures. A lesser number are related to penetrating wounds of the cervical area. This latter group may be related to tracheal or vascular injury as well. Diagnosis is suspected if pain, swelling, dysphagia, or cervical emphysema appears following a procedure. A finding of air in the tissues is a most important sign. Swallowed contrast material, such as iodized oil (Lipiodol), propyliodone (Dionosil), or diatrizoate methyl glucamine (Gastrografin), will usually confirm diagnosis. Endoscopy may also visualize the site of injury. Water-soluble agents, such as diatrizoate sodium (Hypaque), are less satisfactory and are destructive to the lung if aspirated. Barium should be avoided at all times.

Penetrating wounds must be explored if the penetration is deeper than the platysma muscle; however, a contrast study, arteriogram, bronchoscopy, and esophagoscopy may add much information before definitive exploration.

Nonoperative management is periodically recommended by some in selected cases. This course is fraught with risk, and when balanced against the essentially 100% success rate with operative management seems to beg the issue.

Procedure (Fig. 4–18)

An incision is made along the anterior border of the sternomastoid muscle. If the site of injury is clearly lateralized, the incision is made on that side. The deep cervical fascia is incised and the omohyoid muscle is divided. Small anterior cervical veins draining into the internal jugular vein are divided. The carotid sheath is gently retracted laterally, and the visceral compartment is entered. Air in the tissue planes, edema, varying degrees of purulent fluid, foreign material, and necrosis may be seen. The pathologic changes are largely dependent on the interval from injury to operation. The prevertebral space posterior to the esophagus is first developed. Much of the dissection can be done bluntly by the finger.

The posterior plane should be opened as high as possible and well into the superior mediastinum.

The perforation, if identified, should be closed using absorbable sutures in two layers. Excessive necrosis and induration may prevent closure when operative treatment has been delayed.

At least two Penrose drains are placed in the space previously developed, and an active suction drainage tube, such as a Jackson-Pratt tube, is placed near the sutured perforation. All of these drains may be brought out through the lower part of the incision but are probably best brought out through a separate wound posterior to the incision, which should be large enough to permit free drainage.

The entire wound may be left open if the perforation closure is tenuous or if infection is already established. Delayed primary closure may be accomplished 3 or 4 days later if a salivary fistula does not appear and infection is controlled. The final cosmetic result of this is good, and regardless of that consideration, leaving the wound open ensures that fatal mediastinitis will not occur.

Should contamination be minimal and the repair satisfactory, the wound may be closed, loosely suturing the deep fascia, closing the subcutaneous tissue, and leaving the skin open or closed with Steristrips. There should be no hurry in removing drains, and at least one should remain for 7 to 9 days.

A salivary fistula developing after repair should be managed by observation, as all will close spontaneously. Dilatation may be required to prevent or manage stricture formation.

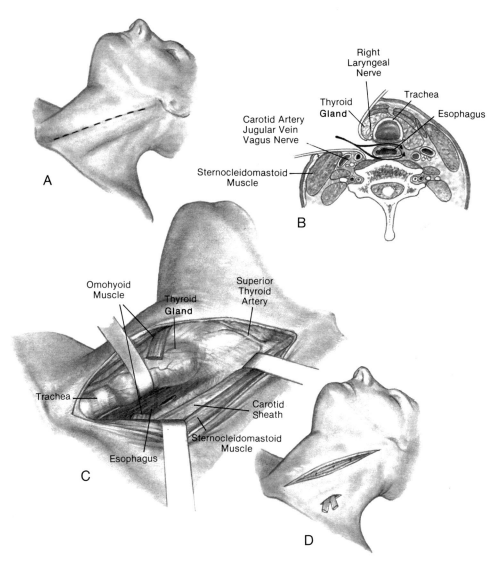

Figure 4–18. Surgical drainage following injury to the cervical esophagus. *A,* The incision position along the anterior border of the sternocleidomastoid muscle. *B,* The plane of drainage, which is posterior to the thyroid and anterior to the carotid sheath and to the sternocleidomastoid muscle. The esophagus must be freed anteriorly, posteriorly, and on the contralateral side. Drains are left in these planes. *C,* An exposed perforation through this type of approach. *D,* Drainage should be via Penrose or Jackson-Pratt type drains through a separate incision; the wound should be left at least partially open.

MANAGEMENT OF INJURIES TO THE THORACIC ESOPHAGUS

The etiology of thoracic esophageal injury is primarily iatrogenic, from esophageal diagnostic instrumentation or from efforts at foreign body removal (65 to 70%). "Spontaneous" rupture of the lower third of the esophagus and penetrating injuries are responsible for most of the remainder of injuries.

Early diagnosis is the key to survival and freedom from protracted illness as a result of mediastinitis and empyema. The number of injuries from manipulative and endoscopic trauma is proportional to the experience and skill of the surgeon. This is particularly true for foreign body extraction. It is necessary to ascertain immediately following the endoscopic procedure if a perforation is present rather than be surprised by the event 12 hours or longer postoperatively. It is my policy to obtain a chest x-ray immediately following foreign body extraction other than that of coins or similar objects and in any patient in whom other injury is suspected.

Symptoms and clinical findings include dysphagia, painful swallowing, substernal, interscapular, or pleural pain, and subcutaneous air in the neck. These are followed quickly by tachycardia, fever, and other evidences of severe sepsis. X-ray findings include mediastinal emphysema, pneumothorax, pleural effusion on either side, widening of the mediastinum, air-fluid level in the mediastinum, and extravasation of ingested contrast material.

Nonoperative management of thoracic esophageal perforation has been advocated from time to time, but it is my opinion that this approach is justified only when the patient is too ill to tolerate an operation and only rarely do patients fit this category.

The operative approach is guided by several principles.

1. **The leak must be terminated by the operative procedure.**
2. **Drainage alone is insufficient and will result in a high mortality rate.**
3. **Extensive mediastinal and pleural drainage is necessary.**
4. **Appropriate antibiotic therapy is required.**

Immediate thoracotomy (Fig. 4–19) with direct suture repair is the procedure of choice when a prompt diagnosis is made. The esophageal mucosa is sutured with absorbable suture followed by interrupted nonabsorbable sutures in the muscular layer. This suture line should be buttressed by a pedicled flap of pleura or preferably a muscle graft with good blood supply. The technique of Grillo (Fig. 4–20), of developing a pedicled flap of parietal pleura which is used to wrap around the injured area of esophagus and sutured in place, is the best procedure available at this time.

Several authors have suggested carrying out a definite procedure, such as resection, if there is an underlying lesion requiring operation, rather than merely repairing the injury. This approach must take into account the patient's overall condition, the duration of perforation, and the extent of soilage of the mediastinum; it is probably applicable only in a minority of patients.

One principle seems valid: Repair of a perforation proximal to an obstructing lesion is usually unsuccessful. Therefore, the surgeon must consider direct management of the obstruction or perform cervical esophagostomy at the same time.

The perforation diagnosed 12 to 24 hours after it occurs is usually associated with such a degree of necrosis, infection, and induration that primary repair is not possible. A number of procedures designed to defunctionalize the esophagus and allow healing over a period of time have been suggested. Various combinations of cervical esophagostomy, ligation, or division of the lower esophagus and extensive drainage all have their advocates. There are insufficient data to recommend one procedure over another. All require prolonged enteral or parenteral alimentation and multiple stages of reconstruction. Therefore, every effort at establishing an early diagnosis of esophageal injury and accomplishing primary repair should be made.

EXPOSURE AND REPAIR OF PENETRATING WOUNDS AT THE BASE OF THE NECK

Gunshot or stab wound victims must be staged into two groups: (1) those who are hypovolemic, unstable, and obviously bleeding, and (2) those whose condition is stable

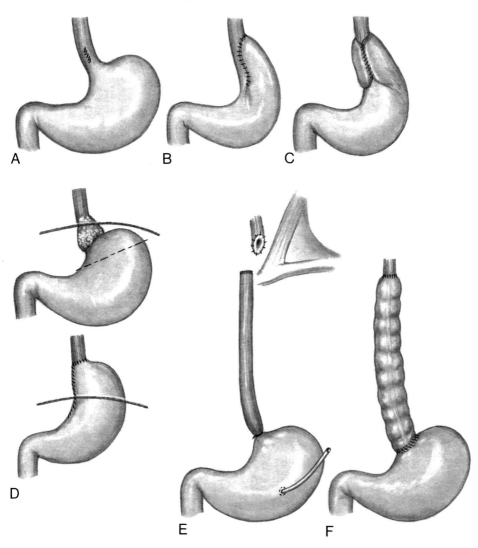

Figure 4–19. Injuries to the lower thoracic esophagus. Various methods can be utilized to manage a perforation of the esophagus in this area. *A,* Simple suture of the injury is possible if diagnosed early. *B, C,* Two techniques of suturing the stomach over the repaired perforation: by simply elevating the fundus and suturing it over the laceration *(B)* and by what is essentially a Nissen procedure *(C). D,* Resection of the esophagus—this is useful when the perforation is related to a condition such as carcinoma of the esophagus, which is not repairable. Primary resection and reanastomosis would be the treatment of choice if diagnosed early. *E,* The method of ligating or stapling the distal esophagus, producing a cervical cutaneous esophagostomy. *F,* In a later stage, colon reconstruction is performed.

and who are without evidence of major hemorrhage. For the latter group there is enough time for diagnostic procedures, such as arteriography, contrast esophagogram, chest and cervical x-rays, and endoscopy. Operative approach must be selected for the procedure indicated.

The patient in unstable condition should be operated upon immediately with adequate blood available. Injuries in or near the midline or the right cervical area are best exposed via a median sternotomy with an extension laterally above and parallel to the clavicle or along the sternocleidomastoid muscle.

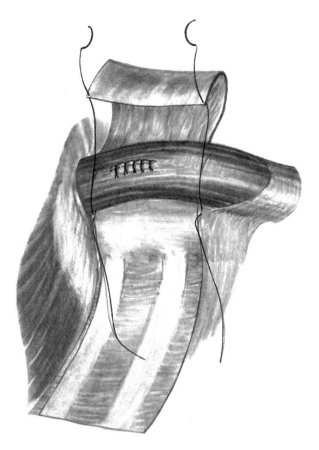

Figure 4–20. The technique of Grillo for mobilizing a pedicled flap of parietal pleura, which is then wrapped about the area of injury and repair as a buttress. (From Hood, R. M., Boyd, A. D., and Culliford, A. T.: Thoracic Trauma. Philadelphia, W. B. Saunders Company, 1989, p. 307. Used by permission.)

This provides adequate exposure for the ascending aorta, innominate artery, subclavian and carotid arteries, and subclavian, jugular and innominate veins.

This incision should be made rapidly. A finger or pack should be used to tamponade the major point of hemorrhage while proximal and distal control is obtained (Fig. 4–21). Only vascular clamps should be used. Primary repair by resection and reanastomosis or replacement by vein graft of injured arteries is accomplished with monofilament vascular suture. Venous injuries are repaired either by direct suture or by ligation.

Vascular repair with associated tracheal or esophageal injury is hazardous, and delayed repair or extra-anatomic grafting is advisable.

Injuries to the left cervical area with arterial bleeding require a left fourth interspace anterior or posterolateral thoracotomy for control of the proximal subclavian artery. A left supraclavicular incision, occasionally with clavicular resection, is then made for the definitive procedure (Figs. 4–22 and 4–23).

A left posterolateral incision is useful if the injury is known to involve the left intrathoracic subclavian artery. A more lateral wound involving the axillary artery can be approached by an incision, as demonstrated in Figure 4–24, which involves severing the pectoralis major and pectoralis minor muscles from their insertion into the bicipital groove and coracoid process. This, with clavicular resection, exposes the distal subclavian artery and the axillary artery.

The ascending aorta is also frequently injured. Most aortic injuries exsanguinate before the patient arrives at a hospital. A median sternotomy is the procedure of choice. Control of the laceration with buttressed sutures, as shown in Figure 4–24, is usually applicable. Through-and-through injuries of the aorta are usually, but not invariably, lethal injuries. Rapid institution of cardiopulmonary bypass via femoral vessels will facilitate repair procedures of the ascending aorta.

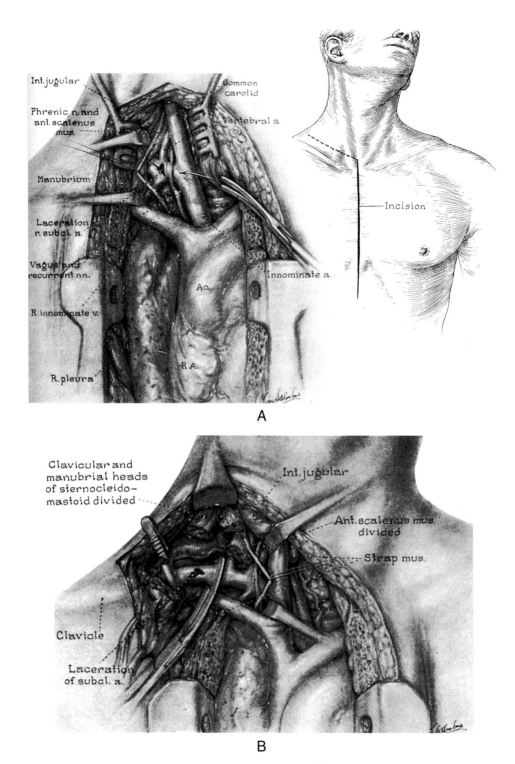

A

B

Figure 4–21. *A,* Exposure of a proximal right subclavian arterial injury obtained through a medium sternotomy incision extended into the right side of the neck. This incision also provides good access to the innominate artery and the proximal right common carotid and vertebral arteries. *B,* The more distal portion of the right subclavian artery is exposed by dividing the sternocleidomastoid, anterior scalene, and strap muscles. (From Brawley, R. K., et al.: Management of wounds of the innominate, subclavian, and axillary blood vessels. Surg. Gynecol. Obstet., *131:*1130, 1970. Reprinted by permission.)

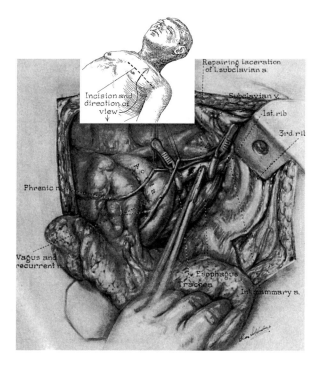

Figure 4–22. The proximal left subclavian artery can be exposed through an anterolateral thoracotomy, allowing for repair of proximal injuries, as seen here, or for temporary vessel control. (From Brawley, R. K., et al.: Management of wounds of the innominate, subclavian, and axillary blood vessels. Surg. Gynecol. Obstet., *131:*1130, 1970. Reprinted by permission.)

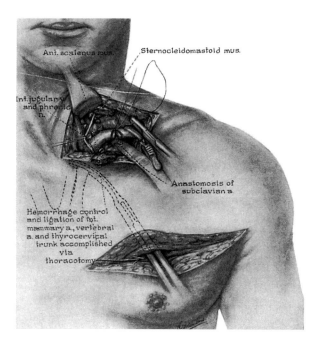

Figure 4–23. An injury to the distal left subclavian artery is repaired via a supraclavicular incision following initial proximal vessel control through an anterolateral thoracotomy. (From Brawley, R. K., et al.: Management of wounds of the innominate, subclavian, and axillary blood vessels. Surg. Gynecol. Obstet., *131:*1130, 1970. Reprinted by permission.)

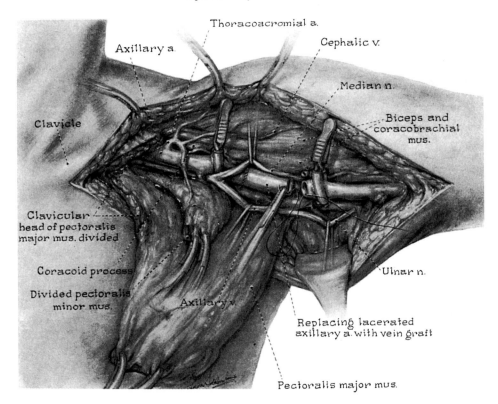

Figure 4–24. With division and inferior retraction of the pectoralis major and minor muscles, wide access is obtained for injuries of the axillary artery. (From Brawley, R. K., et al.: Management of wounds of the innominate, subclavian, and axillary blood vessels. Surg. Gynecol. Obstet., *131:*1130, 1970. Reprinted by permission.)

5

Thoracic Incisions

The selection of an incision for an intrathoracic procedure involves several considerations:

1. **The position that provides the best exposure of the anatomic structures to be dealt with.**
2. **The condition and cardiorespiratory reserve of the patient may preclude a lateral position.**
3. **The location and extent of the pathologic process that may modify the approach and extent of exposure.**
4. **A prior knowledge of the advantages and disadvantages of each incision.**
5. **The preference of the surgeon based on training, experience and ability.**

Numerous papers have advised smaller, anterior or axillary, non-muscle-cutting incisions or other modifications, which usually result in limited exposure and diminished safety. Compromised exposure may allow an uncomplicated procedure to be accomplished, but an extensive pathologic process, an operative mishap involving a major vessel may convert the procedure into a life-endangering nightmare.

Cosmetic considerations and a questionable and usually nonproductive quest for less postoperative pain should be set aside and the incision and its size selected on the basis of maximum safety for the patient and the least likelihood of inducing operative errors based on poor exposure.

MEDIAN STERNOTOMY

Indications

1. **To produce exposure of ascending aorta and great vessels.**
2. **Ideal for anterior mediastinal neoplasms.**
3. **Best exposure for cardiac operations.**
4. **For suspected cardiac trauma.**
5. **For pericardiectomy.**
6. **May also be used if bilateral procedures on the lung are contemplated, such as resection of multiple metastatic nodules.**

Advantages

1. **Is rapid and involves little blood loss.**
2. **Best exposure of the heart and aorta and its branches, except for left subclavian artery.**

3. Less postoperative pain.
4. Provides access to both pleural spaces.

Limitations

1. Poor exposure of descending aortic arch or left subclavian artery.
2. Generally inadequate for pulmonary surgical procedures.
3. Lower trachea is not accessible.
4. Thoracic esophagus is unapproachable.
5. Requires sternal saw.

Procedure (Fig. 5–1)

The patient is placed in a supine position with the arms at the sides. A midline incision is made extending inferiorly from 1 to 2 cm below the suprasternal notch. Carrying the incision high is unnecessary and is cosmetically unattractive. The incision is extended to a point about 2 cm below the tip of the xiphoid process. Utilizing a cautery, the incision is deepened to the periosteal level, taking care to stay in the midline. Hemostasis is produced with the cautery. The periosteum is now incised with the cautery. At the superior portion of the manubrium, blunt and sharp dissection is used to clear the suprasternal notch of tissue. There is usually a transverse vein in the area measuring 3 to 4 mm, which must be ligated and divided. A right angle clamp and the forefinger are used to develop the retrosternal space deep to the manubrium. The midline deep fascia of the abdominal wall is incised with the cautery about 1 to 2 cm below the tip of the xiphoid process. The substernal space is developed with the finger. The sternal saw is introduced at either end of the sternum, and its "foot" should be kept tilted toward the posterior sternal surface and held firmly against it to prevent injury to the pleural or mediastinal structures as the sternum is divided.

Two large vein or Army-Navy retractors are used to elevate one side of the transected sternum while periosteal bleeding points are cauterized. The procedure is repeated for the opposite side. A sternal retractor is then placed and gradually opened to expose the mediastinum.

A variant may be used if only the great vessels are to be exposed. The sternal incision is carried to the third interspace, the sternum is then transected horizontally, and the incision is extended 5 to 8 cm into the third interspace. Both internal mammary arteries must be ligated and divided, and the pleural space is usually opened by this extension. Injuries to the subclavian vessels may also require resection of the medial one half to two thirds of the clavicle if optimum exposure is to be gained.

Closure of the incision after completion of definitive surgery is preceded by careful hemostasis by means of electrocautery. Bone wax may be used on the sternal edges but, because it is a foreign body, it is detrimental to wound healing; its use should be minimized or omitted if possible. A single drainage tube, size No. 28 to No. 36, should be introduced through a midline stab wound below the incision. Tubes should also be placed in either pleural space if they have been entered. These may be introduced through stab wounds near the midline and cross under the mediastinal tube to enter the pleural space and be placed beneath the lower lobe on top of the diaphragm with the tip lying near the posterior chest wall. Tubes should be sutured firmly in place.

The sternum is approximated by No. 22 steel wire with swedged-on needles. These may be driven through the sternum 2 cm lateral to the incised edge, or in advanced osteoporosis, passed completely around the sternum. The sternum may be held approximated by one or two wires while the first one or two are twisted. After all wires are twisted and before the ends are cut, a needle holder is used to twist each wire tightly. Experience will enable the surgeon to carry out this maneuver with minimal wire breakage. The ends of the wires are buried.

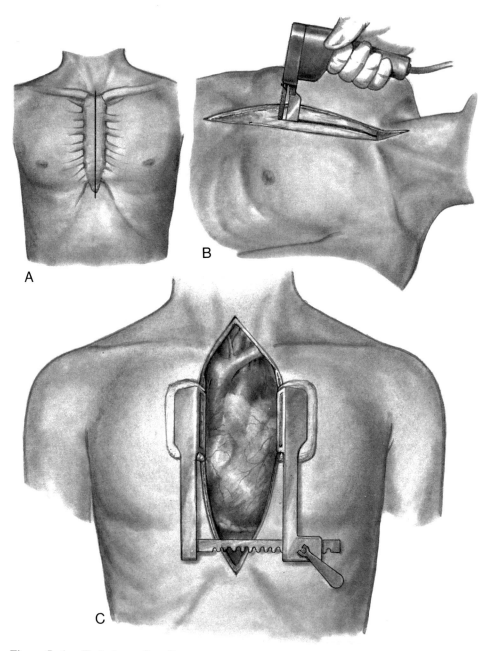

Figure 5–1. Technique of median sternotomy.

The periosteum is then closed. Many suture materials and techniques are used, including continuous monofilament nonabsorbable suture and absorbable types such as Dexon or Vicryl. I prefer a figure-of-eight suture of 2-0 cotton or silk as the best means of preventing secondary sternal separation. The midline abdominal fascia is carefully closed in the same fashion. Many epigastric hernias have resulted from poor closure of this incision.

The subcutaneous tissue is closed with 2-0 or 3-0 absorbable suture and the skin with either subcuticular closure or more usually vertical mattress sutures.

POSTEROLATERAL THORACOTOMY INCISION

Indications

The posterolateral incision is the most frequently used thoracic incision. It is the preferable incision for most pulmonary surgery and for esophageal procedures. Its advantages are obvious. There are some disadvantages under some circumstances. Anterior mediastinal tumors may be poorly visualized and their vascular supply difficult to see. Posterolateral thoracotomy should be avoided in trauma surgery unless the injury is clearly confined to one hemithorax and the patient is hemodynamically stable. The full lateral position is less well tolerated than the supine position when the patient is in unstable condition.

Position

Full lateral.

Procedure (Fig. 5–2)

The patient is turned with the operative side up and the down leg flexed to 90 degrees; a pillow is placed between the legs. Three-inch adhesive tape is used to fix the patient in a vertical position, beginning by attaching the tape to the table anteriorly and then across the patient very firmly to the opposite side of the table. Reversing this order of taping usually results in the patient being too much on his or her face and makes exposure difficult. Place a folded sheet or towel under the axilla to prevent vascular and nerve compression. Leave the up side arm free or supported on a pillow. There is no need to use a support; tape or otherwise fix the position of the arm.

Plan the incision by visualizing a sweeping curve beginning at the level of the middle of the scapula and located midway between the medial border of the scapula and the spinous processes. The incision should swing downward and anteriorly, passing a point 2 inches below the tip of the scapula, then anteriorly to the middle or anterior axillary line to a point 2 inches below the nipple in men or the inframammary fold in women.

The incision may be made with the scalpel followed by electrocautery or made entirely with the scalpel. The principal advantages of the cautery are saving time and minimizing blood loss. The cautery leaves necrosed tissue in the wound but probably no more than that left by multiple ligatures.

If cautery is to be used, make the initial incision with the scalpel through the epidermis only, then complete the skin incision with the cutting current. Use coagulation current for additional hemostasis. Incise the latissimus dorsi muscle with cutting current and produce complete hemostasis, then incise the fascia posterior to the serratus anterior muscle and carry this incision posteriorly and superiorly until the lower margin of the trapezius muscle is encountered. A fourth or fifth interspace thoracotomy will require transection of the lower 3 to 5 cm of the trapezius; a sixth or seventh interspace incision can be made without incision of the trapezius. The rhomboideus major muscle is incised with the trapezius.

Incise inferiorly along the posterior border of the serratus anterior muscle as far as possible, then transect this muscle about one third of its width, keeping the incision as inferior as is practical.

At this point, use a scapula retractor to elevate the scapula, which will permit the surgeon's hand to dissect and open the subscapular space and identify the first rib posteriorly by palation. Count ribs to identify the interspace or rib previously chosen. The bed of the resected fifth rib or the fifth interspace should be used if a pneumonectomy or an upper lobectomy or partial lobectomy is anticipated. The sixth rib or interspace is usually adequate for lower or middle lobectomy.

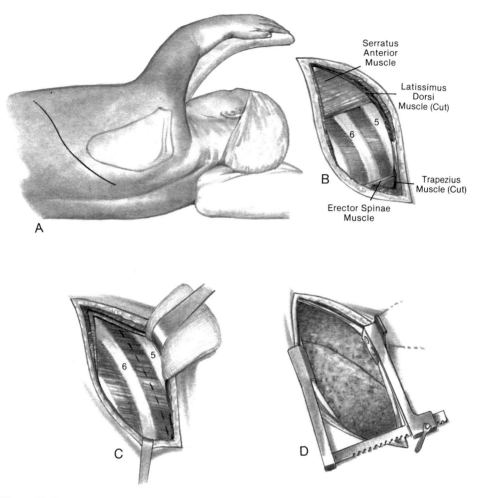

Figure 5–2. Posterolateral thoracotomy (left).

A, Patient is in full lateral position. The incision is begun midway between the scapula and spinous processes, coursing 4 cm below the tip of the scapula and ending about 5 cm below the nipple in the male or the inframammary fold in the female.

B, The incision has been partially made. The latissimus dorsi muscle has been divided; 2.5 cm of the trapezius and rhomboideus major muscles has been severed. The serratus anterior muscle is still intact.

C, The extracostal incision has been completed and the intercostal incision is to be accomplished next.

D, The completed incision with a rib spreader in place.

Illustration continued on opposite page

Incise vertically with the cautery along the lateral edge of the erector spinae muscle and free it for a length of about 8 cm, and then retract it with an Army-Navy retractor, packing the space temporarily with a 4 × 8 sponge.

Rib Resection. Incise the periosteum down the middle of the rib with the cautery and "T" each end. Use a periosteal elevator to push back the periosteum from the external surface of the rib with alternate upward and downward strokes. When the external surface is bared, use the curved sharp end of the elevator to strip the superior edge of the rib, beginning posteriorly and proceeding anteriorly. Then strip the lower edge, beginning anteriorly and exerting force posteriorly. Always keep a sharp edge against the rib. For safety, always use one hand to brace against the chest wall, so that if the instrument slips

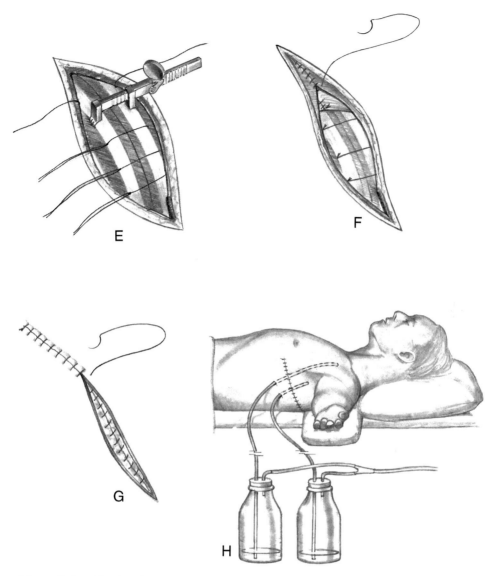

Figure 5–2. *Continued.*

E, Rib cage closure. Pericostal sutures have been placed. A Bailey-Gibbon rib approximator is being used to close the incision while sutures are tied.

F, The extracostal musculature is being closed with continuous Dexon or Vicryl sutures for each muscle.

G, The subcutaneous tissue and skin closures are being completed.

H, The closed incision, showing the relationship of chest tubes to the incision.

it will not result in injury. Considerable force must be used. Getting out of the subperiosteal space and into the intercostal muscle will result in excessive bleeding and make closure difficult.

From this point, use the elevator from above and below to clear the inner surface of the rib. Cut the rib posteriorly within 2 cm of the transverse process with a Bethune rib shear. Next, cut the anterior portion of the rib. Always direct the rib shear from below upwards, never the reverse, to avoid injury to the intercostal vessels and nerve. Carefully incise through the posterior periosteal layer into the pleural cavity.

Intercostal Incision.   Incise the exact center of the intercostal space with the cautery, producing a good hemostasis, and very carefully enter the pleural space. Make an opening large enough to introduce a sponge on a sponge stick. Then, keeping the sponge between the point of cautery and the lung, incise the full length of the space. If an intercostal artery is injured posteriorly, be wary of excessive cautery use in this area for fear of spinal cord damage.

Once the pleural space is entered and found to be free, the remainder of the intercostal space or rib bed can be incised. Otherwise, careful dissection must be begun to free the lung from the chest wall. Occasionally, extrapleural dissection may be necessary to free the lung without damage. Blunt finger dissection may be effective. Generally, it is better to use sharp dissection, utilizing good light and proper scissors. Every injury to the lung will exact a price later in the patient's care, and extensive damage caused by a crude, hurried approach may spell failure for the procedure. Place a suitable rib spreader and open the retractor slowly over 4 to 5 min to minimize the risk of rib fracture.

Closure of the Incision

Rib Resection.   The rib cage should be closed with a series of nonabsorbable sutures. The upper periosteum is included in a simple suture, which actually goes around the periosteum. The lower margin is sutured by catching the lower edge of periosteum, then taking a second suture through the upper periosteal edge. Properly placed, this suture should exclude the intercostal neurovascular bundle. This series of sutures, placed about 1.5 cm apart, provides a strong, air-tight closure that does not require pericostal sutures.

Intercostal Incision.   Pericostal sutures of No. 1 nonabsorbable suture material are required. Wound dehiscence has occurred with catgut and Dexon sutures. Wire sutures are indicated when there is gross wound contamination. However, after 3 to 4 months, most wires break, and once this happens, it will be a source of concern to the patient, and removal may be required because of pain.

The intercostal muscle should be sutured using a running suture of 2-0 absorbable material. This suture is also used to reattach the sacrospinalis muscle to the chest wall. The musculature is then sutured using 2-0 or 0 absorbable sutures. The serratus anterior muscle is repaired first. The full thickness of the muscle may be sutured or only the posterior or anterior fascia coverings may be picked up. The latter technique has the advantage of leaving less suture material in the wound. The thoracic fascia is then closed from the posterior margin of the serratus anterior muscle to the lower margin of the trapezius muscle, which is then repaired with the same suture. The rhomboideus major muscle, if cut, may be sutured as one layer with the trapezius muscle.

A second suture is used to close the latissimus dorsi as just described. The subcutaneous tissue is closed with 3-0 suture, approximating the skin edges accurately. The skin may be closed by any technique; however, I prefer a subcuticular suture of 4-0 Dexon or Vicryl. A light bandage is applied, taking care not to tape too tightly and thereby preventing tape burns.

BILATERAL TRANSVERSE THORACOTOMY (FIG. 5–3)

Indication

This incision gives maximum exposure to the thorax and is the procedure of choice when the anterolateral (submammary) incision is inadequate or when a sternal splitting procedure is likely to be insufficient. It is often the procedure of choice when multiple intrathoracic injuries are present. Turning a trauma patient to a lateral position is usually contraindicated. The exposure to the lower thoracic esophagus is less than ideal.

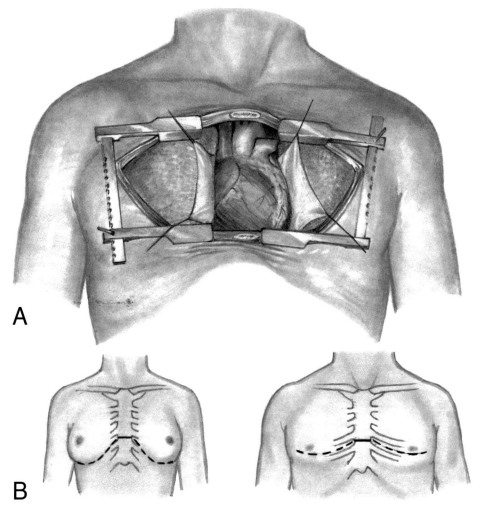

Figure 5–3. *A,* Bilateral transverse thoracotomy. This diagram illustrates the exposure that can be obtained with this incision. *B,* The skin incision may be varied based on the sex of the patient. (From Hood, R.M., Boyd, A.D., and Culliford, A.T.: Thoracic Trauma. Philadelphia, W.B. Saunders Company, 1989, p. 62. Used by permission.)

Position

Supine

Procedure

The skin incision is marked and made, as shown in Figure 5–3. Hemostasis is secured by electrocautery but may be ignored when the procedure is an emergency. The pectoral muscles are incised and/or split. The intercostal space on either side is incised and the pleura entered. The incision is carried medially to the sternal area. The internal mammary vessels are visualized, doubly ligated, and divided. The sternum is then divided with a sternal saw, Stryker saw, or Gigli saw—whatever is available. Two rib spreaders are then placed, one on either side, and the incision widely opened.

The definitive procedure is then accomplished.

Closure of the incision is preceded by meticulous hemostasis by electrocautery. The internal mammary vessels are oversewn with nonabsorbable suture for full security. The sternum is closed by two or three sternal wires. Before these are twisted tightly, pericostal sutures are placed on either side. Usually two or three on each side are sufficient. The sternal sutures are twisted tightly and the pericostal sutures are tied. Pleural and intercostal approximation are not possible and will not be attempted.

The pectoral muscles are then closed with continuous absorbable sutures. The subcutaneous tissue and skin are then approximated by the technique the surgeon prefers.

Chest tubes are placed in both pleural spaces through stab wounds below the incision near the midline or laterally. A third tube may be placed in the anterior mediastinum if desired.

THORACOABDOMINAL INCISION

Thoracoabdominal incision has had many advocates and critics, and even today it probably is not used enough by abdominal surgeons, who do not feel comfortable working in the chest. As a result, they struggle unnecessarily in attempting to do the difficult procedures transabdominally that could more easily be approached by a thoracoabdominal incision. Also, the thoracoabdominal incision is often misused in performing procedures about the esophageal hiatus or fundus, which is better approached transthoracically without the abdominal extension.

The thoracoabdominal incision should be used when necessary to obtain exposure. The diaphragm should not be an artificial boundary, but at the same time it should not be incised indiscriminantly.

Indications

Indications include hiatal hernia repair, resection of the distal esophagus, cardioesophageal junction, or proximal stomach, adrenalectomy, nephrectomy, particularly in upper pole neoplasms, splenectomy if the spleen is grossly enlarged, aortic procedures involving the suprarenal aorta, portocaval, and splenorenal vascular anastomoses, and trauma of the upper abdomen.

Procedure (Fig. 5–4)

The patient may be positioned in full lateral, semilateral, or supine position, depending upon the procedure to be performed. Except in the supine position, the arm on top is suspended from an ether screen or other support.

The surgical incision is begun overlying the sixth or seventh interspace. Hemostasis is produced by electrocautery of the extracostal musculature as it is incised. The skin incision is extended across the costal arch and transversely across the upper abdomen to the midline. The abdominal musculature is incised, including the rectus abdominus muscle. Occasionally it may be necessary to extend the incision across the opposite rectus muscle. The peritoneum is opened to the costal margin.

The diaphragmatic incision is placed in accordance with the procedure to be done. If the operation involves the stomach and cardioesophageal junction, the incision is begun at the hiatus and extended laterally, curving anteriorly to the point of the division of the costal arch. The more lateral the incision, the less muscle will be paralyzed by cutting the branches of the phrenic nerve. An operation not involving the stomach or esophagus may be kept laterally in the plane of the chest wall incision. A rib spreader is used in the thoracic portion of the incision and a Balfour retractor for the abdominal part.

Some use a variation of the abdominal extension. After reaching the midline, the incision is directed inferiorly in the midline as far as the umbilicus or even further. I have not found this incision to have any advantage over the transverse incision unless some procedure involving the lower abdominal organs is anticipated or a pathologic process or injury in the lower abdomen is discovered.

The incision is closed by first closing the diaphragm in two layers, overlapping as described in the discussion on diaphragmatic repair. The three or four sutures nearest the costal arch may be left untied until the arch is sutured. The peritoneum and transversus

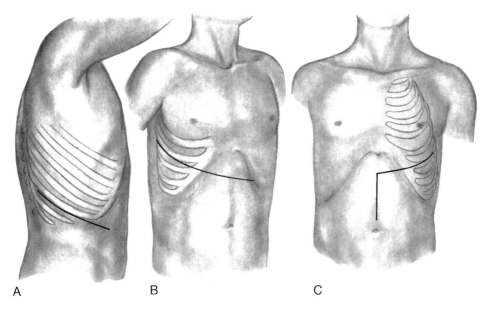

Figure 5–4. Thoracoabdominal incisions. *A,* A tenth interspace approach is suitable for adrenalectomy or nephrectomy. *B, C,* Two varieties of thoracoabdominal incisions that may be used according to preference.

abdominus muscle are then closed with a running Dexon or Vicryl suture. The rib cage is approximated with three or four pericostal sutures of No. 1 absorbable or nonabsorbable material, according to preference. The costal arch cartilage is then sutured with one or two Prolene or wire sutures. Pericostal sutures are tied and the intercostal muscle sutured with running 2-0 Dexon or Vicryl sutures. The abdominal anterior fascia is closed with figure-of-eight sutures of 3-0 steel wire or monofilament Prolene. Subcutaneous tissue is closed with 3-0 absorbable sutures, and the skin is then closed.

A variation of this incision is used for a procedure involving the adrenal gland or kidney. A full lateral position is used. The incision is placed over the tenth interspace. It may not be necessary to enter the peritoneal cavity, and the entire procedure may be kept in the pleural and retroperitoneal spaces.

Drainage of the subdiaphragmatic space is not used routinely and is elected when there is expected drainage of bile or pancreatic secretion or when significant contamination is present. The pleural space must be drained, usually with a single chest tube.

Note

The patient with this incision may have more difficulty with effective coughing. This is because of added pain and impaired diaphragmatic activity.

LEFT ANTERIOR SUBMAMMARY THORACOTOMY

Indications

This incision provides for rapid approach to managing cardiac injury with tamponade if the injury is thought to be on the left side. It may be ideal for forming a pericardial window or in exploring the pericardial sac. A smaller version may be used to implant epicardial pacemaker electrodes. The left anterior submammary thoracotomy can be used for open lung biopsy. The incision provides good access for open cardiac massage when needed. Its principal advantage is that it can be made rapidly and requires few special instruments.

The incision has several disadvantages: (1) it provides very limited exposure of the heart unless the incision is extended, (2) it provides very poor exposure of the lungs except for open lung biopsy, (3) it provides no exposure of the posterior mediastinum.

The incision can be extended to a bilateral anterior thoracotomy, which will provide extensive exposure not only of the heart but also of the entire mediastinum and both lungs.

Position

Most often when this incision is used in an emergency situation, the patient is lying supine with the arm abducted. It is preferable, if there is time, to elevate the left hip and shoulder about 3 inches on a folded sheet or sandbags and to suspend the left arm over the patient on an ether screen.

Procedure (Fig. 5–5)

A 6-inch curved incision is made, generally conforming to the fourth intercostal space in men or following the intermammary fold in women. The pectoralis major and serratus anterior muscles are incised. The fourth intercostal space is incised, exposing the pleura, which is then incised the full length of the wound. At the anterior extremity, the internal mammary vessels are found and may be ligated and divided. This may be ignored momentarily if cardiac arrest has occurred or is imminent, and no attempt at wound hemostasis is made at this time.

A rib spreader is placed, the incision is opened widely, and the pericardium is exposed. The fourth or fifth costal cartilages may be severed near the sternum to gain exposure, and the sternum may also be transected, if necessary. A rib shear is adequate for this purpose.

Closure of the Incision

A single chest tube is required, unless there is air leakage from lung injury. This is placed in the sixth or seventh intercostal space in the midaxillary line. Cartilages that have been cut should be approximated by direct suture through the cartilage. Another alternative is to excise about one inch of each cartilage subperichondrally.

Three or four pericostal sutures are placed, and the adjacent ribs are approximated as well as possible. Intercostal muscle sutures are not possible or necessary anteriorly.

The musculature is approximated with continuous Polyglactin suture material. The subcutaneous tissue is closed with a running suture of the same material. The skin is then closed.

Warning

As stated, this incision is most often used for cardiac tamponade. The operation should not be done in the Emergency Room unless death seems imminent. It should not be undertaken by the inexperienced, or without assistance, adequate ventilatory apparatus, good lighting, and sufficient surgical instruments. The exposure is sometimes less than adequate, particularly for the inexperienced.

AXILLARY THORACOTOMY

Indications

The axillary thoracotomy approach gives limited exposure to the intrathoracic structures but has some usefulness. Cervicodorsal sympathectomy may be accomplished easily by this exposure. Biopsy of upper lobe lesions may also be done.

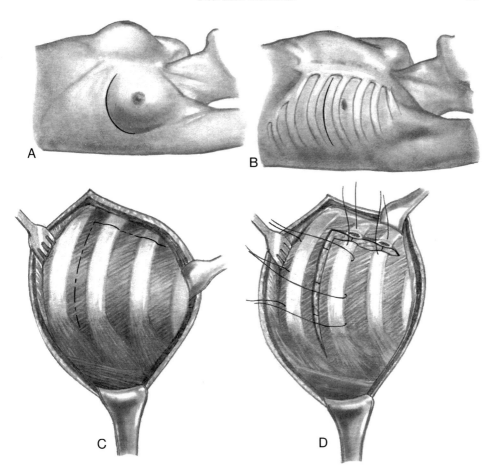

Figure 5–5. Left submammary thoracotomy. *A,* The incision usually employed in female patients. *B,* Incision usually employed in male patients. The fourth interspace is usually the interspace of choice. *C,* Rib cartilages above the incision may be incised and also the inferior cartilages may be severed. *D,* The basic method by which the chest wall is reconstructed prior to wound closure.

Position

Lateral or semilateral.

Procedure (Fig. 5–6)

The patient is positioned with the arm suspended or prepared into the field and covered by stockinette. A 4-to-5-inch incision is made over the third interspace. Retracting the pectoralis major and latissimus dorsi muscles will make the incision possible without transecting any extracostal muscle. The intercostal muscle of the third or fourth interspace is then incised and the pleura opened. Any adhesions present are divided. The sympathetic chain can be visualized by retracting the upper lobe anteriorly and inferiorly. A parenchymal lesion can be incised or excised. Exposure is of necessity limited.

Following completion of the intrathoracic procedure, a single pericostal suture is placed and tied, and the intercostal muscle is sutured. A single chest tube is inserted in the sixth or seventh interspace. The subcutaneous tissues and skin are then closed as in other procedures.

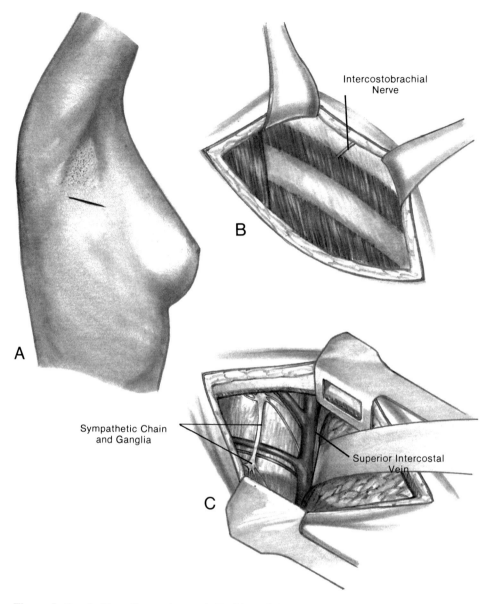

Figure 5–6. Axillary thoracotomy. *A*, Position of the transverse incision in the axilla at the lower margin of the hair line. *B*, Exposure of the third rib and intercostal space through this incision. The intercostobrachial nerve arising from the second intercostal nerve should be preserved. *C*, The surgical exposure obtained. This approach is most useful for cervicodorsal sympathectomy or lung biopsy of the upper lobe.

Note

Use of a headlamp is suggested because of the small incision and limited exposure.

ANTERIOR MEDIASTINOTOMY (CHAMBERLAIN PROCEDURE)

Indications

1. Exploration and securing of tissue for biopsy in bronchogenic carcinoma that is presumed to be nonresectable.

2. Exploration and removal of tissue for biopsy when mediastinal lymphomas or other anterior mediastinal masses are suspected.

Position

Supine, with the arm extended.

Procedure (Fig. 5–7)

An 8 cm incision is made beginning at the lateral sternal border and extended laterally over the third costal cartilage or over the third interspace (the original report described resection of the third cartilage). Hemostasis is produced and the incision deepened (this description will use the intercostal approach), and the intercostal muscle is incised. The internal mammary vessels should be visualized and not injured; if they have been severed, they should be suture-ligated rather than cauterized or secured with hemoclips. The pleura may be dissected from the mediastinum gently and retracted laterally and the pleural space not opened. A more common variant is to incise the pleura and approach the hilum and mediastinum transpleurally. Certainly a greater exposure is obtained, and orientation is easier with this variant.

The mediastinal or hilar mass that prompted exploration is then palpated and inspected. Its relation to the vena cava, aorta, pulmonary artery, and superior pulmonary vein is assessed before an effort is made to incise and remove tissue for biopsy. The degree of vascularity of the neoplasm may be determined by a small incision superficially before a deeper one is made. The surgeon must be certain not to incise a major vascular structure,

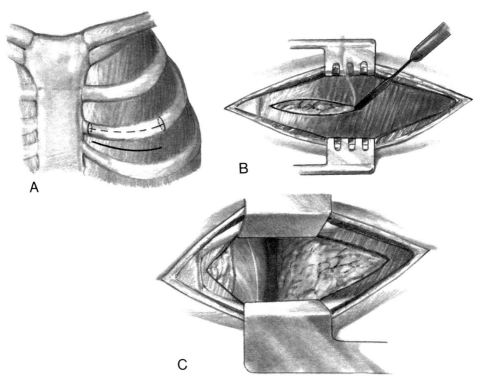

Figure 5–7. Anterior mediastinotomy (Chamberlain procedure). *A,* The location of the incision, which may be over the third costal cartilage and involve resection of the cartilage in the third interspace. *B,* Most of the incision is made by electrocautery. *C,* The exposure gained, which may be intrapleural or extrapleural.

which may be obscured by the tumor. A simple way of securing tissue is to pass a noncutting needle armed with a 3-0 suture about 1 cm deep into the mass; then, using the suture as traction, excise a 1 cm core of tissue about the needle with a No. 15 scalpel blade.

This technique prevents crushing of the tissue and produces a specimen from which the pathologist is more likely to be able to make a diagnosis.

The electrocautery is used to carefully control all bleeding from the biopsy site. The site should be inspected several times over a period of 5 to 10 minutes before closing the incision to be certain of hemostasis. A single chest tube is inserted through the fifth or sixth interspace in the midaxillary line.

Two pericostal nonabsorbable sutures are placed about adjacent cartilages and tied. If a cartilage resection has been done it is only necessary to suture the perichondrium. No attempt is made to suture the intercostal muscle, and the pectoralis major muscle is sutured with a continuous absorbable suture. The subcutaneous tissue and skin are then closed.

Notes

1. **The presence of superior vena caval obstruction makes venous bleeding more likely and more difficult to control.**
2. **The exposure is so limited that great care must be exercised to prevent vascular injury, which may be difficult to manage.**
3. **This is a poor procedure for staging of bronchogenic carcinoma that is thought to be resectable.**

6

Operations Involving the Lung

Pulmonary Surgical Anatomy

THE BRONCHOPULMONARY SEGMENTS

The physician who intends to perform pulmonary surgery must become intimately familiar with topographic, segmental, and hilar bronchopulmonary anatomy. There is no substitute for a nearly perfect knowledge of the anatomy of this area. Topographic anatomy of the lungs is well known and well illustrated in a number of texts and therefore will not be described here.

The bronchopulmonary segments are the functional anatomic subdivisions of the lung. Each contains separate bronchi, arteries, and veins. Occasionally there are incomplete fissures that indicate the segmental plane, but generally the parenchyma is contiguous and therefore, without a prior understanding of the area, the topographic divisions would not be apparent. Normally, no sizable pulmonary vessels cross the intersegmental planes. The pulmonary veins typically lie in the intersegmental plane, whereas the pulmonary arterial divisions accompany the bronchus in the central portion of each segment.

Knowledge of segmental subdivisions is important for two reasons.

First, certain diseases, such as tuberculosis, bronchiectasis, lung abscess, and emphysema, are segmental diseases, even though multiple segments or an entire lobe may be involved. This fact is useful in the differential diagnosis of parenchymal disease.

Second, the bronchopulmonary segments may be managed as separate surgical entities. With the lessening incidence of suppurative disease and tuberculosis, segmental resection has been performed less frequently. Several indications for segmental resection remain, however. There is little value in considering isolated basal segmental resection—that is, separating, for example, the lateral basal segment from the anterior basal segment. Many have concluded that the right upper lobe, except for localized transegmental resection, should be treated as an entity. On the left side, the lingular segments are, for practical purposes, considered a surgical entity.

The bronchoscopist must be thoroughly familiar with bronchial segmental anatomy as seen through the bronchoscope.

Figure 6–1 demonstrates the classification and terminology of pulmonary segments of Jackson and Huber, which has become generally accepted. There is considerable variation in the size and topography of individual segments, which cannot be appreciated by x-ray or at surgery unless preoperative bronchograms have been done.

The anatomic divisions are approximate in the illustrations, and the technique for delineating segmental planes at operation will be discussed in the text dealing with specific resections.

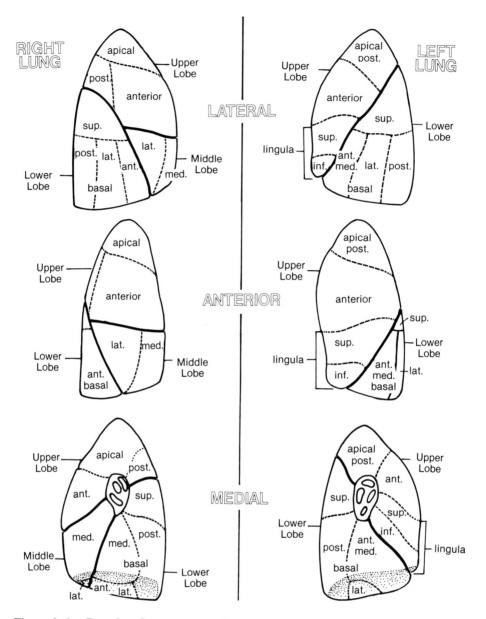

Figure 6–1. Bronchopulmonary segments.

PULMONARY ANATOMY

All drawings in this section and in the section on operations on the lung are drawn as seen by the surgeon standing at the patient's back with the patient in the lateral position and visualized through a posterolateral incision.

Right Lung

The surgeon should be familiar with the nomenclature and topography of the bronchopulmonary segments as demonstrated in Figure 6–1.

The bronchus lies posteriorly in the hilum and maintains this relationship except for the middle lobe bronchus, which passes posterior to the inferior trunk of the pulmonary artery (Fig. 6–2).

The right main bronchus originates at the tracheal bifurcation at a less acute angle than does the left main bronchus. It is only 1 to 1.5 cm in length (Fig. 6–2). The right upper lobe bronchus originates at a 90-degree angle to the main bronchus and is also no more than 1 to 1.5 cm in length. The lobar bronchus trifurcates into apical, anterior, and posterior segmental divisions. A subsegmental anatomy can also be defined, but there is little practical value in this information.

The bronchus from the lower margin of the upper lobe bronchus to the middle lobe orifice is about 3 cm in length and is termed the intermediate bronchus. The middle lobe originates at an angle of about 35 degrees anteriorly and within 1 cm divides into medial and lateral segmental bronchi.

The superior segment of the lower lobe originates from the intermediate bronchus posteriorly at a 90-degree angle, usually directly opposite the middle lobe. The remainder of the bronchus—from the middle lobe to the next branch—is regarded as the basilar division. The medial basal bronchus arises about 1 to 2 cm below the middle lobe orifice. The anterior, lateral, and posterior basal bronchi arise at about 1 cm inferiorly, all at the same level.

Pulmonary Artery. The right main pulmonary artery emerges from the pericardium in a transverse plane. It is anterior to the right main bronchus. Within 2 cm, the artery splits into superior and inferior divisions (Fig. 6–3). The superior division, about 1.5 cm in length, then typically divides into apical and anterior segmental arteries, which enter the upper lobe on its superior and anterior surfaces. The apical segmental vein crosses the anterior artery at a right angle and partially obscures the artery.

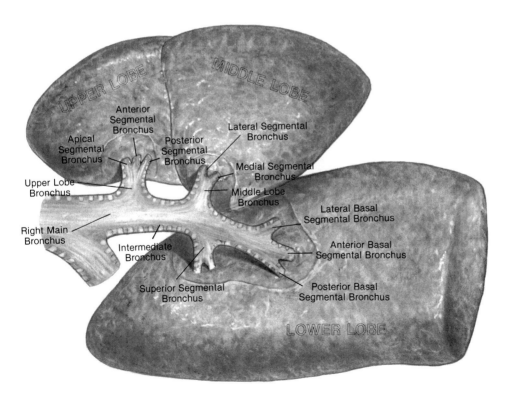

Figure 6–2. Bronchopulmonary anatomy of the right lung.

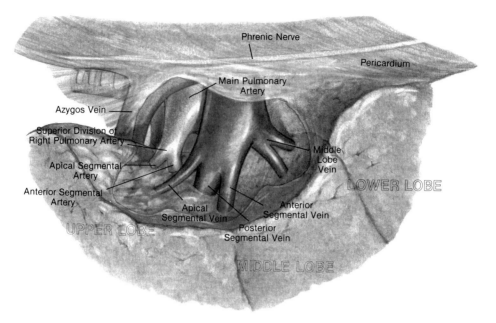

Figure 6–3. Right lung anatomy, anterior hilar view. This view of the anterior aspect of the right hilum is oriented to the lateral position, with the surgeon standing at the patient's back.

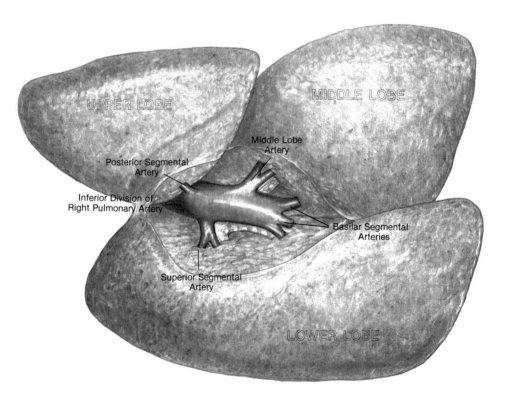

Figure 6–4. Right lung anatomy, interlobar aspect, as seen by the viewer standing at the patient's back. The patient is in the right lateral position, and the upper middle lobe is separated, exposing the pulmonary artery.

The inferior division is 2 to 3 cm in length and enters the interlobar plane in a generally vertical plane directed slightly posteriorly (Fig. 6–4). Its first branch is the posterior segmental artery of the upper lobe, which leaves the parent vessel at a 90-degree angle. One to 1.5 cm distally, the superior segmental artery arises at about a 45-degree angle posteriorly, and directly opposite and anteriorly, one or two middle lobe arteries originate. One centimeter distally, the medial basal segmental artery begins, followed almost immediately by the anterior, lateral, and posterior segmental arteries.

Pulmonary Veins.   The superior pulmonary vein is a large vein that lies in the anterior pulmonary hilum about 1.5 cm posterior to the phrenic nerve (see Fig. 6–3). The undivided vein outside the pericardium is about 1 to 2 cm long. It receives multiple veins from the upper lobe, generally identified as apical, anterior, and posterior segmental veins. There are considerable variations in their number and distribution. The lowermost one or two tributaries drain the middle lobe.

The inferior pulmonary vein lies inferiorly and posteriorly in the most superior portion of the inferior pulmonary ligament (Fig. 6–5). It enters the pericardium transversely, as does the superior vein. It receives a separate vein from the superior segment and several basilar segmental veins with some variation.

Segmental pulmonary veins lie in the intersegmental planes, whereas the segmental arteries are in the central portion of the segment and accompany the bronchi.

Anatomic Variations of Surgical Significance

1. **The apical segmental bronchus may arise separately from the trachea.**
2. **Rarely, the upper lobe bronchus may arise from the trachea.**
3. **The superior segmental bronchus may be represented by two bronchi arising separately.**
4. **There may be from two to four divisions of the superior pulmonary artery trunk.**

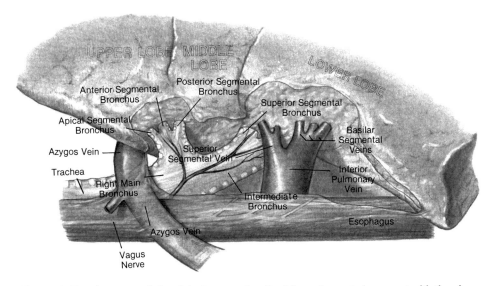

Figure 6–5.   Anatomy of the right lung as visualized from the posterior aspect with the viewer standing at the patient's back. The patient is turned into the full lateral position.

5. **A separate anterior or posterior segmental vessel or both, may arise as the vessel passes beneath the upper lobe and may be difficult to visualize with the superior vein intact.**
6. **There may be a single pulmonary vein.**
7. **Frequently there are interlobar veins traversing the fissures.**

Left Lung

Bronchi. The left main bronchus lies more inferiorly than does the right main bronchus and appears in the posterior hilum below the level of the main pulmonary artery. The main bronchus has a more acute angle with reference to the trachea and is about 5 cm in length.

The left upper lobe bronchus arises from the anterolateral surface of the left main bronchus at a 90-degree angle (Fig. 6–6). This origin is obscured by the main pulmonary artery as the bronchus passes medial to the artery. The left upper lobe bronchus is no more than 1 cm in length and immediately divides into apical posterior, anterior, and lingular segmental divisions. The lingular bronchus is the largest segment and divides again into superior and inferior divisions. Surgically speaking, the left upper lobe bronchus and its branches are not clearly visible until pulmonary arterial branches to the upper lobe have been divided.

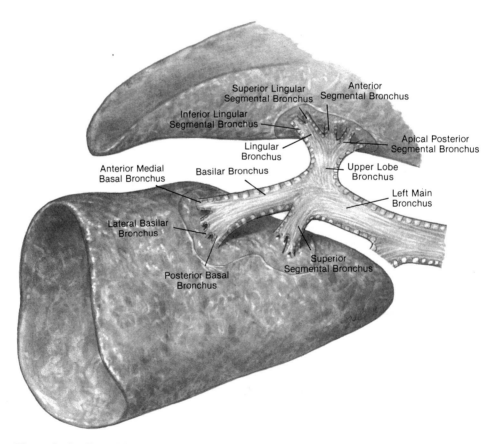

Figure 6–6. Bronchial anatomy of the left lung, demonstrating the location and structure of the left lung as viewed from the interlobar aspect with the viewer at the patient's back and the patient in the lateral position.

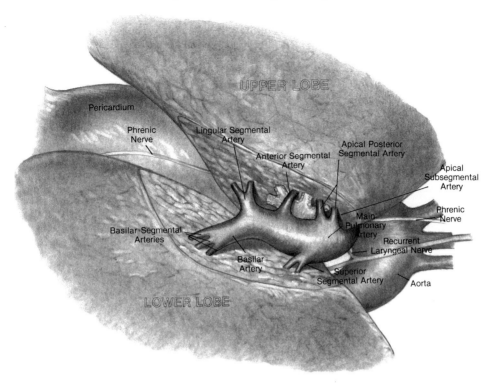

Figure 6–7. Left lung anatomy, interlobar view. The pulmonary artery and bronchus are seen from the interlobar aspect with the patient's back at the bottom of the picture, as would be seen in a left lateral thoracotomy.

The lower lobe bronchus gives origin to the superior segment about 1.5 cm from the upper lobe orifice. Again it arises at a 90-degree angle from the posterior wall. The basilar bronchus extends about 3 cm and divides into anteromedial, lateral, and posterior segmental branches.

Pulmonary Artery. The left main pulmonary artery leaves the pericardium in a transverse plane (Fig. 6–7). Just at the pericardial reflection, the ligamentum arteriosum can be found. The recurrent laryngeal nerve arising from the vagus nerve as it crosses the aorta turns and passes under the ligamentum and then ascends superiorly. The pulmonary artery is the most superior structure of the left hilum.

About 1.5 to 2 cm distally, a large branch arises from the anterior surface. This represents the apical posterior segmental artery. It typically divides into two branches after a distance of 0.5 cm. The artery descends inferiorly and enters the interlobar fissure anterior to the bronchus. The first branch just as the fissure is entered is the superior segmental artery of the lower lobe, which originates from the posterior surface at about a 45-degree angle. At about the same level anteriorly, a vessel to the anterior segment arises. The lingular artery arises anteriorly 1 to 2 cm inferiorly. The anteromedial, lateral, and posterior basilar segmental arteries arise about 1 cm distally.

Pulmonary Veins. The superior pulmonary vein lies in a transverse position in the anterior aspect of the hilum (Fig. 6–8). The undivided vein is about 1 cm in length outside the pericardium. An apical vein that curves superiorly over the apical posterior artery is a constant feature. One or two lingular tributaries are also present inferiorly. Usually two other veins arise from the upper lobe.

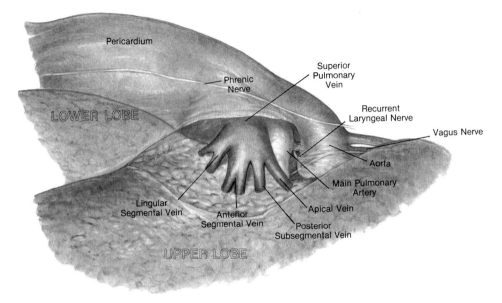

Figure 6–8.   Left lung anatomy, anterior view. The surgeon is standing at the patient's back with the patient in the lateral position, reflecting the lung posteriorly, and viewing the anterior hilum.

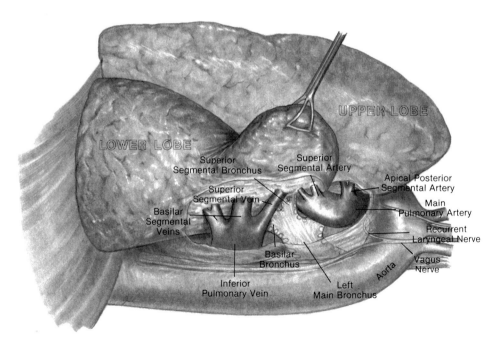

Figure 6–9.   Left lung anatomy, posterior view. The patient is in the lateral position; the surgeon is standing at the patient's back and the lung is reflected anteriorly.

The inferior pulmonary vein is almost identical with the right (Fig. 6–9), lying posteriorly and inferiorly. It also lies in a transverse plane and is about 1 to 1.5 cm in length. The most superior tributary is from the superior segment. Two or three other veins drain the basilar segments. These veins, as in all other areas, lie in the intersegmental planes.

Anatomic Variations of Surgical Significance

1. **The lingular bronchus may arise separately from the main bronchus.**
2. **The upper lobe arterial branches are variable and may number from three to seven.**
3. **The anterior segmental artery may arise from the lingular artery.**
4. **There may be arterial branches from the lingular artery to the anteromedial segment, or the reverse may occur.**
5. **Two superior segmental arteries may be present.**
6. **There also may be two separate lingular segmental arteries.**

Bronchial Arteries. Bronchial arteries vary in size and location. Most often there is a single bronchial artery lying on the posterior wall of the right main bronchus with branches to all lobes and segments. On the left there are usually two bronchial vessels, one anteriorly and one posteriorly. Unless some vascular anomaly exists or there is some form of cyanotic heart disease, these vessels do not represent a special surgical problem.

Basic Surgical Techniques

DISSECTION OF PULMONARY VESSELS

The dissection and ligation or stapling of pulmonary arteries and veins require a different technique than for systemic vessels. The pulmonary vessels are thin-walled and fragile. They tear easily and cannot be clamped with standard hemostats. The following suggestions may be helpful.

A perfect knowledge of hilar anatomy is a basic necessity. This should result in a three-dimensional concept so that the location of any vessel is in mind at all times, even though it is not visible. The relationship of the artery to the bronchus and pulmonary veins must also be kept in mind.

There is almost always a perivascular plane that permits rapid, safe dissection in an avascular area. This plane must be sought and identified. Except in some acute suppurative states and when long-standing tuberculous disease or other granulomatous disease is present, this plane is present. When it is absent, it may be wise to begin dissection by encircling the main pulmonary artery proximally with a large suture strand before the more hazardous dissection is started, so that if injury occurs, control is assured.

Three sides of each artery should be dissected completely before an attempt is made to pass a right angle forceps beneath the vessel. If this is not done, perforation is likely. Pulmonary vessels should not be grasped with thumb forceps, even those with vascular jaws. Only the adventitia should be grasped. The vessel may be held or retracted with "peanut" dissectors safely.

Pulmonary vessels should be ligated with nonabsorbable sutures, such as silk, cotton, or polyester. Ligature of a main pulmonary artery can be accomplished using 0 silk ligature; however, it is much safer to clamp the vessel with an angled or curved vascular clamp, ligate the artery distally, and transect the vessel, leaving a 0.5 cm cuff of arterial wall. Size 4-0 Prolene is used as a running horizontal mattress suture, followed by a continuous, simple, over-and-over suture across the end of the vessel (Fig. 6–10).

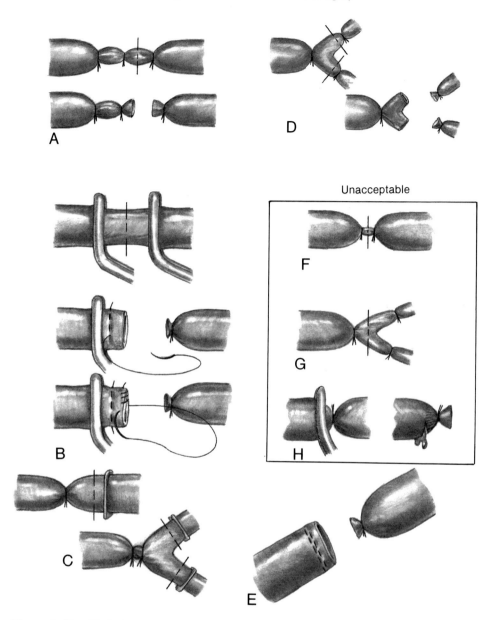

Figure 6–10. Variation and techniques of dividing and ligating pulmonary arteries.

A, The technique of triple ligation with division of the artery, leaving two proximal ligatures separated from each other with an adequate vascular stump.

B, The technique for applying vascular clamps and dividing the artery, first using a primary row of horizontal mattress sutures by a second row of simple continuous suture across the vessel. This is most useful in managing the main pulmonary artery rather than lobar segmental divisions.

C, An alternative technique using a proximal ligature. Preferably two ligatures should be used, and the distal vessel should be secured by hemoclip application division.

D, The technique of ligating proximal to a bifurcation and severing the vessel distal to the bifurcation to produce a large cuff, from which the ligature is unlikely to escape.

E, The technique of using vascular staples to close the proximal artery.

F, G, and *H,* Demonstrate unacceptable techniques. *F,* Unacceptable technique of dividing between ligatures too close together, leaving a stump that is too short and that favors ligature slippage. *G,* Ligating after a bifurcation and severing the vessel proximal to the bifurcation, producing a stump that is too short. *H,* The technical error of using a crushing clamp and attempting to ligate the pulmonary artery proximally. Either distally or proximally the crushing clamp usually causes tearing of the vascular structure.

Lobar or segmental pulmonary arteries can be ligated with 2-0 nonabsorbable suture proximally and distal ligatures or hemoclips beyond a point of division. A suture-ligature should be used, or at least a second proximal ligature (Fig. 6–11). It is always safer to transect a vessel distal to a bifurcation to gain length and to produce a proximal cuff larger than the ligated area. Several variations are possible, as shown. The principal pitfalls of pulmonary arterial dissection and ligation include: (1) attempting to pass an angled clamp

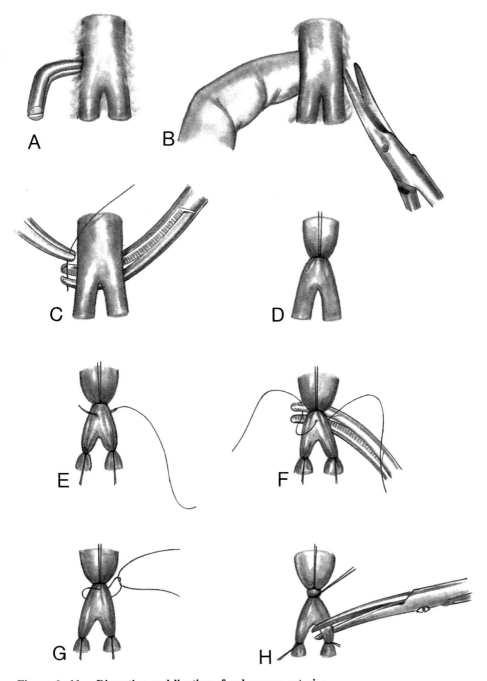

Figure 6–11. Dissection and ligation of pulmonary arteries.

around an incompletely dissected vessel; (2) clamping with a crushing hemostat prior to ligation; (3) leaving too short a stump of vessel distal to a single ligature; (4) ligating a major vessel with suture material of too small a caliber or using too much force and cutting the fragile wall; (5) using excessive traction during dissection, which can easily tear a vessel at a point of branching; (6) penetrating a vessel unwittingly at a "crotch" or bifurcation (Fig. 6-10).

Pulmonary veins can be managed similarly, although ligature of a major vein may be accomplished more safely than that of a major artery.

The stapling instrument is considered preferable for securing the main pulmonary artery and veins. It is simple; the suture line is more accurately done than is possible with manual suturing; and at times, the length of vessel available is so short that safe ligation is not possible. "V" size staples are best. It is my experience that stapling of pulmonary vessels is safe, rapid, and effective.

Inadvertent injury to a major pulmonary artery requires rapid, safe control and repair. Digital pressure is utilized first while the field is cleared of blood. Then the situation is evaluated calmly and the method of control selected.

Should the injured vessel be a major one, it may be wisest to encircle the main artery proximally or, if this is not possible, open the pericardium and clamp the intrapericardial portion of the artery while repair is accomplished.

Sometimes the exposure may be sufficient for application of either a partial occlusion vascular clamp, or the entire vessel may be cross clamped with a vascular clamp.

Suture of a laceration may often be accomplished safely by exposing a small segment of the injury and suturing sequentially as more of the laceration is uncovered.

A major loss of blood volume should be managed by digital control while the hypovolemia is corrected before attempts at repair are made, which may result in further loss.

Suture material should be 4-0 or 5-0 Prolene.

PERIPHERAL ADHESIONS

The freeing of the lung from the chest wall is a necessary part of any intrathoracic procedure, whether the definitive procedure involves lung or not. The degree of success with which this is accomplished has much more to do with the final result than is generally supposed.

Far too often, hurried, crude, or inept separation of adhesions has resulted in major injury to the lung, phrenic or vagus nerve, and vascular structures in the apex of the chest and mediastinum. The most common source of postoperative bleeding is from vascular adhesions in the chest wall.

The first entry into the pleura may result in lung damage when total pleural obliteration is present. If extensive pleural disease is known or suspected, a rib resection is preferable to an intercostal incision. This gives added exposure to visualize the proper plane of dissection. Dissection is usually easier in the interpleural plane rather than the extrapleural plane (Fig. 6-12).

Once the proper plane is identified, blunt finger dissection may be found adequate for filmy nonvascular adhesions. There may be only a few dense vascular adhesions, which can be separated by sharp dissection or by electrocautery (Fig. 6-13). Occasionally the lung is totally fused and requires slow, painstaking, sharp dissection. A hurried or crude approach here will result in multiple injuries to the lung.

As the surgeon approaches the mediastinum anteriorly and posteriorly, he may fail to "turn the corner" and carry the dissection plane posterior to the aorta or esophagus. Blind dissection of the mediastinal surface of the lung above the hilum may result in transection of the phrenic or vagus nerve; therefore, the apex of the lung should be freed first, so that this area can be dissected under direct vision.

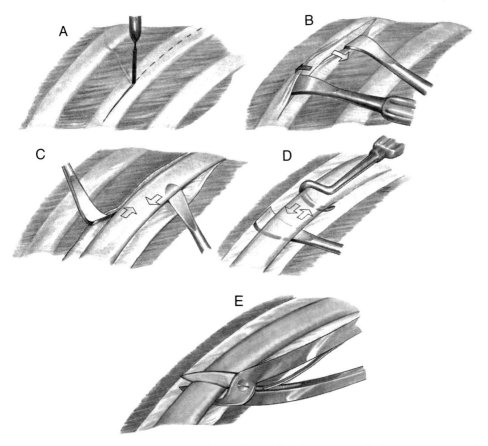

Figure 6–12. Technique of rib resection. Rib resection for empyema drainage, or as a part of thoracotomy, is a technique rarely mastered by young surgeons. It should be accomplished with no damage to adjacent intercostal muscle and without injury to the pleura.

A, Incision of the periosteal surface in the middle of the rib by electrocautery and transverse cut lines at the point of rib transection.

B, Removal of the periosteum from the rib surface by alternately pushing and pulling the elevator without tearing the periosteum.

C, Use of the sharp edge of the elevator for stripping the periosteum from the superior margin of the rib, *always* directing the force *anteriorly* and stripping the inferior edge with the flat end of the elevator in the position shown and applying force in the *posterior direction only.*

D, Technique of removing the periosteum from the posterior surface of the rib with the Haight elevator, or as an alternative, using the Doyan rib stripper.

E, Cutting the rib with a Bethune rib shear in the proper position.

Occasionally in malignancy, tuberculosis, or lung abscess, the pleural involvement may defy dissection. Then a localized extrapleural dissection is desirable, leaving a patch of pleura on the lung. Rarely, the entire dissection may have to be extrapleural. Bleeding from extrapleural dissection may be severe and require considerable time with the cautery at more than one time during the procedure.

Tuberculosis, actinomycosis, and histoplasmosis may result in dense pleural disease that destroys even the extrapleural plane. Dissection in the apex is particularly difficult and dangerous. Injury to the subclavian vessels and brachial plexus is an ever-present threat. Occasionally the surgeon must leave an area of dense, thickened pleura or even some lung tissue rather than injure the apical structures.

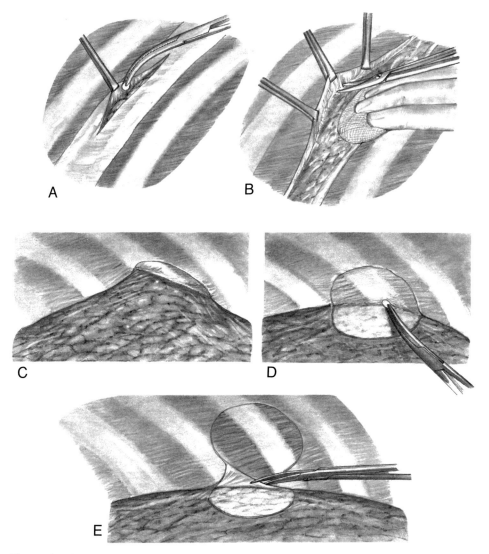

Figure 6–13. Techniques of dissection of pleural adhesions. *A,* Beginning dissection with "peanut" dissector through the bed of a resected rib. *B,* Sharp dissection with countertraction may be necessary. *C–E,* Extrapleural dissection over a limited area (as shown) or over an extensive area may be required. This is desirable when the parietal pleura is invaded by neoplasm or in the area of a lung abscess or tuberculous cavity.

Control of bleeding following extrapleural dissection is almost impossible without the extensive use of the electrocautery, and even then the areas of dissection must be reinspected repeatedly because an area of eschar may separate and allow further bleeding. Any bleeding that is obviously under arterial pressure should be oversewn rather than relying upon cautery. Diaphragmatic vessels are particularly prone to rebleed.

CLOSURE OF THE BRONCHUS

Closure of the bronchus (Fig. 6–14) has been the subject of many publications in earlier years. Many complex methods of suture closure were devised. Before automated

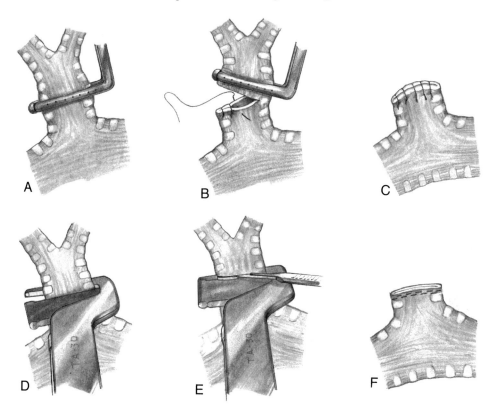

Figure 6–14. *A* to *C,* The technique of bronchial division and suture closure. *D* to *F,* The technique of bronchial stapling.

stapling devices became available, it was apparent to most surgeons that the more complex the suture technique, the higher the incidence of bronchial disruption. Conversely, the more satisfactory bronchial closure has, to most surgeons, been a simple suture technique.

The technique of bronchial dissection should involve careful, gentle handling. It is unwise and unnecessary to strip the bronchus bare of all peribronchial tissue, which will deprive the bronchus of most of its blood supply. For the same reason, be sure to keep a length of bronchus proximal to the intended site of closure. Similarly, ligating the bronchial vessels proximally at a distance is unwise.

The technique of stapling has been the most significant advance in this field of surgery. I have used staple closure in over 700 bronchial closures without a single postoperative bronchial disruption. Two fistulas occurred at 6 months and over 1 year later, both related to recurrent neoplasms. The stapling device can be misused, and poor results may follow. It was possible with the first-generation instruments to apply too much pressure and crush the bronchus. With the currently available instruments, this is not likely to occur, because the instrument will not close if too much compression is required. Experimental data show that the current devices do not exceed a pressure of 300 lb/sq in. This design removes the possibility that an unexperienced surgeon will close the instrument too tightly.

Several points are important in staple closure: (1) The proper site must be determined accurately before the instrument is closed, so that only one site will be subjected to compression. (2) The closed instrument should be left in place for as short a time as possible. (3) The remaining lung should be inflated as soon as the instrument is closed to be certain that the lumen of the remaining bronchus is not compromised. In this context, it is frequently better to staple the basal bronchus and superior segmental bronchus separately rather than risk compromising the middle or upper lobe bronchial lumina. (4) Never use a staple size smaller than 4.8 mm. (5) Be certain that the plane of closure approximates the anterior wall of the bronchus to the posterior wall. (6) All instruments should be inspected periodically by a manufacturer's representative to be sure that they are properly adjusted.

Several stapling devices are now marketed. I prefer those manufactured by the United States Surgical Company because of the basic design principles, particularly because crushing pressure is controllable and preventable. The disposable versions are excellent but more expensive. The quality of stapling devices is steadily improving.

Size 4.8 mm staples are best used for bronchial closure; 3.5 mm or "V" staples are best used for vascular closure.

Should a suture technique be chosen, the surgeon should avoid grasping the cut end of the bronchus with any instrument.

The suture technique involves clamping the bronchus distal to the intended point of transection. This may be omitted if the bronchus is a main bronchus or if there is insufficient room because of the disease process. The bronchus is cut transversely for 4 to 5 mm, and the cut end is sutured as illustrated with 4-0 nonabsorbable suture, which should be tied very carefully to avoid cutting or unnecessary devascularization. After two sutures, the cut is extended and additional sutures are placed. The sutures should be 2 to 3 mm apart. For a main bronchus, seldom are more than six sutures required; for a lobar bronchus, three or four sutures are usually enough. Too many sutures devascularize. After the closure is complete, the suture line is immersed in saline and up to 45 cm of inflation pressure is applied by the anesthesiologist. Additional sutures are placed if there is an air leak between sutures. Should there be leakage through needle holes, either the surgeon used too large a needle or the needle was passed using force away from the direction of the needle, which enlarged the tract unnecessarily.

Covering the bronchial stump with a pleural flap is a time-honored technique, but is of unproved value. The pleural tissue is probably of little use because its vascularity is minimal. Pedicled muscle is probably superior, but its use makes the procedure more time-consuming and complicated. Coverage of the bronchus has not been used with the stapling technique, and no fistulas have occurred.

SUTURE MATERIAL IN PULMONARY RESECTION

Each center has devised methods of suturing, wound closure, and suture use. Often these techniques become the rule even though there may be little rational basis for them. Almost every suture material has been used by some authority at some time with apparently satisfactory results. Much usage is provincial, and this attitude frequently thwarts all consideration of varying methods or techniques. Therefore, this section can only reflect my prejudice and experience and may not necessarily represent the best. The techniques described have been modified from time to time as new suture materials have become available.

The surgeon should adopt a routine based on sound reason and should know the advantages and limitations of various suture materials.

Bronchial Suture

Automated stapling is preferred over all other techniques, but there are instances in which suture closure of a bronchus is necessary. A 4-0 synthetic material, such as Tev-Dek, is preferred, using a fine vascular needle. This is considered less likely to produce granuloma formation than silk or cotton. Recently, Grillo has suggested that Vicryl and Dexon may be better. The newer monofilament absorbable suture (PDS) has proved to be excellent for this purpose.

Vascular Suture

It is often necessary to suture an injured pulmonary artery or to close a transected vessel. Prolene (6-0, 5-0, or 4-0) seems to serve this purpose better than other vascular sutures. It is not without its hazards and the user must be familiar with them. Tev-Dek can be easily substituted and has some advantages, among them being that it provides a more secure knot and is less likely to break at a site of stretching or torsion. A disadvantage is the roughness of the material, which may tear a vessel if poor technique is used.

Closure of main pulmonary arteries and veins may also be accomplished by automated stapling using "V" staples. Although it is not as widely accepted as for bronchial closure, I believe that this method is preferable.

Ligatures for pulmonary vessels are largely a matter of choice, but 2-0 silk or cotton is quite adequate. Larger vessels are best ligated with 0 size material to minimize the cutting quality of smaller sutures.

Wound Closure Suture

Pericostal sutures are preferred by most. I prefer size No. 1 Tev-Dek, Ticron, and Mersilene. Many other surgeons use Dexon or Vicryl. Catgut should not be used. Occasionally, in a grossly infected field, No. 22 stainless steel wire is acceptable, and does not carry the risk of becoming a foreign body. Wire eventually breaks, probably from structural fatigue, and should not be used routinely.

Suture of Musculature

Muscle suture may be accomplished with a wide variety of materials. Dexon and Vicryl seem to be most satisfactory, although silk and cotton have been used for many years with minimal problems.

Skin closure is largely a matter of preference. I use 4-0 Dexon or Vicryl as a subcuticular suture.

7

Pulmonary Procedures

PNEUMONECTOMY, BASIC CONSIDERATIONS

Pneumonectomy is a procedure of such magnitude that the operation must receive full consideration before committing the patient to the procedure. It may not be possible to predict whether pneumonectomy can be tolerated by a particular patient before operation. The surgeon may gain additional information by using a double-lumen intratracheal tube; and after the pulmonary artery is exposed, ventilation is stopped on the side to be resected and a pressure recording needle placed in the central pulmonary artery, which is then occluded distally. There should be no drop in Po_2 or rise in pulmonary pressure. Should either occur, it is a serious question whether to proceed or not. For purposes of this discussion, it is assumed that the resection is being performed for carcinoma.

When the thorax is opened, a systematic exploration is performed. This should have two primary purposes: (1) to confirm the diagnosis and by direct vision assess the severity of pulmonary dysfunction, assuming that the contralateral lung, by probability, will manifest a similar situation; and (2) to establish whether resection is possible and to what degree an extended procedure is necessary. Establishing resectability involves several considerations.

1. **Is there any regional extrapulmonary disease? If so, is it technically resectable (pleura, pericardium, diaphragm)?**
2. **Are hilar nodes involved?**
3. **Is there evidence of mediastinal extension? Are all grossly involved mediastinal nodes resectable without leaving any gross disease behind?**
4. **Can the resection be performed extrapericardially? If not, after opening and exploring the pericardial sac, is the lung resectable intrapericardially?**
5. **Evaluate each vein and the pulmonary artery individually beginning with the vascular structure most heavily involved. Then assess the main bronchus. Is it possible to divide the bronchus in an area free of tumor?**

The surgeon should not be committed to a course of action by dividing a major vessel or bronchus, only to find another structure that cannot be divided or must be divided through tumor. Considerable experience is required to be able to make an accurate appraisal and not make the error of attempting an impossible resection. Make a mental checklist before beginning definitive resection.

When resection apparently is possible, I prefer to begin with the pulmonary vein draining the area of neoplasm, hoping to diminish tumor cell embolization produced by manipulation.

106

RIGHT PNEUMONECTOMY

Position

Lateral.

Incision

Posterolateral thoracotomy.

Procedure

The thorax is opened through the fifth interspace or via the periosteal bed of the resected fifth rib. Rib resection generally permits an airtight closure, which in turn results in better mediastinal stabilization. Loss of air from the pleural space through the incision from the pleural space may produce acute mediastinal shift to the operated side. Pleural adhesions are divided, and the lung is completely mobilized.

Main Pulmonary Artery (Fig. 7–1A, B).   The lung is retracted inferiorly, exposing the superior surface of the hilum. The dissection is begun close to the pericardium, exposing the superior surface of the artery. It is necessary to find and dissect the relatively free perivascular plane. The dissection may be completed with the finger or by means of a large curved clamp, such as a Haight or a curved DeBakey aortic clamp.

The vessel may be stapled with 30-V staples, or clamped temporarily with a curved vascular clamp while its branches are ligated with 2-0 nonabsorbable suture material. The artery may then be transected, leaving at least a 0.5 cm cuff. The vessel is closed with 4-0 Prolene or Tev-Dek sutures in two layers. The suture nearest the clamp should be a continuous horizontal mattress suture and the second should be continued with the same suture material in a simple running suture over the end of the vessel. The clamp should be opened slowly while the stump is held with the thumb forceps to ascertain if hemostasis is complete. Care should always be taken with the needle, using gentleness and always drawing the needle through the vessel in a curve; otherwise the fragile pulmonary artery may be torn. The superior and inferior divisions may be treated separately if the main trunk appears unusually short or of large caliber.

Superior Pulmonary Vein (Fig. 7–1B).   Retract the lung posteriorly, exposing the anterior hilar structures. Incise the mediastinal pleura longitudinally. Care must be taken to find and protect the phrenic nerve. Reflect the pleura laterally, exposing the vein. Dissect carefully until the anatomic perivascular space is found, then by blunt and sharp dissection isolate each tributary and the main trunk. Encircle the vessel with a 0 silk or cotton ligature. Then, either ligate the vessel as proximally as possible or staple the vessel with a TA 30 instrument using V staples. A second suture ligature is used proximally if ligature is chosen. The tributaries can be ligated with a 2-0 nonabsorbable suture or closed with medium or large hemoclips. The vessel should be transected over a right angle clamp, leaving as much proximal stump as possible.

Inferior Pulmonary Vein (Fig. 7–1C).   Dissection is begun by dividing the inferior pulmonary ligament from the diaphragm to the inferior margin of the inferior pulmonary vein. There are usually several small vessels in this pleural reflection, which require cauterization, hemoclip, or ligature. Reflect the lung anteriorly, exposing the posterior hilum, and continue the pleural incision superiorly to the bronchus level.

Dissect the inferior pulmonary vein as described above, and finally ligate or staple and transect the vein. The surgeon must remember that the esophagus is immediately posterior and if the primary tumor extends to this level, great care must be exercised to prevent injury to this structure.

Contrary to common supposition, dividing the pulmonary vein first does not result in engorgement of the lung, as it might with the spleen. The pressure-flow relationship in the lung is linear, and blood flow is merely diverted to the opposite lung.

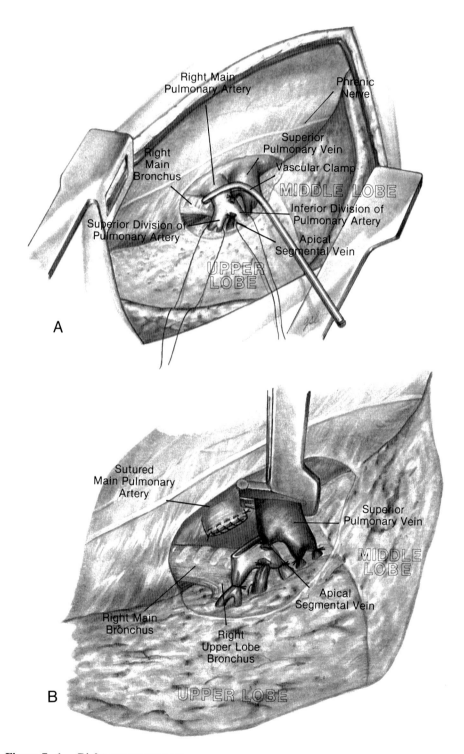

Figure 7–1. Right pneumonectomy.

A, The view with the lung reflected inferiorly and posteriorly, exposing the main pulmonary artery. A vascular clamp has been applied to the artery and distal branches are being ligated. The apical pulmonary vein has been ligated and divided.

B, A later view of the procedure with the lung reflected more posteriorly, showing the sutured stump of the main pulmonary artery. A TA 30 stapling instrument is being applied to the superior pulmonary vein. The distal tributaries of the vein have been ligated.

Illustration continued on opposite page

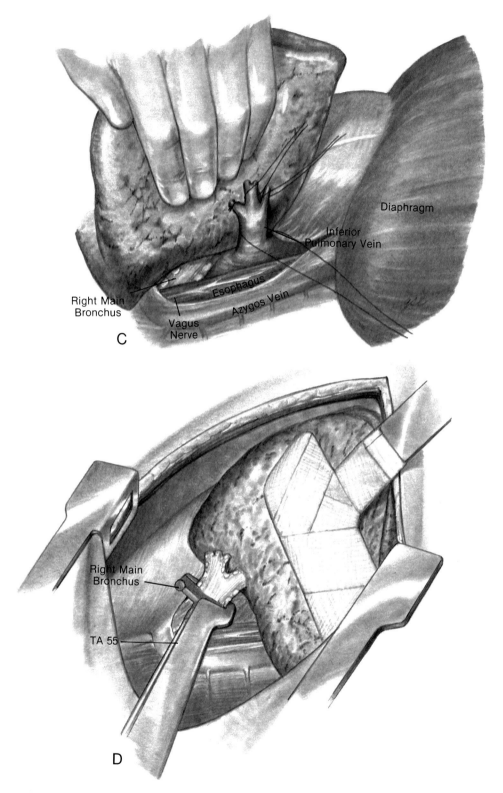

Figure 7–1. *Continued.*

C, The lung has been retruded anteriorly. The inferior pulmonary ligament has been divided and the inferior pulmonary vein has been dissected free. Ligatures are encircling the undivided vein and its tributaries.

D, The lung is reflected anteriorly and inferiorly. The right main bronchus has been dissected free and is being stapled with a TA 55 instrument using 4.8 mm staples.

Bronchial Dissection (Fig. 7–1D).   The lung is retracted anteriorly and elevated from the mediastinum. The bronchial artery, lying on the posterior surface, is first secured by ligature or hemoclip; then the peribronchial tissues are separated by blunt and sharp dissection. Because all vascular structures have been severed, there is little risk to bronchial dissection. Subcarinal nodes may pose a problem, and although they should be removed en bloc, they still must be dissected free at the level to be transected. The site of bronchial transection should be as high as possible, preferably within 1 cm of the carina.

The bronchus may be closed with a TA 55 stapling instrument using 4.8 mm staples. This is the preferable method. The bronchus should be placed in the stapling instrument so that the anterior and posterior walls are approximated. Suture closure may be elected, and in this case the bronchus must be clamped distal to the site of division and incised on its superior margin. The partially opened bronchus is then closed with 4-0 Tev-Dek or Prolene with simple sutures through the wall and tied across the open end. Finger tamponade may be necessary momentarily to control air leakage. Sutures must be tied firmly, but not tightly enough to necrose the bronchus, which has limited blood supply at best. The incision is alternately made and sutured until the transection is completed. The lung is removed and the pleural space is partially filled with saline solution while the anesthesiologist exerts a tracheal pressure of up to 45 cm H_2O by manual ''bagging'' to identify any air leaks.

A stapled suture line does not require pleural or muscle coverage, but a sutured bronchial stump should be covered with a pedicled, vascularized pleural flap or muscle graft. This should be carefully sewn into place (see description of an alternative procedure under *Left Pneumonectomy*).

The mediastinum and chest wall should be inspected for bleeding points. I prefer to irrigate the pleural cavity and wound with 2 liters of warm distilled water in an effort to destroy neoplastic cells which may have been scattered.

The wound is then closed, making every effort to make the closure as airtight as possible.

A needle is used to aspirate 1000 to 1200 cc of air to reduce the volume of pneumothorax. The patient is turned into the supine position and a portable chest film is made to assess mediastinal position. If it is not midline, additional air should be removed or instilled and, if necessary, a second film made. Some prefer to leave in a chest tube for periods up to 24 hours to adjust the pleural volume.

RIGHT UPPER LOBECTOMY

Incision

Posterolateral thoracotomy.

Procedure

A standard posterolateral incision is made and the pleural space is entered through the fifth intercostal space. Any pleural adhesions are dissected by sharp and blunt dissection.

Superior Hilar Dissection (Fig. 7–2A).   The lung is retracted inferiorly, exposing the superior surface of the hilum. A semilunar pleural incision is made in the mediastinal pleura 1 cm below the azygos vein, and several small lymphatics and vessels are transected after control by ligature or hemoclip. The right main bronchus and its upper lobe division are identified. Just anterior to the bronchus, the superior division of the right pulmonary artery can be seen. The perivascular sheath is entered and the artery dissected free. The main trunk is about 1 cm long and typically branches into the apical and anterior divisions. Often the apical vein overlies the artery and may require transection before the arterial dissection can be completed. The artery and each of its tributaries are ligated and the right superior pulmonary artery is divided distal to its division.

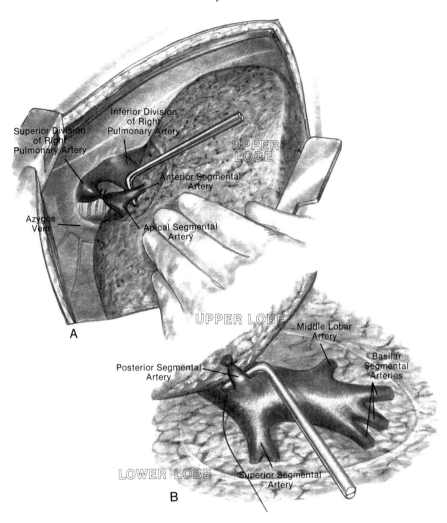

Figure 7–2. Right upper lobectomy.

A, The lung is seen from the superior and anterior aspects. The superior division of the pulmonary artery has been dissected free and doubly ligated. Its apical and anterior divisions are being dissected.

B, Interlobar view of the same procedure demonstrating passage of the ligature about the previously ligated posterior segmental artery. The relationship to the other pulmonary artery divisions is seen.

Illustration continued on following page

Anterior Dissection (Fig. 7–2C). The lung is displaced posteriorly, exposing the anterior hilar area. The pleural incision made earlier is extended inferiorly, posterior to the phrenic nerve. The superior pulmonary vein can then be seen. The perivascular plane is entered and the apical, anterior, and posterior tributaries are doubly ligated and divided. The middle lobe tributaries must be identified and preserved.

The surgeon must keep in mind that the posterior vein wall is intimately related to the inferior division of the pulmonary artery and that dissection outside the perivascular plane or careless technique can result in arterial injury.

Interlobar Dissection (Fig. 7–2B). The interlobar fissure is entered and the lower lobe retracted inferiorly while the upper lobe is displaced superiorly. Dissection is begun at the point of convergence of the horizontal and oblique fissures. The pulmonary artery

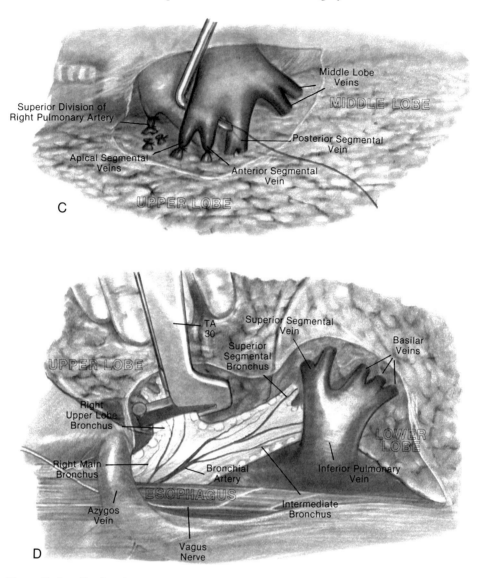

Figure 7–2. *Continued.*

C, View of the anterior aspect of the hilum as viewed from the patient's back. The pulmonary artery dissection has been completed and the tributaries of the superior pulmonary veins are being ligated prior to division.

D, Posterior view of the hilum following dissection of the interlobar fissure and the anterior hilum, and stapling of the right upper lobe bronchus prior to its transection. Sufficient bronchial stump must be left to avoid compromise of the remainder of the bronchial lumen.

Illustration continued on opposite page

will frequently be partially obscured by a lymph node, which must be removed or dissected free. The perivascular plane is entered and 1 to 1.5 cm of the artery is exposed. Orientation is accomplished by identifying the superior segmental artery and the middle lobe artery or arteries. Then the dissection is extended superiorly about 1.5 cm, at which point the posterior segmental artery will be seen leaving the main trunk at a 90 degree angle. The posterior segmental artery should be carefully exposed, then doubly ligated and divided after sufficient length is available. The remainder of the fissure between the

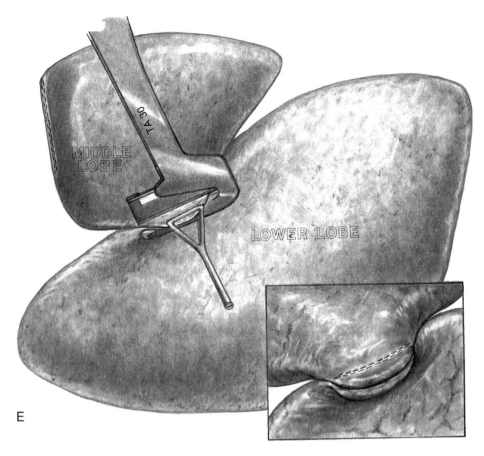

Figure 7–2. *Continued.*
E, A technique of stapling the edges of middle and lower lobes together to prevent volvulus of the middle lobe. (Part *E* is from Hood, M. D.: Stapling technique involving lung parenchyma. Surg. Clin. North Am., 3:June, 1984.)

lower and upper lobes is separated. Should it be incomplete, the lung should be reflected anteriorly and the pleural incision extended inferiorly; then, working from both posterior and anterior directions, a small opening is made. Through this, the TA 55 stapling instrument with 4.8 mm staples is inserted, and the parenchyma is stapled, then divided.

Posterior Dissection (Fig. 7–2D). The lung is reflected anteriorly and the pleural incision extended, if this has not already been done. The peribronchial tissue is dissected by sharp and blunt dissection. This dissection should continue until all segmental bronchi are exposed. The anterior surface of the bronchus is cleared, and the bronchus is completely exposed. A TA 30 stapling instrument with 4.8 mm staples is then positioned and oriented to close the bronchus, opposing the anterior wall against the posterior wall within 0.5 cm of the origin of the bronchus. Manual lung inflation is used to be certain that the main bronchus is not compromised. The bronchus is then stapled, severed, and tested for air leakage.

At this point, only the horizontal fissure, which is more often incomplete, remains. A TA 90 stapling instrument with 4.8 mm staples is carefully placed; the fissure plane is stapled and the upper lobe severed. The lobe should now be free and can be removed. However, the surgeon must be wary of another upper lobe artery originating between the origin of the superior division and the posterior segmental artery; if this is not sought, it may be torn or result in a tear in the main vessel.

Should the fissure between the lower and middle lobes be complete, it is preferable to fix the two lobes together by (1) stapling the two edges together (Fig. 7–2E) or (2) grasping the edges of both lobes with an Allyce clamp and ligating the tissue at two or three points. This will prevent volvulus of the middle lobe.

Two tubes are placed, with the anterior one in the apex of the pleural space sutured in place and the other more inferiorly and posteriorly. The chest wall is closed as described.

RIGHT MIDDLE LOBECTOMY

Indications

The middle lobe is the lobe least frequently removed as a unit. Most often it is removed with the upper or lower lobe because of cross fissure involvement or hilar involvement by neoplasm. At present, carcinoma is the most common indication, although any benign tumor may also originate in the middle lobe. Bronchiectasis, now becoming an uncommon disease, often involves the middle lobe. The middle lobe syndrome, once fairly common, is now unusual. Compression or erosion of the middle lobe bronchus by an enlarged or calcified lymph node can produce atelectasis, infection, and bronchiectasis.

Position

Right lateral or anterolateral.

Incision

Right posterolateral or anterolateral.

Procedure

The pleural space is opened through the fifth intercostal space. Pleural adhesions are separated and the lung is fully mobilized. The interlobar fissure is opened. All dissection except for the middle lobe vein is carried out via the interlobar fissure. The lobar lobe is retracted posteriorly and the middle lobe anteriorly. Some retraction of the upper lobe superiorly will aid exposure.

Arterial Dissection (Fig. 7–3A). Dissection is begun at the base of the interlobar fissure where the posterior tip of the middle lobe ends and the horizontal fissure begins. The inferior trunk of the pulmonary artery lies in a vertical plane. Enter the perivascular plane. The middle lobe artery arises anteriorly. Frequently two separate middle lobe arteries are present. The vessel to the posterior segment of the upper lobe arises from the lateral side of the artery 1 to 1.5 cm superiorly and is easily injured. The superior segmental artery arises posteriorly, directly opposite the middle lobe vessel. The middle lobe vessel or vessels are doubly ligated or secured distally with hemoclips and divided.

Bronchial Dissection (Fig. 7–3B, C). The middle lobe bronchus arises from the anterior surface of the intermediate bronchus at an obtuse angle directly beneath the pulmonary artery. Once the middle lobe branches are transected, the artery is retracted posteriorly, and the bronchus may be easily palpated. Enlarged, vascular lymph nodes may be present in the bronchiectatic patient. Nodes involved with granulomatous infection, such as tuberculosis or histoplasmosis, may be difficult to free from the bronchus and adjacent vessels. Once the bronchus is free, it may be stapled with 4.8 mm staples or transected and oversewn, as described elsewhere. One must be certain not to amputate or staple too close to the intermediate bronchus and narrow it.

Venous Dissection (Fig. 7–3D). The lung is reflected posteriorly, exposing the anterior hilum. The pleura overlying the superior pulmonary vein is incised, and all of the

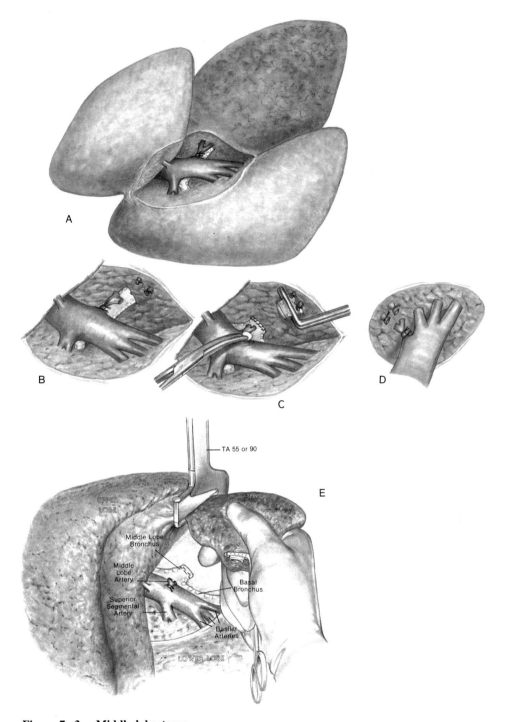

Figure 7–3. Middle lobectomy.

A, Interlobar view. The middle lobe artery has already been doubly ligated. Note the relationship of the middle lobe artery to the superior segmental artery.

B, C, Arterial division is complete and provides access to the middle lobe bronchus, which is clamped, transected, and oversewn with interrupted sutures.

D, Anterior view. The middle lobe veins feeding to the superior pulmonary veins have been ligated and severed, leaving only the usually incomplete horizontal fissure to be divided.

E, The vascular and branchial dissection and division have been completed. The incomplete fissure between the upper and middle lobes is being stapled. A TA 55 or TA 90 stapling instrument may be chosen, depending on the amount of tissue to be divided 4.8 mm staples are used.

tributaries of the vein are exposed. The most inferior vein is the middle lobe vein. Occasionally there are two. When there is more than one middle lobe vein, ligate and divide only the most inferior one.

The horizontal fissure between the upper and middle lobes is rarely complete; it is best divided by stapling. The area of dissection in the fissure is extended at the hilar level to communicate anteriorly with the area of vein ligation by blunt dissection, producing a tunnel-like passage (Fig. 7–3F). A TA 90 stapling instrument with 4.8 mm staples is used to close the upper lobe surface. Care should be taken to staple in the interlobar plane and if necessary to err on the middle lobe side.

The fissure between the middle and lower lobes is separated. Usually it is complete. If not, it may be also divided after being stapled. The lobe is then removed.

I usually do not cover the bronchial stump if it has been stapled.

There is no difficulty with the lung filling the space created by middle lobectomy.

Two chest tubes are inserted, and the chest is closed.

RIGHT LOWER LOBECTOMY

Position

Right lateral.

Incision

Posterolateral thoracotomy.

Procedure

The pleural space is entered through an incision in the sixth intercostal space or through the bed of the resected sixth rib.

Pleural adhesions are divided by blunt and sharp dissection with control of bleeding from vascular adhesions by electrocautery, hemoclip, or ligature. The entire lung should be mobilized. The surgeon may choose venous division first if the procedure is being done for malignancy.

Arterial Dissection (Fig. 7–4A, B). The oblique fissure is entered using blunt and sharp dissection and electrocautery for hemostasis. The central portion of the fissure is deepened at the juncture of the minor or horizontal fissure. A lymph node may be encountered first, but at this point the inferior trunk of the right pulmonary should be encountered. The perivascular space should be sought and entered, and the remainder of the arterial dissection carried out in this plane. One should immediately identify the middle lobe artery or arteries arising from the anterior aspect of the vessel. Directly opposite the middle lobe division, the superior segmental artery is seen arising from the posterior surface of the artery. This vessel should be doubly ligated and divided.

The basilar division should then be dissected free and the basilar segmental vessels also freed. The main vessel is then doubly ligated: The individual branches are each ligated and the branches severed after all ligatures are completed, leaving a generous cuff of the basilar artery. Take care not to obstruct the middle lobe artery by ligating the basilar division too close to the middle lobe division. The lower portion of the oblique fissure is separated. Occasionally this fissure is incomplete and requires stapling, taking care not to encroach on the middle lobe or injure the middle lobe vein.

The superior or posterior portion of the oblique fissure is usually incomplete and may be divided at this point or following division of the inferior pulmonary vein. It may be approached first posteriorly by incising the mediastinal pleura longitudinally, beginning at the level of the upper lobe bronchial origin. Then, by blunt finger dissection, working posteriorly and from the previously opened interlobar fissure, the two fields are connected

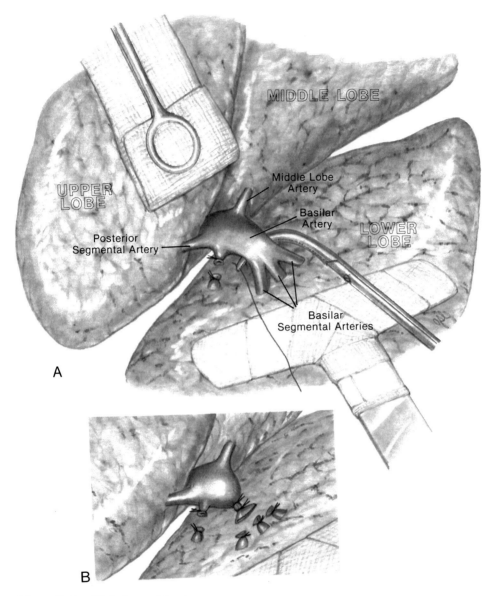

Figure 7-4. Right lower lobectomy.

A, Interlobar view. The superior segmental artery has been ligated and divided, and a ligature is being placed about the basilar division. The relationship of the posterior segmental and middle lobe arteries to the lower lobe vessels should be noted.

B, A later sequence: all lower lobe arteries have been ligated and severed.

Illustration continued on following page

at the bronchial level. A TA 55 stapling instrument using 4.8 mm staples is used to suture the fissure, erring if necessary on the lower lobe side. Two rows of staples may be used, one on either side; or the GIA stapling device may be used if preferred. The fissure is then completely opened.

Venous Dissection (Fig. 7-4C). The lobe is reflected anteriorly, exposing the posterior hilar surface. The pleural incision just made is extended to a point below the inferior pulmonary vein.

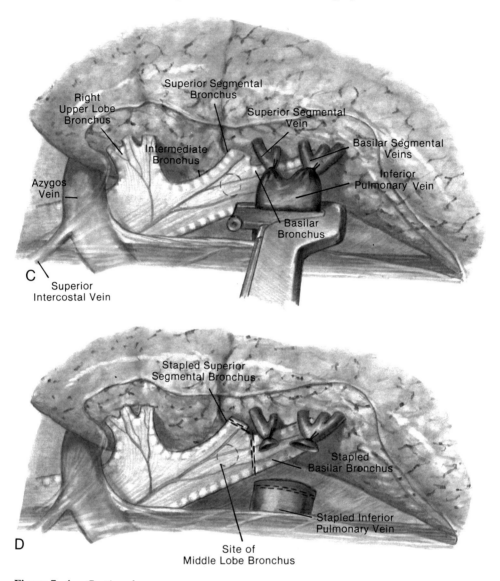

Figure 7–4. *Continued.*

C, The tributaries of the inferior pulmonary vein have been ligated and the main trunk is being stapled with a TA 30 instrument and V staples.

D, All vascular structures have been divided and the superior and basilar bronchi have been stapled separately to prevent occlusion of the middle lobe bronchus.

The pulmonary ligament is then divided, beginning at the diaphragm and extended until the vein is seen. There are small arteries in the ligament that will require ligation or hemoclips.

The vein is then exposed and the perivascular sheath is defined and entered. The undivided vein is dissected free, producing sufficient space anterior to the vein so that a TA 30 stapling instrument can be passed around the vein. The segmental tributary veins are dissected free and individually ligated as distal as possible. Then the undivided vein is stapled as close to the pericardium as possible using V staples, after which the segmental veins are transected. Alternative methods of securing the vein proximally include clamping the vein with a curved vascular clamp and oversewing the vein after division with 4-0 vascular suture, or, less desirably, ligating the vein. A second suture ligature is advisable, but ligatures are always more hazardous.

Bronchial Dissection (Fig. 7–4D). The only remaining structure is the bronchus. It is freed from surrounding tissue by blunt and sharp dissection, clearly exposing the superior segmental bronchus and the middle lobe bronchus. Usually it is necessary to handle the superior segmental bronchus and the basilar bronchus separately to avoid compromising the lumen of the middle lobe bronchus. The bronchus preferably is stapled with a TA 30 stapling instrument using 4.8 mm staples; the stapled bronchus is then severed. After both bronchi have been transected, the lobe is removed from the pleural space. Alternatively, the bronchus may be transected and closed by the suture technique described previously. Bronchial arteries should be ligated before or after dividing the bronchus. The horizontal fissure between the upper and middle lobes may be complete. This feature leaves the middle lobe free to undergo volvulus on its pedicle. The middle lobe should be securely attached to the remaining upper lobe by stapling the free edges together or by grasping a small portion of both lobes with an Allyce clamp and ligating the tissue held. If the latter method is used, two or three points of fixation are preferable.

Chest tubes are placed and the chest wall is closed.

LEFT PNEUMONECTOMY

Position

Lateral.

Incision

Posterolateral thoracotomy.

Procedure

The thorax is opened via the fifth interspace or the bed of the resected fifth rib. The lung is mobilized by freeing it from any existing pleural adhesions by blunt or sharp dissection, and hemostasis is produced by patiently applied electrocautery.

Arterial Dissection (Fig. 7–5A). The lung is retracted inferiorly and posteriorly to expose the main pulmonary artery as it emerges from the pericardium. Dissection is begun on the superior surface of the artery, and once the perivascular space is entered, the entire vessel is encircled by blunt dissection. Many times the forefinger is the instrument of choice. Once this has been accomplished and the recurrent laryngeal nerve is carefully exposed and protected, one of the three methods of arterial division is utilized. Preferably the vessel is stapled with a TA 30 stapling instrument using V staples. The artery is not transected at this time. Occasionally, the branch to the apical posterior segment is ligated separately and transected to gain additional length. The artery may be clamped with a vascular clamp after being ligated distally. The vessel is then transected and oversewn as described elsewhere. Ligation is the least safe method.

Venous Dissection (Fig. 7–5B). The lung is reflected posteriorly, exposing the anterior aspect of the hilum. The mediastinal pleura is incised posterior to the phrenic nerve. The superior pulmonary vein is clearly seen and the perivascular plane is entered, and the vein and its tributaries are dissected free. The proximal vein is then stapled using a TA 30 stapling instrument with V staples. The tributary veins should be ligated separately.

The lung is then retracted anteriorly, exposing the posterior hilum. A vertical incision is made anterior to the esophageal plane; the inferior pulmonary ligament is divided and small vessels lying in the ligament are controlled by hemoclips or ligatures. The inferior pulmonary vein should be clearly visible. The tributaries are individually dissected free and either ligated or occluded with hemoclips distally. The undivided vein is dissected and

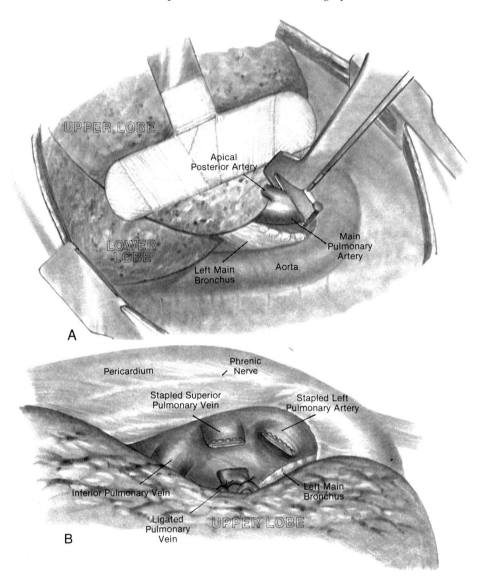

Figure 7–5. Left pneumonectomy.
A, The lung is retracted inferiorly and the main pulmonary artery has been completely dissected free. A TA 30 stapling device is shown being applied to the vessel.
B, A view of the anterior aspect of the left hilum showing the stapled and divided superior pulmonary vein and the stapled and divided main pulmonary artery.

either stapled with 30 V staples or doubly ligated as close to the pericardium as possible. The vein may be severed if stapled, or its tributaries divided to give greater length if ligated. It may also be clamped with a vascular clamp and oversewn.

Bronchial Dissection.   The lung is retracted anteriorly as described for inferior vein dissection. The vagus nerve should be visualized and protected. Two or three vagus branches to the lung are seen in the area and should be severed after proximal and distal hemoclip application, because they are usually accompanied by small arteries. There are usually two bronchial arteries accompanying the left main bronchus. They should be

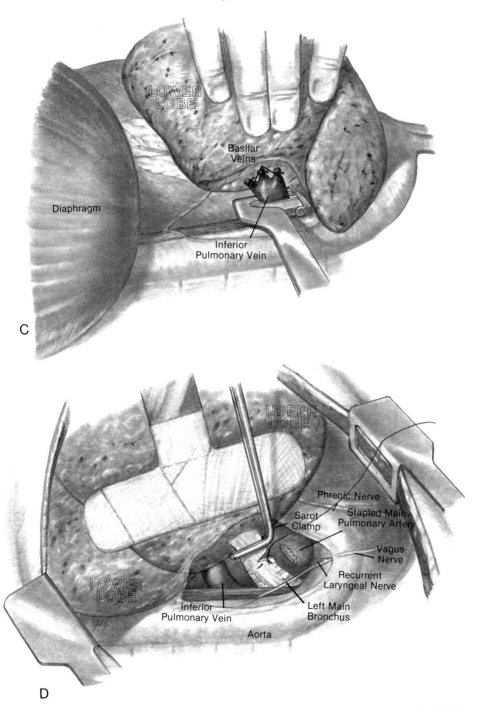

Figure 7–5. *Continued. C,* The lung is retracted anteriorly and superiorly. The inferior pulmonary ligament has been divided and the inferior pulmonary vein dissected free. It is being stapled using a TA 30 instrument with V staples. *D,* The lung has been reflected anteriorly, exposing the posterior hilum. The left main bronchus has been dissected free, clamped distally, and is being transected and closed with interrupted 4–0 prolene sutures. The stapled main pulmonary artery stump is seen.

dissected and ligated or controlled by hemoclip. Then, using blunt finger dissection, the bronchus is encircled. The left hand is used to elevate the lung, placing traction on the main bronchus and exposing the portion lying deeper in the mediastinum.

An area of bronchus 1 to 1.5 cm distal to the carina is cleared by blunt and sharp dissection, and the TA 55 stapling instrument with 4.8 mm staples is placed transversely across the bronchus. Care must be taken to orient the instrument so that the anterior and posterior walls are apposed. The stapler is closed and fired and the bronchus amputated as close to the instrument as possible.

The mediastinum is immersed in saline solution, and the anesthesiologist is asked to apply up to 45 cm H_2O ventilation pressure manually to be certain that the bronchial stump closure is airtight.

The lung is removed from the pleural space. A careful search is made for uncontrolled bleeding points. After hemostasis is ascertained, the thoracic wall is closed without drainage, as described elsewhere.

A thoracentesis is done as soon as closure is completed, and 1000 to 1200 cc of air is removed from the pleural cavity. The patient is turned into the supine position, and a portable chest x-ray film is made to note the mediastinal position. Additional air may be removed or instilled until a midline position of the mediastinum is attained.

Alternative Procedure

A pneumonectomy for bronchogenic carcinoma may be difficult or impossible with the technique just described because of the proximity of the neoplasm to the mediastinum. Before deciding that a neoplasm is nonresectable, the surgeon should open the pericardium and examine the intrapericardial pulmonary vessels. The pericardium is a natural barrier to the spread of neoplasm, and tumor may involve the external surface of the pericardium but spare the inner surface and the vessels.

A vertical incision is made just posterior to the phrenic nerve; however, if the nerve is obviously involved, the incision may be made anterior to the nerve. After exploration has revealed no intrapericardial involvement, the incision is extended superiorly over the pulmonary artery.

Before any vessel is divided, it is necessary to determine that the bronchus can be transected at a point free of tumor and that there is no esophageal or aortic involvement. The surgeon should evaluate lymph node involvement at this point. I consider it unwise to carry out pulmonary resection for carcinoma and leave gross neoplasm in the mediastinum. On the other hand, subaortic or anterior mediastinal node involvement does not contraindicate resection if these nodes can be removed without evidence of any residual neoplasm.

The superior pulmonary vein is encircled and then stapled with a TA 30 stapling instrument and V staples. The pulmonary artery is then dissected free and as much of its length as possible secured and stapled with TA 30 V staples. A similar maneuver is carried out for the inferior pulmonary vein after the pericardial incision is extended posteriorly and then superiorly to the bronchial head.

The length of vessels may not permit distal ligation; therefore, after all the vessels have been stapled, they are severed distal to the staple lines. This results in blood spillage into the surgical field but does not represent a greater blood loss over that which would have been contained in the specimen.

The bronchus is then dissected, stapled, and transected as described previously. The pericardial incision is completed and the specimen removed with a window of pericardium measuring about 8 cm by 5 cm. No attempt is made to close the pericardium unless the defect is sufficiently large to permit herniation of the heart. Generally, it is unnecessary to excise sufficient pericardium that herniation is a risk.

It is under these circumstances that stapling becomes a most valuable method, because usually there is insufficient length of vessel available to permit any other type of closure with safety.

LEFT UPPER LOBECTOMY

Position

Left lateral.

Incision

Posterolateral thoracotomy.

Procedure

An incision is made and the pleural space is entered through the fifth intercostal space. All pleural adhesions are freed by blunt and sharp dissection and complete hemostasis produced by electrocautery.

Arterial Dissection (Fig. 7–6A, B). The lung is retracted inferiorly, exposing the superior area of the hilum. A curved pleural incision is made about 1.5 cm below and parallel to the arch of the aorta. Several small vessels, lymphatics, and vagus nerve branches are severed after control with hemoclips. The recurrent laryngeal nerve should be visualized and protected. The main pulmonary artery will be seen paralleling the aorta and curving inferiorly to enter the interlobar fissure. From the pulmonary side, a fairly large branch arises and immediately divides into apical and posterior arteries. The perivascular plane is entered over the main artery, and this branch is dissected free and ligated proximally; each of its branches is then ligated or secured with hemoclips, after which the branches are transected. Occasionally, the apical tributary of the superior pulmonary vein overlies the artery and must be divided before completing arterial dissection. The remainder of the main arterial trunk is cleared to its entry into the interlobar fissure.

Excessive traction on the hilum, displacing it inferiorly, may easily result in tearing the intima of the apical posterior artery or avulsion of the vessel with the result of serious hemorrhage, particularly in the older patient. Rapid encirclement of the main artery by finger dissection may be necessary for control and repair. Attempts at clamping are ill-advised because the vessel may be injured irreparably.

The interlobar fissure is separated by blunt and sharp dissection. Arterial dissection is begun at about the junction of the upper third with the middle third of the fissure. The artery is exposed, the perivascular plane is entered, and the dissection extended superiorly. The remainder of the fissure is separated using the TA 55 stapling instrument, if necessary. This should connect the initial dissection field with the interlobar field.

The pulmonary artery dissection is continued. The first branch in the fissure is the superior segmental artery or arteries arising posteriorly. Almost directly opposite this vessel are one or two arteries to the anterior segment of the upper lobe. They are usually small and rise anteriorly. These vessels should be doubly ligated and divided.

Further inferiorly and anteriorly, the lingular artery arises. It branches quickly into superior and inferior divisions. Occasionally, both branches arise separately. The artery and its branches are doubly ligated and divided distal to the bifurcation. Hemoclips may be used distally. The inferior portion of the fissure is then separated using the stapling instrument if necessary.

Venous Dissection (Fig. 7–6C). The lung is reflected posteriorly and the mediastinal pleura is incised posterior to the phrenic nerve. The superior pulmonary vein and its tributaries are then completely dissected. Each tributary is ligated or hemoclipped distally. The main trunk can be stapled with a TA 30 instrument with V staples or ligated. The peripheral divisions are then divided. Should the pulmonary pathologic process extend very close to the pericardium, precluding stapling or ligating, the vessel may be clamped with a curved vascular clamp, transected, and closed with vascular sutures as described. Alternatively, the pericardium may be entered and the vein stapled and transected and sutured intrapericardially.

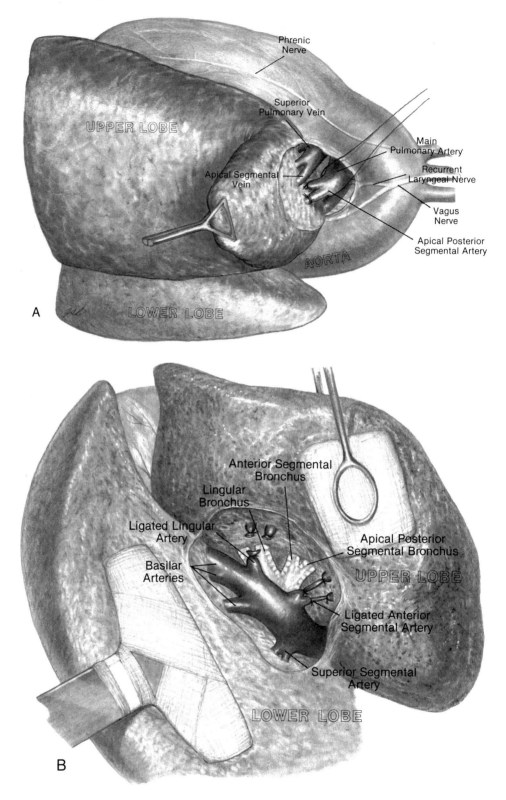

Figure 7–6.   Left upper lobectomy. *A*, The lung is retracted inferiorly and posteriorly. The main pulmonary artery is seen. The apical posterior segmental artery is being ligated. The distal branches have been ligated. The relationship to the superior pulmonary vein should be noted. *B*, The lingular artery and its divisions have been ligated and divided, and the anterior segmental arteries have been ligated and await division.

Illustration continued on opposite page

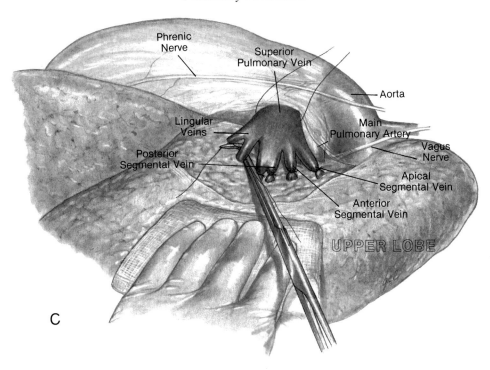

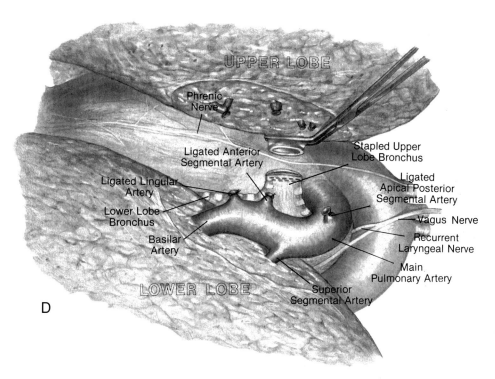

Figure 7–6. *Continued. C*, Anterior view. The superior pulmonary vein is seen. Its tributaries are being individually ligated before ligation or stapling of the main venous trunk which is encircled with a suture. *D*, Interlobar view. All vascular structures have been transected. The upper lobe bronchus has been stapled with 4–8 mm staples and amputated.

Bronchial Dissection (Fig. 7–6D).   The interlobar fissure is again entered, and the upper lobe bronchial can be identified emerging anteriorly from beneath the pulmonary artery. The artery is freed from the bronchus and retracted using a "peanut" dissector. The bronchus is dissected free and a TA 30 stapling instrument with 4.8 mm staples is placed across the bronchus, taking care not to compromise the lumen of the main bronchus or to leave a stump more than 1 cm in length. The bronchus is stapled and amputated. This should allow the lobe to be removed. The bronchial closure and the parenchymal closure sites are submerged in saline solution to test for air leakage. Hemostasis is assured. Anterior and posterior chest tubes are placed and sutured in place, and the incision is closed.

LEFT LOWER LOBECTOMY

Position

Left lateral.

Incision

Posterolateral thoracotomy.

Procedure

An incision is made, resecting the sixth rib or using the sixth intercostal space. Pleural adhesions, if present, are freed by blunt and sharp dissection, and the inferior pulmonary ligament is divided to the level of the inferior pulmonary vein. Small vessels in this area are controlled by cautery or hemoclips.

Arterial Dissection (Fig. 7–7A).   The lung is allowed to resume its normal orientation and the interlobar fissure is entered in its midportion. The pulmonary artery is found at the base of the fissure lying in the same plane of orientation as the fissure. Once the artery is exposed, the perivascular plane is entered and dissection is extended superiorly. Usually two upper lobe branches (the anterior segmental artery and the lingular segmental artery) arise in the interlobar fissure. There may be two separate lingular vessels, and the origin of the anterior segmental artery is inconstant; it may arise from the lingular artery. There may be as many as seven separate vessels to the upper lobe.

The superior segmental artery arises posteriorly 1 to 2 cm cephalad to the lingular artery origin. Occasionally, there are two vessels to the superior segment.

Before proceeding with arterial dissection, connect the interlobar plane of dissection along the artery with the posterior pleural incision. If it is not complete, the fissure is divided with a TA 55 stapling instrument using 4.8 mm staples.

The fissure is now complete except for an inferior area between the anterior basal area and the lingula. This area may be completely free but usually requires separation by dissection or stapling.

The superior segmental artery is then isolated and doubly ligated with 2-0 nonabsorbable suture and transected.

The basilar artery is then dissected free just inferior to the origin of the lingular segmental artery. It is ligated with 2-0 or 0 nonabsorbable ligature. The basilar segmental branches may be individually ligated or closed by hemoclips distally. The basilar artery or its branches are severed, leaving a generous cuff proximally.

Venous Dissection (Fig. 7–7B, C).   The lung is reflected anteriorly, exposing the posterior hilum. The mediastinal pleura is incised from a point where the inferior ligament dissection ended to a point opposite the main bronchus. The mediastinal tissue is dissected free over the inferior pulmonary vein, and the perivascular plane is entered. Using blunt and sharp dissection, the main trunk of the vein is freed and encircled with a 0 silk ligature. Each tributary is dissected free and either ligated as distally as possible with 2-0

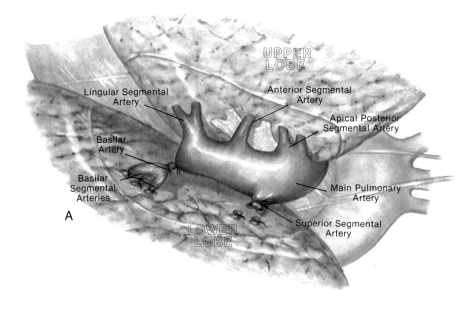

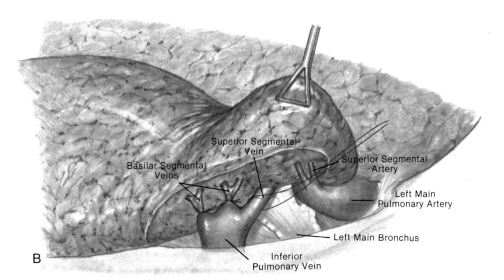

Figure 7–7. Left lower lobectomy.

A, Interlobar view. The superior segmental artery and its divisions have been ligated and divided. The basilar artery and its branches have been ligated but not yet transected. The relationship of these vessels to the lingular and anterior segmental arteries must be kept in mind.

B, Posterior view. The segmental veins to the lower lobe are being ligated. The superior segmental artery is shown intact. Note the relationship of these vessels to the lower lobe bronchus.

Illustration continued on following page

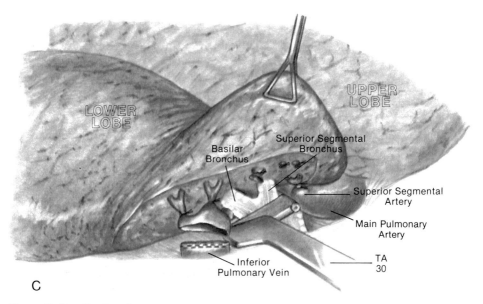

C

Figure 7–7. *Continued.*
  C, The inferior vein has been stapled and divided. A TA 30 stapler with 4.8 mm staples is being applied to the left lower lobe bronchus. Note the divided superior segmental artery.

suture or secured by hemoclips. The main trunk is stapled with a TA 30 stapling instrument with V staples. The tributary veins are then severed. The main trunk of the vein may be clamped with a vascular clamp, transected, and oversewn with 4-0 vascular suture.

Bronchial Dissection (Fig. 7–7C). The remaining pulmonary artery is then dissected free of the underlying bronchus to permit bronchial dissection. The lower lobe bronchus is dissected free by blunt and sharp dissection, identifying the origin of the upper lobe bronchus. The surgeon must remember that the anterior wall of the bronchus is intimately related to the superior pulmonary vein, which can be easily injured (Fig. 7–7C).

The bronchus is temporarily occluded at the level to be transected to be certain that the upper lobe bronchus is not compromised. Observing the upper lobe as the lung is being inflated will establish this fact. A TA 30 stapling instrument with 4.8 mm staples is used to close the bronchus, which is then transected. This should permit the lobe to be removed from the thorax. A careful search for controllable air leaks and points of bleeding is now made. The bronchial stump may be covered with a pleural or muscle flap if a suture closure has been used.

Two chest tubes are inserted, as described elsewhere. The chest is then closed in the manner described under *Posterolateral Thoracotomy.*

Note

Occasionally, there are sizable veins from the lower lobe draining to the superior pulmonary vein and these will traverse the interlobar fissure.

The origin of the superior segmental bronchus may be so close to the upper lobe that it may have to be divided separately from the basilar division.

A carcinoma that involves the vein as far as the pericardium may still be resectable if the pericardium is opened and the vein is transected at that level, removing a 4 cm by 5 cm area of pericardium.

SUPERIOR SEGMENTECTOMY (EITHER LOWER LOBE)

Resection of this segment may be accomplished by either of two approaches. One is to use the method described by Overholt, which involves hilar dissection and division of segmental arteries and bronchi followed by blunt finger separation of the intersegmental plane while traction is applied to the divided bronchus. The other is to remove the segment by stapling in the general location of the segmental plane, following division of hilar vessels and bronchus. The first procedure is more anatomic but leaves a raw parenchymal surface with multiple air leaks and with a shape that does not conform anatomically to the pleural space; it therefore has a high incidence (15%) of persistent air leak and resultant space problems. It does preserve, if uncomplicated, the maximum pulmonary function.

The stapling procedure compromises expansion of the remaining lung and distorts it, but does minimize operating time, blood loss, and development of bronchopleural fistulas.

Position

Lateral.

Incision

Posterolateral thoracotomy.

Procedure

Make a standard thoracotomy incision using the fifth or sixth interspace.

Arterial Dissection (Fig. 7–8A). Begin dissection in the interlobar fissure. The inferior division of the pulmonary artery will be found at the juncture of the horizontal and oblique fissures. Dissection should be blunt and sharp, with the use of cautery and hemoclips for control of small intersegmental vessels. Once the artery is identified, dissect until the perivascular space has been entered. The point of approach will be within 1 cm of the superior segmental artery posteriorly and the middle lobe artery anteriorly. The branch to the posterior segment of the upper lobe arises about 1 to 1.5 cm cephalad from the lateral aspect of the artery, perpendicular to the main trunk. It is vulnerable to injury by traction and blind scissors dissection superiorly.

Isolate the superior segmental artery and its two divisions. Ligate the artery at its origin with 2-0 nonabsorbable suture and either ligate the branches as distally as possible or secure these divisions with medium hemoclips. Cut each branch over a right angle clamp rather than transecting the segmental artery. A suture ligature may also be used.

Bronchial Dissection (Fig. 7–8B, E). The dissection and division of the superior segmental bronchus may be approached through the interlobar fissure as shown in Figure 7–8B or posteriorly as in 7–8D. The following describes the posterior approach. Reflect the lung anteriorly, exposing the posterior hilum. Incise the pleura over the bronchus and inferior pulmonary vein. Begin bronchial dissection over the intermediate bronchus. The first bronchial division will be the superior segmental bronchus, which should be isolated by blunt and sharp dissection. Do not make an attempt to pass an instrument around the entire bronchus at this point for fear of injuring the middle lobe bronchus anteriorly (right) or lingular bronchus (left). Once the surgeon is certain that the segmental bronchus is identified and freed, a right angle clamp may be passed around the bronchus and, by blunt instrumentation, a large space developed.

At this point, attention should be diverted to that portion of the oblique fissure between the superior segment and the upper lobe. If the fissure is incomplete, it is best divided at this time by introducing a TA 90 or TA 55 stapling instrument with 4.8 mm staples, completing the separation between the two lobes. Stapling will minimize the air leakage from the upper lobe.

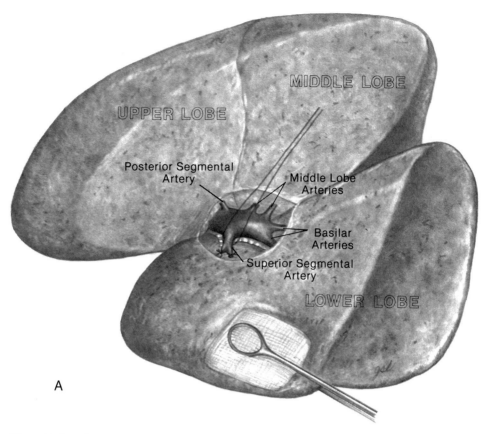

A

Figure 7–8. Superior segmentectomy, right interlobar view.
A, The superior segmental artery has been dissected free and the distal branches have been ligated. A ligature has been passed about the superior segmental artery.

Illustration continued on opposite page

A TA 30 stapling instrument using 4.8 mm staples is used to staple the superior segmental bronchus, taking care not to leave a stump more than 0.5 cm in length or to compromise the lower lobe bronchus.

All dissection is now complete except for the intersegmental plane and the division of the inferior pulmonary vein from the superior segment (Fig. 7–8D, E). This vein or some of its tributaries may be ligated at this point.

The intersegmental plane may be determined in part by inflating the lower lobe and observing the margin between aerated and nonaerated segments. Then, place a hemostat on the severed bronchus and, using the bronchus as a guide, sweep the finger gently through the parenchyma, seeking a plane of least resistance. The finger will come to the pleural surface and the pleura may be incised. Do not incise the pleura first because it will be done inaccurately.

Remove the segment and pack the raw segmental surface of the lower lobe with a warm pack for 5 to 10 minutes. Remove the pack, identify small intersegmental bleeding points, and ligate or oversew each. Small bronchi may be identified using increased ventilatory pressure and saline irrigation. Each should be oversewn with 5-0 Prolene or similar material.

The intersegmental plane may be managed alternatively by using a TA 55 or TA 90 stapling instrument with 4.8 mm staples. This distorts the lung and limits lower lobe expansion but minimizes air leaks.

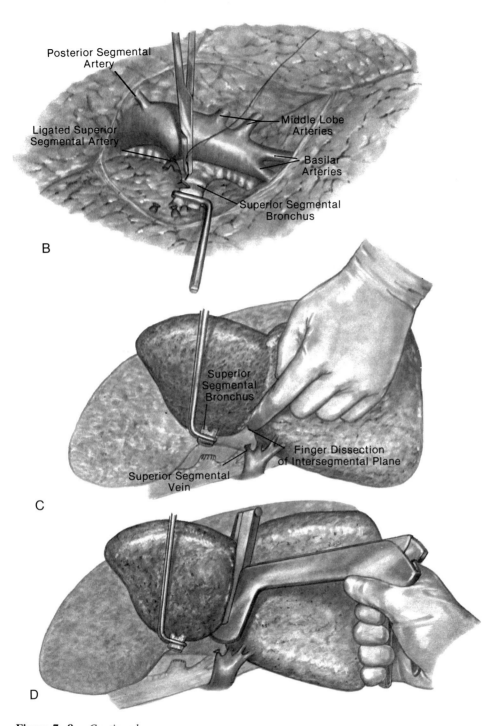

Figure 7–8. *Continued.*

B, Interlobar view with the artery to the superior segment ligated and transected. The bronchus has been clamped and is being divided and closed by sutures simultaneously.

C, Superior segmentectomy, right-sided, posterior view. The inferior pulmonary vein has been dissected free and the tributary from the superior segment has been ligated and divided. The superior segmental bronchus has been divided and sutured.

D, Alternative technique of stapling the right lower lobe in the general plane of the interlobar fissure and closing the fissure. This results in some loss of volume of the basal segments but controls almost all air leakage from the segmental surface.

Illustration continued on following page

131

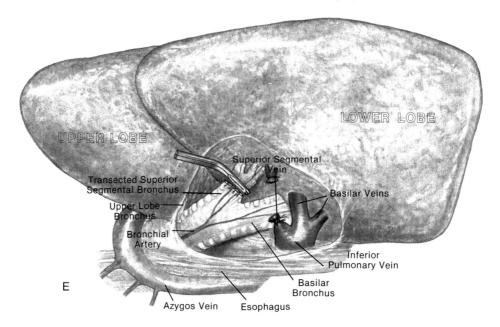

Figure 7–8. *Continued.*
E, Superior segmentectomy, right posterior view. The inferior pulmonary vein has been dissected
and the tributary of the superior segment has been ligated and divided.

Illustration continued on opposite page

The segmental surface may be left as is, or the edge of the remaining lower lobe may
be approximated to the inferior surface of the upper lobe by sutures or by staples. This will
minimize the space and probably terminate leaks much sooner.

Chest tubes are placed in the usual manner, and the chest is closed.

LINGULAR SEGMENTECTOMY

Lingulectomy is probably more often accomplished by stapling without prior isolation
and division of bronchial and vascular structures. Although this is simple and may be done
rapidly, the remaining portion of the upper lobe is severely distorted and restricted from
full expansion.

Indications

1. Localized inflammatory disease, i.e., bronchiectasis.
2. Benign or malignant neoplastic disease that can be excised by a lesser resection than
   a lobectomy.

Position

Left lateral.

Incision

Posterolateral thoracotomy.

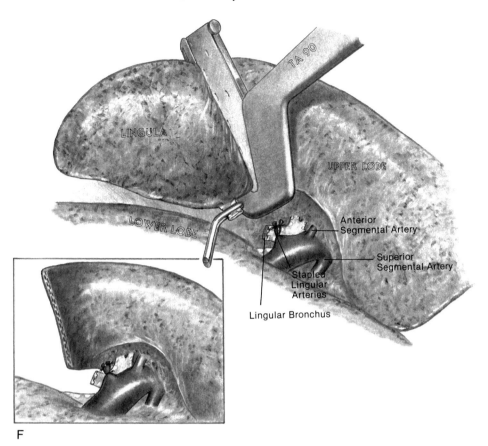

F

Figure 7–8. *Continued.*

F, **Lingular segmentectomy, interlobar view.** The ligated and severed lingular artery is sewn. The lingular bronchus has been stapled and divided. A TA 90 stapling instrument is being applied, conforming generally to the intersegmental plane. *Inset,* The completed resection. Some distortion and compression of the remaining upper lobe parenchyma are unavoidable if staples are used. (From Hood, M. D.: Stapling technique involving lung parenchyma. Surg. Clin. North Am., 3: June, 1984.)

Procedure

The incision is opened widely and exploration of the lung, hilum, and mediastinum is carried out after all pleural adhesions are separated.

The surgeon must be certain that the lesion to be resected lies clearly in the segment and that a more major resection is not required.

Arterial Dissection (see Fig. 7–7A). Open the interlobar fissure and expose the pulmonary artery. The arterial anatomy is more variable in this area than in any other. The first branch of the artery in the fissure arises from the posterior aspect of the vessel and supplies the superior segment. Anteriorly, at about the same level, is a branch to the anterior segment of the upper lobe. The next inferior branch arising anteriorly should be the lingular artery. It is usually about 4 to 5 mm in diameter and about 1 cm in length before dividing into the superior and inferior divisions. These two vessels may arise separately from the pulmonary artery, however. The artery is ligated proximally with 2-0 nonabsorbable material. The distal branches are either ligated or secured with medium hemoclips and the branches transected. The anterior segmental artery may arise from the lingular artery.

Bronchial Dissection.   The lingular bronchus is dissected free using the same exposure. The bronchus is found anterior to the pulmonary artery. It is not well visualized until the artery has been divided. The lingular division is the most inferior and largest branch. It may be exposed by blunt and sharp dissection. The anterior surface of the bronchus lies in close association with the superior pulmonary vein anteriorly. A TA 30 stapling instrument with 4.8 mm staples may be used to staple the bronchus. Care must be taken not to compromise the remaining segmental bronchi. The bronchus is severed and the distal stump grasped with a hemostat.

Venous Dissection.   The lung is then reflected posteriorly, exposing the anterior hilar surface. The pleura is incised vertically about 1 cm posterior to the phrenic nerve. The main trunk of the superior pulmonary vein is exposed. The most inferior tributary is the vein from the lingula. Occasionally there will be two veins draining the lingular segments. The vein is doubly ligated or ligated proximally and secured with hemoclips distally.

The Intersegmental Plane.   All bronchial and vascular structures have now been divided and the surgeon is now ready to dissect the intersegmental plane. First the lung is inflated and the juncture between atelectasis and aeration is noted as the approximate segmental division at the pleural level. The hemostat holding the divided bronchus is now placed on traction laterally and superiorly. Using the bronchus as a general guide, the forefinger is swept transversely from medial to lateral, arriving at the pleural surface usually very close to the site determined by inflation.

The pleura is then cut with the dissecting scissors and the segment is removed. A warm, moist pack should be placed against the raw segmental surface with the lung only partially inflated. After a period of about 5 minutes, the pack is removed. Small bleeding points are ligated and small bronchial leaks are oversewn with 5-0 monofilament suture.

The raw surface may be left open, oversewn, or sutured to the lower lobe. Generally, the area is left exposed.

The pleural space is irrigated. Two chest tubes are placed, and the wound is then closed.

Alternatively, the segmented plane may be stapled, using a TA 90 instrument with 4.8 staples (Fig. 7–8F). This results in some distortion of the remaining lobe.

Note

Segmental resections have approximately a 15% bronchopleural fistula incidence leading to prolonged chest tube requirement or empyema. Therefore, before selecting this procedure, the surgeon must weigh this risk against the value of upper lobe preservation.

Segmental resection techniques are best not applied to lungs involved with emphysema.

RESECTION OF BASAL SEGMENTS (EITHER LOWER LOBE)

Indications

Bronchiectasis was formerly the principal indication for performing basal segmentectomy; however, with the striking decrease in suppurative pulmonary disease, this procedure is now infrequently performed. When bronchiectasis does occur, it is still a reason for resecting basal segments. It should be established that the disease is localized to segments unilaterally or bilaterally, so that the removal of these segments will totally eradicate the disease and at the same time leave sufficient lung to enable the patient to sustain resection and have minimal symptoms of respiratory insufficiency. Bronchogenic carcinoma may represent an indication if a peripheral lesion is present in the basilar area, pulmonary function is severely limited, and the patient is not thought to be a candidate for lobectomy.

Pulmonary sequestration might be a third indication.

Position

Lateral.

Incision

Posterolateral thoracotomy.

Procedure

The patient is anesthetized and turned into the full lateral position. An incision is made, all pleural adhesions are divided, and hemostasis is obtained.

Dissection is begun using the interlobar exposure described previously. Once the fissure is completely separated, the arterial dissection is begun. Arterial anatomy differs on the right and left; therefore, this part of the dissection is described separately for each side.

Right Side

Arterial Dissection (Fig. 7–9A).   Dissection is begun at the point of origin of the transverse or horizontal fissure. The artery is encountered and the perivascular plane is entered. The surgeon should become oriented by identifying the middle lobe and superior segmental arteries. The arterial dissection is extended inferiorly, exposing the basilar arterial divisions. The main basilar artery is encircled and ligated with 2-0 nonabsorbable sutures. Each segmental branch is ligated separately or secured with a hemoclip. Each segmental artery is then transected.

Bronchial Dissection (Fig. 7–9B).   Division of the basilar artery exposes the basilar bronchus lying posteriorly. It may be dissected free and stapled or closed with sutures about 0.5 cm from the middle lobe and superior segmental bronchus. The surgeon must be careful in either stapling or suturing not to compromise the middle lobe or superior segmental bronchus.

Left Side

Arterial Dissection.   The main fissure is separated in its midportion, and the main pulmonary artery is found lying in the base of the fissure following the direction of the fissure. The lingular artery is identified arising from the anterior surface. The artery is dissected free inferior to the lingular artery and ligated with 2-0 nonabsorbable sutures.

Each of the three basilar segmental branches is ligated separately or closed with a hemoclip and severed.

Bronchial Dissection.   The basilar division of the lower lobe bronchus will be exposed and should be dissected free using the origin of the superior segmental bronchus as a guide. The bronchus is stapled or otherwise closed and transected 0.5 cm distal to the superior segmental bronchus. One may close the stapling instrument and inflate the superior segment if there is any question of closure site.

Either Side

Venous Dissection (Fig. 7–9C).   The lung is reflected anteriorly, exposing the posterior surface of the hilum. The mediastinal pleura is incised vertically from the diaphragm to the level of the upper lobe bronchus. The pulmonary ligament is divided and small arterial vessels are secured.

The inferior pulmonary vein should be seen clearly. The perivascular plane is entered, and dissection of segmental veins is carried out extending well into the parenchyma. The superior segmental vein with its most superior tributary is identified and preserved. All other tributary veins are doubly ligated and transected.

EXTRAPLEURAL PNEUMONECTOMY (FIG. 7–10)

Indication

This procedure was relegated to obscurity by most internists and surgeons because of the effectiveness of antituberculosis antibiotics. However, with the resurgence of the disease, this procedure is still required, and although it is a procedure of considerable risk, it can be curative and allow full rehabilitation. It is indicated in the patient with a chronic mixed-tuberculous empyema associated with extensive destructive parenchymal disease, to the degree that lung expansion is not possible if complete decortication were accomplished.

Position

Lateral

Anesthesia

General, using double-lumen tube.

Procedure

A posterolateral incision is made and hemostasis accomplished with the electrocautery. The extracostal musculature is incised and hemostasis again produced. A long length of the fifth rib is removed subperiosteally. The thick parietal wall of the empyema space is then encountered. Dissection may be begun extrapleurally or between the empyema peel and the parietal pleura. The dissection plane is advanced posteriorly, anteriorly, superiorly, and inferiorly. The empyema wall may be rigid because of thickness and calcification and great force may be required to separate it from the chest wall.

As the mediastinum is approached posteriorly, the surgeon must use great care to "turn the corner" to the mediastinal pleura and not blindly carry the dissection behind the aorta on the left or the esophagus on the right.

This error can result in injury to the aorta or disruption of intercostal arteries or esophageal injury. Once the dissection plane is over the mediastinum, almost all evidence of inflammation and adhesion is absent and hilar dissection can be done as in any other pneumonectomy.

The adherence to the apex of the pleural space may be extreme, and it may be impossible to dissect the empyema wall away without injury to the subclavian vessels and brachial plexus. In this situation, it is wiser to leave a small area of the peel in the apex rather than incur this risk.

The adherence to the diaphragm is also dense and requires slow, meticulous dissection to avoid excessive injury to the muscle or to the phrenic nerve. Again, it is necessary to "turn the corner" from the chest wall to the diaphragm and not inadvertently detach the diaphragm from the chest wall altogether. Also, as in the apex, it may be necessary to leave some peel in the costophrenic sulcus. It will do no harm.

The volume and bulkiness of the empyema and the attached lung may be such that visualizing the hilar structures may be difficult. A simple maneuver (Fig. 7–10B) may help.

A 50 cc syringe with an 18-inch gauge needle may be used to empty the empyema cavity of most of its contents and thereby diminish its size. However, in empyema of many years duration, calcification may negate the value of this procedure.

The mediastinal dissection can be done as described in the section on pneumonectomy. It is preferable to divide the bronchus first to stop the flow of infected secretions into the contralateral lung. Once the lung and empyema cavity are removed, the surgeon is usually surprised by the small size of the pleural cavity. It is wise to cover the bronchial stump

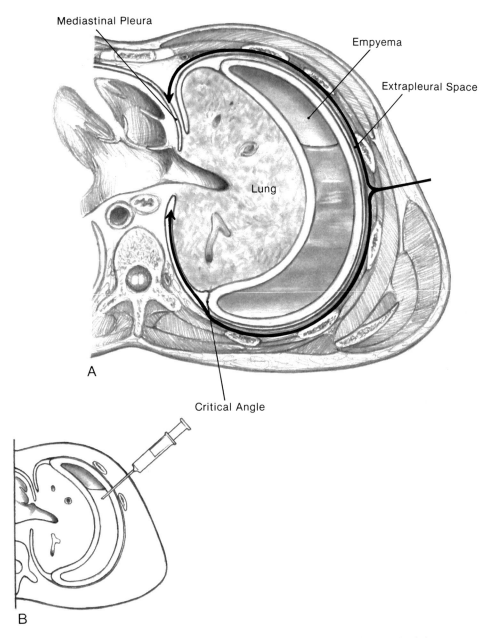

Mediastinal Pleura

Empyema

Extrapleural Space

Lung

Critical Angle

A

B

Figure 7–10. Principle of extrapleural pneumonectomy. *A,* Through a standard thoracotomy incision, the dissection is begun in the extrapleural plane and carried to the mediastinal level. Usually, although lightly fused, the pleura in this area is not involved in the empyema. Pulmonary vascular and bronchial dissection can be accomplished in a relatively normal fashion. *B,* Technique of aspirating the contents of the empyema to reduce its bulk and facilitate dissection. (From Hood, R. M., et al.: Surgical Diseases of the Pleura and Chest Wall. Philadelphia, W. B. Saunders Company, 1986. Used by permission.)

with a vascular structure such as intercostal muscle. The pleural cavity is irrigated with large amounts of saline, and antibiotic solution may be advantageous.

The wound is closed as with any posterolateral incision. After the chest wall is closed, it is best to remove most, if not all, of the air from the cavity, and it may be possible to obliterate it altogether.

Note

Patients who are candidates for this procedure have been ill for years. They are often cachectic and anemic. Their organisms are often resistant to most of the antituberculous antibiotics. A period of carefully supervised hyperalimentation can be a major factor in the success of the surgical procedure. At least one month's therapy with carefully chosen antibiotics is also critical in preventing contralateral spread and bronchial disruption.

One point to remember is that, even with the use of a double-lumen intratracheal tube, the anesthesiologist must be much more aggressive in keeping both sides of the bronchial tree free of secretions. Also, a separate suction tube should be used on the contralateral side. A major postoperative spread of tuberculosis usually proves to be a fatal complication.

RESECTION OF SUPERIOR SULCUS TUMORS

A superior sulcus tumor represented a hopeless lesion for treatment until the pioneer work of Shaw, Paulson, and Mallams demonstrated that preoperative radiation based on clinical diagnosis, followed by en bloc resection of the involved chest wall and upper lobe, would result in a significant number of long-term survivors. The amount of radiation is usually 3000 rad given over 2 to 3 weeks, with a 3 to 4 week interval elapsing before resection. The addition of chemotherapy may also be of value in management.

Procedure (Fig. 7–11)

A posterolateral thoracotomy incision is made with the skin incision carried much higher than is usual posteriorly. The pleural space is entered in the fourth intercostal space. Exploration is carried out to determine hilar and mediastinal involvement. Also, the extent of chest wall involvement is determined, and the area of resection is outlined with the cautery.

A rib spreader is then placed with one blade resting on the fifth or sixth rib and the other under the scapula. Adequate exposure is thus consistently obtained. The highest attachments of the serratus anterior muscle are separated from the second and third ribs, and the scalenus medius muscle is also divided. The electrocautery is used for this dissection. The scalenus anterior muscle is then separated from the first rib using extreme care to protect the subclavian artery and vein and the cords of the brachial plexus. Should neoplasm be encountered encasing the artery or vein or more than the T1 or C7 nerve roots, a decision must be made as to the value of further effort at resection. These nerve structures can be sacrificed with maintenance of adequate arm innervation but with disability, and an extra-anatomic graft will permit the artery to be resected. However, survival in this group of patients is not high.

The anterior ribs, beginning with the third one, are cut with the rib shears; then the posterior rib is cut after exposing the transverse process. An osteotome is used to sever the transverse process and to remove some of the vertebra if necessary to remove the tumor and detach the rib at the same time. The line of bone incision must be in a flat plane from back to front, and the bone cutting instrument must not be angled medially, which will risk injuring the spinal cord. The T1 nerve root near the foramen is usually excised, if neoplasm involves this root, it may be preferable to have a neurosurgeon perform a laminectomy and resect the root inside the epidural canal to give a wider margin of resection. Each rib and process is similarly cut. Except for a few soft tissues, the chest

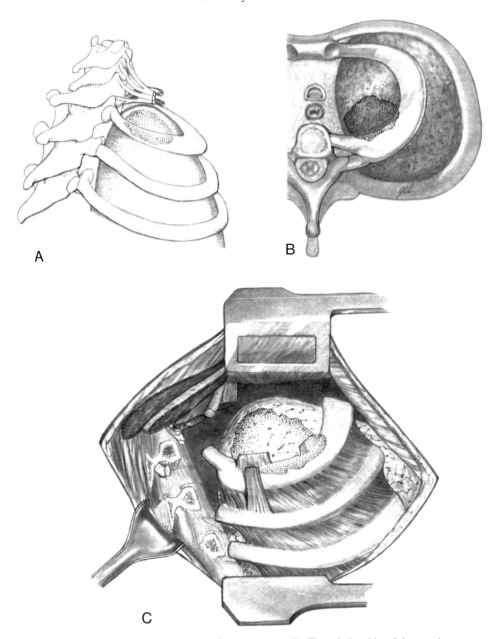

Figure 7–11.   Resection of superior sulcus tumor. *A, B,* The relationship of the usual tumor to the rib cage and the thoracic outlet structures. *C,* Skeletal resection is carried out by transection of the upper two or three ribs posteriorly at the level of the transverse process, which may be also be resected. Portions of the vertebrae may be included. Resection of the T1 nerve root is also shown. Resection may be extended farther if indicated, but this is not the usual procedure. The upper lobe is then resected in the usual way, or the surgeon may choose to remove the upper one third to one half of the lobe by transegmental stapling if there is no extension of the tumor to the hilum.

wall and the neoplasm should be free and attached only to the upper lobe. Hemostasis should be carefully secured. The surgeon should be careful in cauterizing intercostal vessels close to the dura, as the transmitted heat may injure the spinal cord. Suture ligature or oxidized cellulose packing is preferable.

A lobectomy is then performed, as elsewhere described. The neoplasm is often small and involves only a small area of the apical segment. It is acceptable to resect only the segment rather than the entire lobe. The remaining lower lobe or lower and middle lobes are usually adequate to fill the pleural space, so that it is usually unnecessary to use any prosthetic material for the chest wall defect. The paradox is minimal, and the cosmetic result is adequate without reconstruction. The pleural space is drained in the usual way with two tubes and the incision is closed.

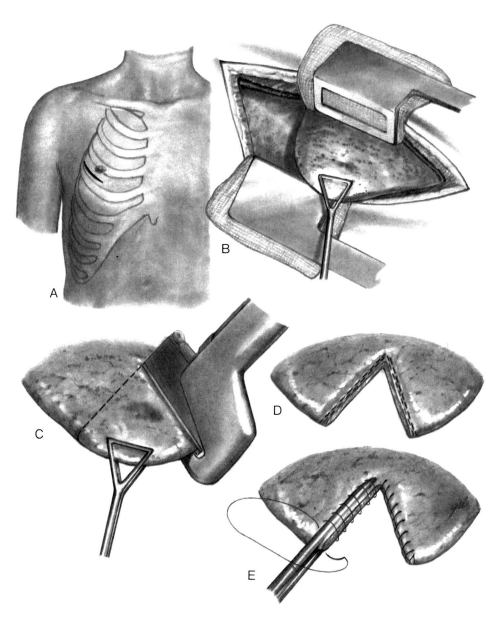

Figure 7–12. *A*, Site of incision for lung biopsy. The patient is usually in the supine position. *B*, A limited exposure is available through this incision. The edge of the middle lobe or occasionally the upper lobe is grasped with a Duval forceps. *C* and *D*, A TA 55 stapling instrument is used to remove a 4 cm wedge-shaped piece of lung. *E*, A similar procedure can be accomplished using a suture technique.

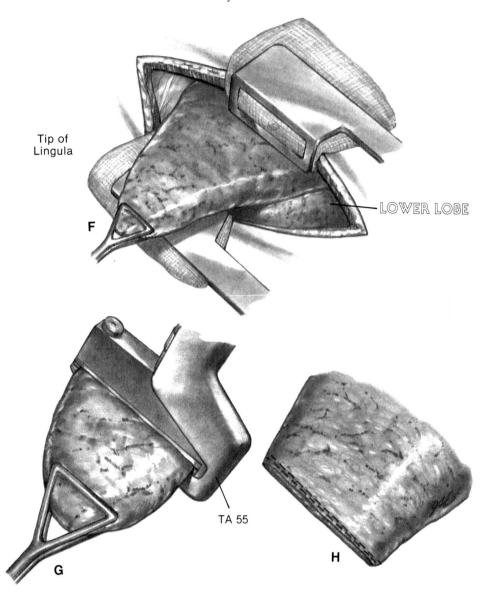

Figure 7–12. *Continued. F* through *H,* A similar technique can be applied to the lingular segment on the left side. (From Hood, M. D.: Stapling technique involving lung parenchyma. Surg. Clin. North Am., 3: June, 1984.)

WEDGE OR LOCAL EXCISION

Indication

This limited form of pulmonary resection can be chosen for (1) removing tissue for biopsy (Fig. 7–12) in diffuse lung disease; (2) resection of a peripheral circumscribed lesion that appears benign for examination; (3) resection of metastatic malignant lesions, particularly when multiple; and (4) resection of a primary bronchogenic carcinoma that is peripherally located in the patient who is very old (i.e., over 75 years) or who has severe pulmonary dysfunction. The use of these techniques for the diagnosis of lesions thought to be primary malignant lesions that appear to be resectable has been unwise and considered poor technique. Increasing experience seems to indicate clearly that limited resection of bronchogenic carcinoma is acceptable when the patient's respiratory status is marginal or poor. Data are insufficient at present to demonstrate that a local, wedge, or segmental excision has the same survival rate as lobectomy in comparable lesions and patients. There is a definite trend toward lesser resection based on similar survival data from lobectomy compared with segmental or local excision. However, the lobectomy series include patients with tumors too large or too central to be removed by segmental resection. All of those resected locally are shown, by the fact that they were resectable by less than lobectomy, to be smaller, more peripheral tumors and therefore not comparable.

Procedure

A posterolateral, anterolateral, or anterior thoractomy may be selected, as desired. The surgeon must be wary of selecting an incision that provides limited exposure, only to discover that a major resection is required. At least four techniques are applicable. A wedge resection using the TA 30, TA 55, or GIA stapling instrument is the simplest technique. The lesion must be peripheral and located near a fissure for this technique to be used. A peripheral lesion not near a fissure may be grasped with a Duval lung forceps, the lobe deflated, and a TA 55 staple instrument applied as shown in Figure 7–13. Alternatively, a suture technique (Fig. 7–14) may be utilized if stapling instruments are not available. A vascular clamp is applied and the lesion is excised. The area is loosely oversewn, the clamp is removed, and the suture is tightened and oversewn with a second suture line.

Any lesion can also be removed by incision and dissection followed by suture closure. This is less desirable and more likely to result in significant blood loss or postoperative air leak.

Wedge excision should not be attempted when the lesion lies deeply in the lung. Any of the techniques described here may result in injury to major pulmonary vessels or segmental bronchi, and the suture or staple line may devascularize a large area of parenchyma or occlude the bronchus to a significantly large area of lung.

Hemostasis is ensured and drainage tubes inserted; the chest is then closed. The surgeon may be tempted to close the incision without drainage, but this is often an unwise decision, resulting in pneumothorax or a collection of fluid requiring later intubation.

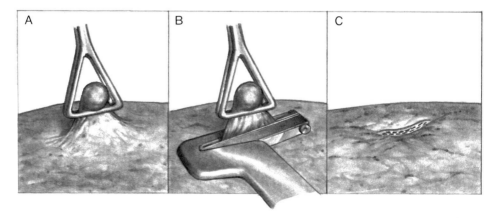

Figure 7–13. *A* through *C*, A subpleural nodule can be excised by grasping it with a Duval forceps and applying a TA 55 stapling instrument, as shown. This minimizes the amount of lung resected, but it is not adequate for a malignant lesion. (From Hood, M. D.: Stapling technique involving lung parenchyma. Surg. Clin. North Am., 3: June, 1984.)

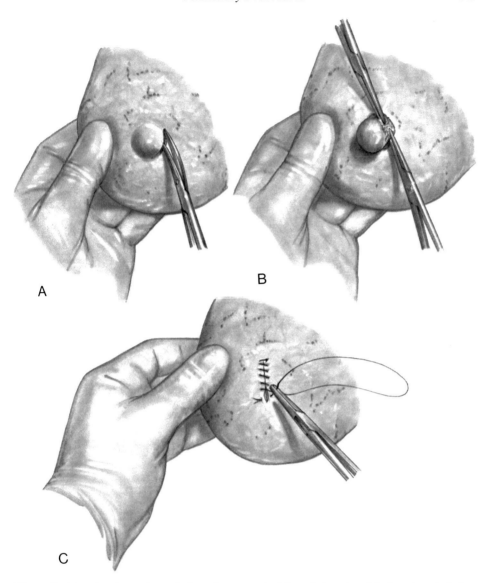

Figure 7–14. An alternative technique for removal of the subpleural nodule by suture technique without use of stapling devices. *A, B,* The pleura is incised with scissors. The nodule is being pressed anteriorly by the hand applying pressure posteriorly. The nodule is dissected free with vascular components clamped and later ligated. *C,* The defect is closed by continuous suture of 2-0 or 3-0 catgut. This is most applicable to a nodule that is in a subpleural plane.

BRONCHOPLASTIC PROCEDURES

A small group of patients with centrally located adenomas and carcinomas present a challenge to the surgeon. Figure 7–15 shows several possible resections and reconstructions for these tumors. The procedures become applicable when lobectomy or pneumonectomy is not possible because of limited pulmonary function or when the disease is localized and situated so that a bronchoplastic procedure can preserve the maximal amount of functioning lung and yet accomplish an adequate tumor resection.

The suture techniques are the same as described in the operative procedure for tracheobronchial injury. Ventilation techniques require considerable ingenuity and are

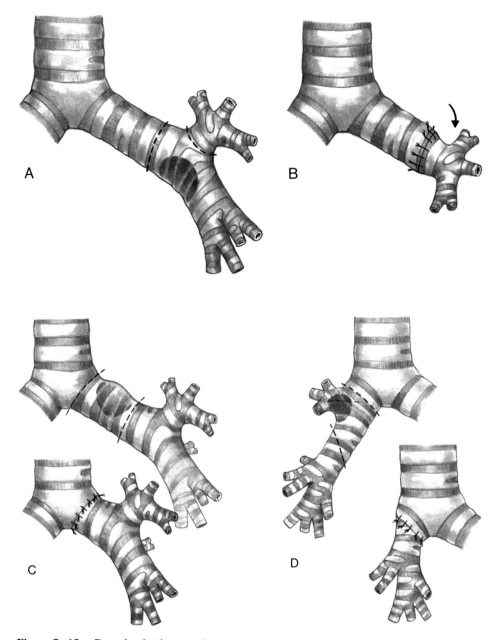

Figure 7–15. Bronchoplastic procedures. Simplified presentation of some techniques used for the preservation of functioning normal lung tissue where neoplastic lesions are small and located in or near main bronchi. Bronchial adenomas are more likely to be managed by these techniques. These procedures may be applied to resection of carcinoma when the tumor is small and when the patient's pulmonary reserve does not permit pneumonectomy. Careful preoperative planning, close cooperation, and often improvisation are necessary to accomplish a satisfactory procedure. Suture material may be Dexon, Vicryl, Prolene, or steel wire.

Illustration continued on opposite page

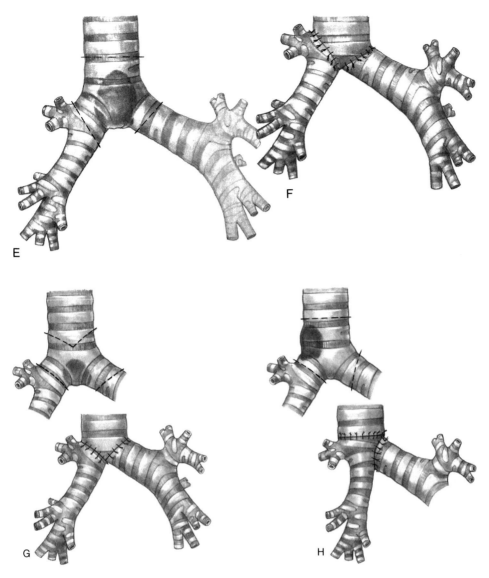

Figure 7–15. *Continued.*

subject to individual modification based on the anatomic and physiologic states encountered.

Postoperatively, bronchoscopy should be performed daily for several days to provide secretion control and to keep the anastomotic area clear of encrusted secretions.

A detailed operative procedure is not a practical approach and is not presented.

RESECTION OF TRACHEAL STRICTURE (FIG. 7–16)

Tracheal stricture following prolonged intubation with an endotracheal tube or a cuffed tracheostomy tube has become a relatively common complication of prolonged ventilation. A high-pressure inflatable cuff, excessive pressure in a low pressure cuff,

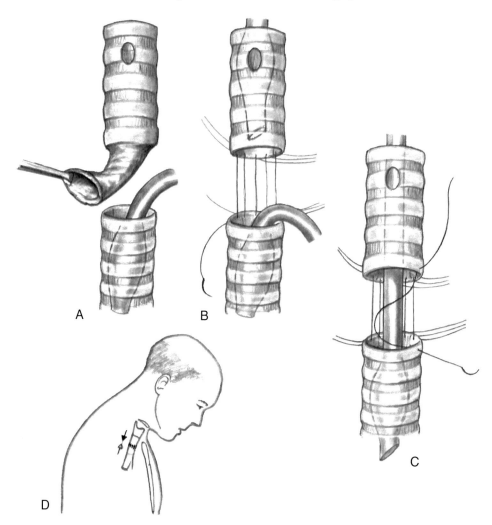

Figure 7–16. *A,* A cervical incision has been made. The cervical trachea has been dissected free and transected distal to the stricture. This has been accomplished under local anesthesia. An endotracheal tube has been inserted into the distal trachea for general anesthesia and ventilation.

B, The posterior row of sutures has been placed. The sutures are full thickness, with the tying to be extraluminal.

C, An endotracheal tube has been introduced transorally and advanced into the distal trachea. The anterior row of sutures is being placed.

D, The head must be sharply flexed during the approximation of the two segments. This position should be maintained for several days postoperatively.

failure to change tubes often, and infection are contributing factors. These strictures usually become apparent in the late postintubation period, and the diagnosis is often delayed unnecessarily.

Strictures vary in length, severity, and location. Most can be managed through a cervical incision. Some require a proximal sternal split of the manubrium. Those nearer to the carina may require a full sternal split.

The procedure shown is of the common variety.

Position

Supine.

Anesthesia

If the stricture is severe, the procedure can be begun under local anesthesia and converted to general anesthesia after the distal trachea has been opened. The entire procedure can be completed under local anesthesia in most patients. High-frequency jet ventilation can be used if available. Complete cardiopulmonary bypass has been used for lower and more complex strictures.

Procedure

An initial transverse cervical incision is made and hemostasis produced by electrocautery. The anterior cervical muscles are separated and the visceral compartment entered. The trachea is exposed and its mobilization begun. There are by varying degrees of peritracheal inflammatory reaction and fibrosis requiring tedious dissection. The thyroid isthmus may be divided if necessary, and inferior thyroid veins require division. A careful search for and identification of the recurrent laryngeal nerves must be carried out.

The extent of the stricture is usually apparent externally, although not certainly. The initial transverse incision into the distal trachea should be made about 1/2 cm distal to the apparent stricture. The entire trachea is transected. If general anesthesia is to be instituted at this point or, if it is already in progress, an endotracheal tube is inserted through the operative field into the distal trachea and ventilation established. Two sutures placed laterally can be used to stabilize the trachea. Sharp and blunt dissection is then used to free the trachea to the carinal level.

The proximal trachea and the strictured area are then mobilized completely and transected above the stricture. Both ends should be inspected to be certain that no mucosal stricture remains, and further excision is done. The surgeon must be careful to excise no more trachea than necessary. The total length of trachea that may be excised with reanastomosis is about six tracheal rings. This amount requires considerable tension. Proximal mobilization is carried out and laryngeal release can be done if necessary.

An endotracheal tube is then introduced orally through the proximal trachea, and after the tube in the distal trachea has been removed it is advanced into the distal segment.

Suture material may be Prolene, Vicryl, or PDL. All of these and fine steel wire have been successfully used. A posterior row of simple, full-thickness sutures is placed so that the knots will be on the outside, but left untied until all the sutures are in place. The distal trachea is then elevated to meet the proximal end and sutures are tied. The tension must be maintained at this time to protect the posterior sutures. The lateral and anterior sutures are then placed and tied. The suture line should be tested with pressure and saline and additional sutures placed if necessary. It is usually necessary because all sutures are being tied to flex the neck anterior to minimize tension.

The flexion should be maintained continuously.

The decision as to establishing tracheostomy for the postoperative period must be made at this point. Most surgeons have preferred tracheostomy. The author has consistently performed this procedure without a postoperative tracheostomy with no adverse sequelae.

The wound is then closed without drainage, using absorbable material. Skin closure by subcuticular suture or skin clips or staples is done.

Flexible bronchoscopy should be done at 2 and 4 days to inspect and debride the anastomosis area.

DRAINAGE OF LUNG ABSCESS

Indication

A surgical procedure for acute lung abscess is rarely necessary. Antibiotic therapy is usually successful in managing the acute abscess. Resection is preferred for the chronic abscess or the acute abscess not responding to antibiotic therapy.

Transthoracic drainage may be indicated in patients who are extremely toxic and who are not responding to therapy. These patients would also include those considered unfit for anesthesia and resection. Usually the abscess requiring drainage is large and the organisms are resistant staphylococci or gram-negative organisms. Frequently, the patients are elderly, debilitated, alcohol or drug abusers, and anergic.

Procedure (Fig. 7–17)

The abscess must be peripheral, close to the visceral pleura, and at least 5 cm in diameter. Localization by chest x-ray, fluoroscopy, and computed tomography (CT) scanning must be accurate.

After the site of drainage has been determined, a vertical incision about 8 cm in length is made. A 5 cm segment of overlying rib is resected subperiosteally. The intercostal vessels and nerve are doubly ligated and a segment is excised. A 2 to 3 cm disc of periosteum and parietal pleura is excised, and the area is explored carefully to be certain that fusion of parietal and visceral pleurae has already occurred. The wound is packed with gauze if fusion has not occurred, and the skin and subcutaneous tissues are closed. A chest tube may be necessary to evacuate pneumothorax.

After 72 hours the wound can be reopened and again inspected.

If pleural fusion is present a needle is first used to enter the cavity to ascertain that the drainage site has been properly selected. An electrocautery tip is used to traverse the lung parenchyma until the cavity is entered. The tract is widened to produce an adequate opening, and the abscess cavity is packed loosely with gauze. The wound is left completely open. A chest x-ray is made immediately to be certain that there is no pneumothorax.

Wound packing should be changed about every 2 days. This type of procedure usually results in a permanent bronchocutaneous fistula.

Note

An attempt at drainage of an abscess deep in the parenchyma, and to a lesser extent drainage of all abscesses, carries the risk of entering a major pulmonary artery with the cautery. Rapid control by pressure and suture is necessary.

Should a pneumothorax appear after drainage of an abscess, a chest tube for dependent drainage must be inserted to prevent pyopneumothorax.

SCALENE LYMPH NODE BIOPSY

Indications

Scalene lymph node biopsy is used as a diagnostic approach to pulmonary diseases, such as sarcoidosis and various pneumoconioses, and as a diagnostic and staging procedure for bronchogenic carcinoma.

This procedure has been avoided by many surgeons if nodes are not palpable. Involved nodes are not necessarily enlarged and because of their position are usually not palpable when there is enlargement.

A common mistake is made in removing supraclavicular nodes rather than mediastinal nodes from the paratracheal area. A low yield will thus occur.

Approximately 30% positive nodes are recovered in patients with bronchogenic carcinoma. Sarcoidosis involves these nodes in about 90% of cases.

Anesthesia

Local or general.

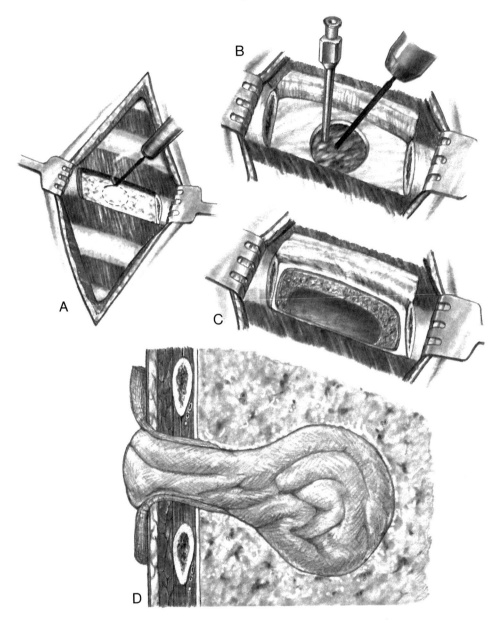

Figure 7–17. Drainage of lung abscess. *A*, The completed rib resection with a disclike incision being made in the posterior periosteum and pleura. *B*, After pleural synthesis has been demonstrated, a needle is used to explore and identify the abscess cavity. A cautery instrument is used to cut through the pulmonary parenchyma and enter the abscess cavity, producing adequate hemostasis. *C*, The abscess exposed. *D*, Abscess loosely packed with gauze.

Procedure (Fig. 7–18)

The patient should be supine with the head turned away from the operative side. Anesthesia is produced by local infiltration and is progressively extended as the dissection is deepened. A 5 cm incision is made just above and parallel to the clavicle. The center of the incision should be over the division between the sternal and clavicular heads of the

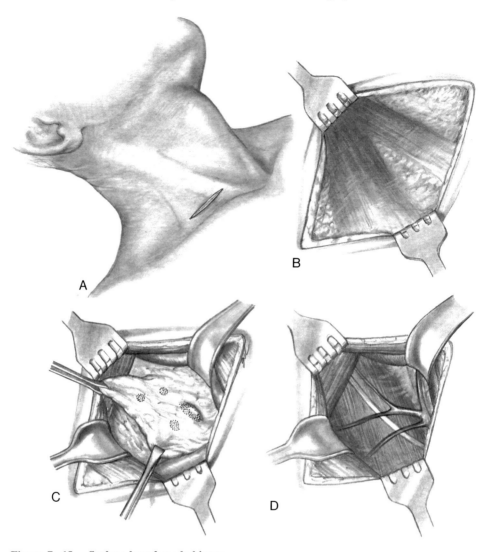

Figure 7–18.   Scalene lymph node biopsy.

A, Position of the patient and location of the incision, above and parallel to the clavicle and centered over the separation between the sternal and clavicular divisions of the sternocleidomastoid muscle.

B, The skin incision is completed; the division between the two heads of the sternocleidomastoid muscle is seen. This space is opened longitudinally and the muscle is retracted.

C, The fat pad has been resected and the remaining structures are noted. The demonstrated vessels can bleed seriously if injured, and the phrenic nerve is vulnerable to injury.

D, The scalene fat pad lying on and medial to the scalenus anterior muscle is being delivered from the mediastinum. Several small lymph nodes are noted.

sternocleidomastoid muscle. The two muscle divisions are then split longitudinally and retracted using phrenic retractors. The omohyoid muscle can be seen traversing the superior portion of the surgical field. The position of the scalenus anterior muscle can be ascertained by palpation at this point. The internal jugular vein is then identified and freed along its lateral border for about 3 cm and retracted medially. A Babcock or Allyce clamp is used to grasp the fatty tissue overlying the scalenus anterior muscle and extending medially and inferiorly into the mediastinum along the trachea. A mixture of very cautious sharp and blunt dissection is used to free this pad of tissue. The transverse scapular and transverse cervical arteries lie in the field and must be sought and either ligated or avoided. The phrenic nerve lies on the scalenus anterior muscle, running from lateral to medial, and therefore is vulnerable to injury. Should a single obviously abnormal lymph node be encountered, it may be removed without removing the entire fat pad. Hemostasis must be meticulous. The finger or mediastinoscope may be used to explore the mediastinum further. The subclavian vein forms the lower margin of the surgical field where it joins the internal jugular vein and is also easily injured.

The thoracic duct lies in the surgical field on the left side and joins the subclavian vein on its superior surface near the vein's termination; it should be identified. Appearance of chylous fluid in the field indicates injury, and the duct must be ligated.

The wound is carefully inspected for hemostasis and lymph drainage. A single suture is used to approximate the sternocleidomastoid muscle. The platysma muscle is closed with a continuous 3-0 absorbable suture, and the skin is sutured with a subcuticular 4-0 absorbable suture. A drain is not usually required.

Note

The small incision and limited exposure in an area of major vascular structures demands good lighting, assistance, and careful technique.

The venous distention that is present when the superior vena cana is obstructed increases the risk of bleeding, and many surgeons consider this circumstance a contraindication to this procedure, as well as to mediastinoscopy.

MEDIASTINOSCOPY

Indications

Mediastinoscopy is a diagnostic and staging procedure useful in patients with bronchogenic carcinoma. Some believe that it should be performed routinely prior to thoracotomy. However, the necessity of general anesthesia and operative risk should require that this operation be utilized only when indicated and not performed routinely. The significance of identifying involved nodes is controversial at this time. It is doubtful that the operation will provide useful information if the CT scan is negative. Mediastinoscopy may establish the diagnosis when it is not otherwise available. It may establish inoperability when there is gross mediastinal invasion and when involved nodes are invading the trachea, vena cava, or other structures. In my opinion, the finding of isolated small, positive nodes should not be a contraindication to thoracotomy. This is particularly true for squamous cell carcinoma. The procedure has limited usefulness for lesions on the left side.

Position

Supine with the head slightly extended.

Procedure (Fig. 7–19)

A transverse skin incision, about 4 cm in length, is made just above the superior edge of the sternum. The incision is deepened and the anterior cervical muscles are separated by a vertical incision. This divides the pretracheal fascia and permits entrance into the visceral compartment of the neck.

Finger dissection is then used to create a space anterior to the trachea and posteriorly to the innominate vessels. The mediastinal tissues are palpated to detect enlarged nodes, and the dissection is carried to the carinal level. The mediastinoscope is introduced into the dissected space. Nodes that were palpable are sought, and either they are excised or

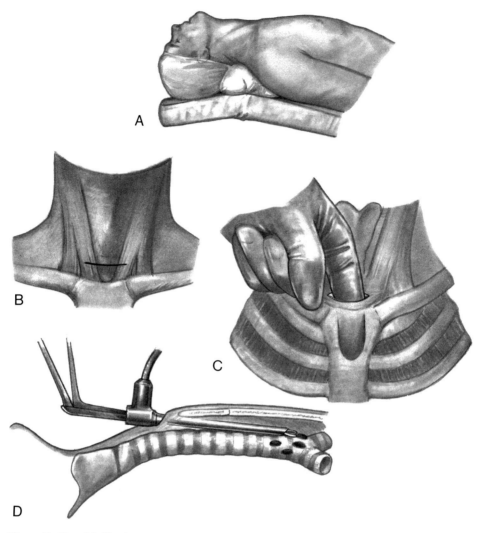

Figure 7–19.   Mediastinoscopy. *A,* The position of the patient on the operating table. *B, C,* The location of the incision with finger dissection of the pretracheal fascia. The mediastinoscope is then introduced. *D,* Taking a sample of an anterior tracheal node near the carina.

a piece is removed for biopsy. If a larger mass is encountered, it is safer to aspirate it with a needle first or perform needle biopsy rather than use biopsy forceps.

The dissection may be carried beyond the carinal area on the right, but this seems unnecessary.

Bleeding may be controlled with the electrocautery or by temporary packing. Hemoclips may be useful on occasion. When full hemostasis has been attained, the subcutaneous tissues and skin are sutured.

Note

The findings must be evaluated in light of all clinical information. Contralateral node involvement should preclude further surgery.

Fixation of tumor to the trachea or vena cava is also a finding indicative of inoperability. The performing of either scalene node biopsy or mediastinoscopy in the presence of a superior vena caval obstruction is to be questioned.

TECHNIQUE OF BEDSIDE BRONCHOSCOPY

Bronchoscopy in the recovery room or intensive care unit is required occasionally. Indications for bedside endoscopy include the following:

1. **Retention of secretions producing atelectasis.**
2. **To clear secretions in a patient with an endotracheal tube in whom routine suctioning has been ineffective.**
3. **To remove encrusted secretions from a tracheal or bronchial anastomosis.**
4. **To assist in re-expanding a lung when an endotracheal tube has been inadvertently introduced into a main bronchus and left for several hours.**
5. **To clear the bronchial tree following aspiration of vomitus.**

Selection of Bronchoscope

Either the flexible fiberoptic bronchoscope or the rigid ventilating bronchoscope may be used. Selection should be based on the problem to be managed, not on the lack of skill of the surgeon.

Usually secretions can be removed adequately using the flexible bronchoscope, and because this instrument is better tolerated by the patient, it is preferable. Also, in the intubated patient rigid bronchoscopy requires extubation and reintubation, as it does in the tracheostomy patient.

However, particulate food particles from aspiration or thick, tenacious secretions cannot be removed except with the ventilating bronchoscope. A complete lobar or total lung atelectasis can be managed better and more quickly with the rigid instrument.

Anesthesia

The intubated patient usually requires no anesthesia, nor does the tracheostomized patient.

Bronchoscopy in the awake, unintubated patient requires a topical anesthetic. The following technique is useful. The agent may be 0.5% tetracaine hydrochloride (Pontocaine), 1% lidocaine, or 4% cocaine.

Spray the mouth, pharynx, and nasal passages with an ordinary atomizer. Repeat this procedure about every minute for 4 to 5 minutes. A Jackson laryngeal forceps wrapped with cotton soaked in the anesthetic agent is used to anesthetize the tonsillar fossae and the posterior one third of the tongue. A curved malleable cannula and syringe are then used to inject 2 mL of anesthetic into the larynx and trachea. This is repeated once. One should expect adequate anesthesia in about 10 minutes from the beginning of the procedure. The total amount of anesthetic should not exceed 15 to 20 mL because most reactions are dose-related.

Procedure (Fig. 7–20A to C)

The head of the bed is elevated about 30 to 35 degrees, and the headboard of the ICU bed is removed. The surgeon stands at the head of the bed. The bronchoscope is introduced into the right side of the mouth. As the epiglottis is approached, the tip of the bronchoscope should be in the midline. The instrument is advanced about 1 cm past the tip of the epiglottis and elevated, bringing the arytenoid cartilages and vocal cords into view. The instrument is turned sidewise to enter the laryngeal opening, and the trachea is

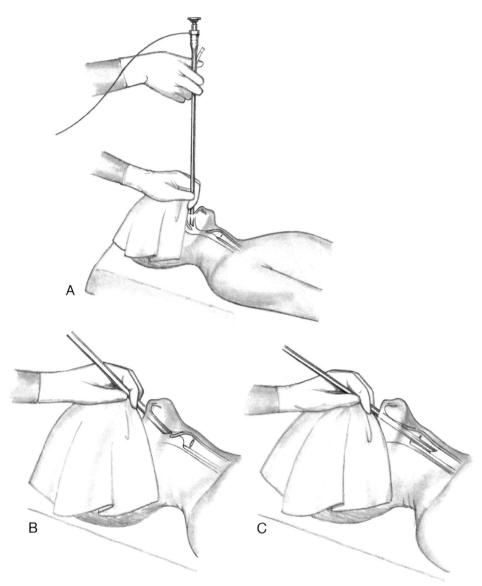

Figure 7–20.   Bedside bronchoscopy (rigid bronchoscope and topical anesthesia). *A,* The position of the surgeon and patient for introduction of the bronchoscope. *B,* The epiglottis is elevated and the vocal cords are seen. *C,* The bronchoscope is advanced into the trachea for aspiration of secretions.

then entered. Usually, copious secretions are encountered, and must be suctioned. Adequate time should be allowed for removal of secretions and the patient should be encouraged to cough, bringing secretions out of smaller bronchi. Suctioning should be intermittent to avoid hypoxia. Someone should listen with a stethoscope to assess the reappearance of breath sounds and disappearance of rales and rhonchi. The instrument is then removed.

The flexible bronchoscope can be introduced through the nose and, once the posterior pharynx is reached, the larynx can easily be seen and cannulated.

More time should be spent when the flexible bronchoscope is used because of the small size of the suction port. One should use copious amounts of saline solution to thin secretions so that their removal becomes possible.

The next hour after bronchoscopy should be spent in assisted coughing, which will probably produce more secretions than the bronchoscopy.

MANAGEMENT OF SPONTANEOUS PNEUMOTHORAX

Spontaneous pneumothorax may be divided into three general varieties: (1) pneumothorax occurring in young, otherwise healthy people without evidence of pleural or pulmonary disease; (2) pneumothorax resulting from rupture of a bullus in patients with pulmonary emphysema; and (3) pneumothorax secondary to rupture of a pulmonary cavitary lesion that is a part of a pulmonary infection, such as tuberculosis or lung abscess. Only the first two categories will be discussed here.

The most common form of spontaneous pneumothorax is the first category. Treatment is generally based on three factors: (1) whether the episode is the first, second, third, or one of multiple events; (2) the extent of collapse; and (3) presence of persistent bronchopleural fistula or prompt recurrence.

The following protocol is mine, based on experience with over 2500 patients, and in general it correlates with the opinion of a majority of thoracic surgeons.

Management of First Episode.   The patient is managed in the emergency room or outpatient area of the hospital. A patient with a collapse involving the apex only or estimated to be less than 15% is sent home to return for daily follow-up x-ray films. Unless there is progression of collapse, nothing is done. If the collapse is greater, a No. 12 trocar chest tube (or large Intracath) is inserted into the pleural space anteriorly and connected to waterseal apparatus and suction. The patient is observed for 1 hour, and if air leakage does not persist, the tube is clamped for an hour and an x-ray made at the end of this period. If complete expansion has been maintained, the tube is removed and the patient is sent home but asked to return in 24 hours. Should there be recurrence during this period, the patient is admitted and a No. 20 to No. 24 chest tube is inserted and maintained until the lung has been completely expanded, with no air leakage for 24 hours. The tube is then removed.

A major collapse (70 to 100%) is treated by admission to the hospital and chest tube insertion as just described.

Management of Repeated Episodes.   A documented second episode is managed the same as the first. A third, or repetitive, pneumothorax is subjected to thoracotomy, stapling of blebs, and pleurodesis, which consists of abrading the parietal pleural surface, including the diaphragm and mediastinal pleura, with a dry sponge.

An uncommon complication is concomitant hemothorax. This results from a pleural adhesion to a vascular structure pulling away and injuring the vessel or just the tearing of a vascular adhesion. The source of bleeding may be an intercostal vessel, the subclavian vessels, or vena cava, and hemorrhage may be rapid and even massive, requiring urgent thoracotomy.

Spontaneous Pneumothorax Related to Emphysema

Pneumothorax as a complication of pulmonary emphysema is a greater problem. The patient with advanced chronic pulmonary disease tolerates the collapse and loss of functioning lung poorly. The nonelastic lung may show only 40 to 50% collapse on x-ray, yet a tension pneumothorax may actually be present. Extreme respiratory distress is common. Chest tube insertion is almost always necessary, and a bronchopleural fistula is frequently large. It closes very slowly or not at all, and recurrence is common.

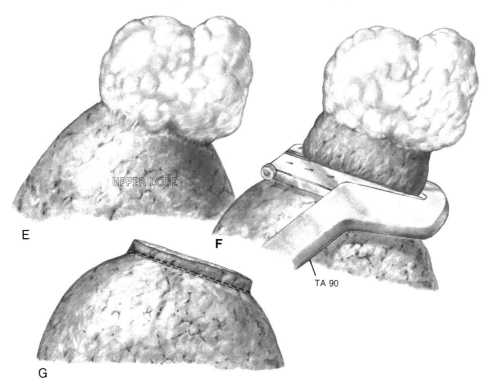

E

F

TA 90

G

Figure 7–21. *Continued.*

E, A diagrammatic illustration of a less frequent cause of pneumothorax, rupture of an area of bullous formation in a lung involved with emphysema.

F and *G,* A TA 90 stapling instrument is being applied. It should be applied to an area of more normal lung and not to the bulla, so that staples will be less likely to tear out with lung expansion. (Parts *E, F,* and *G* from Hood, M. D.: Stapling technique involving lung parenchyma. Surg. Clin. North Am., 3: June, 1984.)

8

Single Lung Transplantation

John H. Calhoon

Pulmonary lung transplantation is a new and evolving field. Much of this chapter reflects personal experiences with our own program in San Antonio. Single lung transplantation is a discipline that requires a great deal of intensive effort by the thoracic surgeon to effect a reasonable outcome. Unlike the routine pulmonary patient, who receives good preoperative selection, has appropriate technical success in the operating theater, and vigilant management in the postoperative period and goes on to a speedy and full recovery, the lung transplant patient can, even with the same attention to pre-, intra-, and postoperative management, have a devastatingly rapid demise from either rejection or infection at any time after their surgery.

Pulmonary transplantation, unlike its cousin, cardiac transplantation, has no easy way of accurate frequent end organ biopsy and surveillance. Routine bronchoscopy is not well tolerated by the pulmonary transplant recipient and, when he or she is doing well, it is difficult to get the patient to comply with routine bronchoscopic surveillance and biopsy. Even when bronchoscopic biopsy tissue is obtained or bronchoalveolar lavage pursued, the data gathered are difficult to interpret and often leave one puzzled as to how to prevent infection or rejection or both on the basis of the study. Lung transplantation also poses unique challenges to the thoracic surgeon because of the frequency of impaired bronchial healing, the constant exposure of the end organ to outside pathogens (unlike any other transplant) via the airway, and the performance of the transplant operation in the face of a contaminated field and specimen. Added to these concerns are the rather unique difficulties of ventilation-perfusion mismatch frequently seen with early donor lung dysfunction, recipient lung, ventilatory abnormality, and/or relative increased vascular resistance. Despite all these obstacles, pulmonary transplantation has become an established and accepted mode of therapy in the past few years.

A brief historical perspective reveals that, since Dr. Hardy's first report of a successful pulmonary transplant in 1963, over the ensuing 20-year period 38 transplants were performed worldwide with no long-term survivors. Dr. Joel Cooper and his group in the late 1970s became interested in lung transplantation, and in the mid-1980s reported on a successful series initially of seven clinical patients with five long-term survivors. Their success has spurred our group and others to pursue clinical lung transplantation vigorously and with success.

INDICATIONS

Indications for single lung transplantation vary from center to center and surgeon to surgeon. Most surgeons agree that indications include primarily pulmonary disease, i.e., a lack of other significant systemic illness such as diabetes or coronary disease, hypertension, renal insufficiency, and the like. Patients should be less than 60 years, and severe irreversible pulmonary dysfunction should be present. We have not found it necessary to completely wean patients from prednisone or other immunosuppressants before transplantation. Emphysema and pulmonary fibrosis have been our most common pulmonary diseases treated by transplantation. Contraindications to single lung transplantation include active infections; severe life-limiting systemic disease; renal or hepatic failure; drug, alcohol or tobacco abuse; and a history of poor medical compliance. Although initial success with pulmonary hypertension has been reported by our group, our current feeling is that pulmonary hypertension is probably best not treated by single lung transplantation at this time. Another relative contraindication in our experience is a history of steroid intolerance manifested by emotional, gastrointestinal, or skeletal complications. In particular, vertebral osteoporosis and a tendency to compression fractures have led to poor long-term results despite adequate pulmonary function. Septic lung disease must be considered a strong contraindication to single lung transplantation and is probably the one clear-cut indication for bilateral single lung transplantation at this time.

INDICATIONS FOR
SINGLE LUNG TRANSPLANTATION
- **Age $<$ 60 years**
- **Otherwise healthy**
- **Infection-free**
- **Pulmonary fibrosis**
- **Emphysema**

Note: **Exceptions to these indications may be made,**
but lead to increased morbidity and mortality.

DONOR SELECTION

Donor selection is an area that the successful lung transplant surgeon will not overlook. Time spent in ensuring that the donor has excellent lung function and no sign of infection, and ensuring appropriate donor management before and during procurement of a good lung graft is well spent. Ideally, the donor is a nonsmoker and relatively young. We use no preset age cut-off in the potential donor, but do tend to reserve grafts from older donors for older patients.

Selection should be based on careful review of the potential donor's history, physical examination, laboratory data, diagnostic test, and culture results. The potential donor should be scrutinized with the same care as the potential recipient. The first step is a good history. The nursing notes from the emergency room, the admission physical examination, or the emergency medical service record might all reveal a history of suspected aspiration. Any donor with probable aspiration should be discarded. Other factors in the history include the age of the donor, smoking and social history, intravenous drug abuse, previous pulmonary surgery, and any significant thoracic trauma and/or pulmonary contusion. The caretaker's assessment of the character and volume of the potential donor's secretions are useful. Grossly purulent secretions or a Gram stain with many white cells or fungi rule out lung donation. Po_2/Fio_2 ratio of greater than 300 is very important. Should the ratio be less than this and the patient have signs of volume overload or be without PEEP at the time of measurement, diuresis and/or PEEP can be used to improve the oxygenation ratio and recruit a potential donor. Should the ratio not improve, the other causes of interstitial water leading to a low ratio are aspiration, infection, and contusion, and all preclude lung donation.

Bronchoscopy has been used as a screening measure for potential lung donors, but when the history for lung injury is negative and pulmonary function is excellent, it seems unnecessary. If aspiration and/or infection is suspected, bronchoscopy is warranted. Adverse bronchoscopic findings of information or purulence preclude use of the lung.

Bronchoscopic lavage may show cultures or findings suggestive of mouth flora. These findings have led to adverse results. Length of intubation is associated with colonization of the tracheobronchial tree, and a period of longer than 3 days is a relative contraindication.

A complete serologic panel should be obtained, screening for HIV, hepatitis B and C, cytomegalovirus (CMV), syphilis, and ABO blood group. ABO incompatibility is an absolute contraindication for transplantation. Positive titers for hepatitis B and C, CMV, and syphilis are relative, whereas antibodies to HIV are an absolute contraindication. CMV-matched donor and recipient probably lead to decreased CMV related morbidity in the transplanted patient. Where possible, CMV donor recipient match is desired and transfusion of donor with CMV negative products and leukocyte filters is preferred.

Once a potential donor has been screened for serologic infectious or functional contraindications, size considerations should be studied. X-ray measurements of horizontal and vertical lung size, as well as chest circumference below the nipple line, are helpful. Predicted total lung capacity and vital capacity of the donor and recipient may be evaluated using measured height and weight. Recipient indication should be considered in donor selection because patients with COPD have different thoracic cavity size relative to body surface area from those with restrictive lung disease. Size discrepancies seem to be tolerated better than expected and are not absolute contraindications to transplantation and use of a donor. In general, the lung capacity of the donor should be the same as or slightly larger than the recipient's predicted total lung capacity. Occasionally the surgeon finds a particularly sick recipient on the list and considers the use of a marginal donor with deficiencies in one or several of the criteria aforementioned. **Use of a marginal donor should be approached with caution because it can lead to early morbidity and increased mortality.**

Donor Management

Once a potential donor meets brain death criteria, management commences. Brain death is associated with an outpouring of vasoactive substances, capillary permeability changes, and fluctuation in the hormonal regulation of the body's homeostatic mechanisms that make pulmonary and other organ donation difficult. Serum glucose, cortisol, and ADH levels may be very labile. Temperature regulation is also lost. A successful pulmonary donation can be obtained without detriment to other organ systems. Colloid blood volume replacement, inotropic support, physiologic amounts of PEEP, temperature control, and chest physiotherapy can maintain other organ systems while optimizing lung function. Specific donor measures should include nasogastric tube drainage to prevent aspiration, frequent tracheobronchial lavage, and probably prophylactic antibiotics.

Donor Procurement

Once a potential donor has been identified and pulmonary function optimized, the donor should be taken into the operating theater for procurement as soon as possible. An anesthesiologist should be in attendance to monitor the donor with attention to ventilator settings, fluid replacement, electrolytes and hemodynamics.

The most commonly used method of lung donor harvesting is that of static cold crystalloid flush. Most centers use Euro-Collins solution with or without minor changes. A variety of agents in addition to a Euro-Collins flush solution are being evaluated with respect to improve preservation. Promising agents include glutathione and other antioxidant compounds admixed with balanced salt solutions similar to Euro-Collins.

Donor lungs may be taken in conjunction with cardiac harvest. The right, left, or both lungs may be removed. The standard median sternotomy incision is performed with the aorta and both vena cava completely dissected. The pleura is opened longitudinally on the appropriate side(s) and the entire pericardium is excised from the diaphragm to the pleural apex, extending posteriorly through the phrenic nerve. The inferior pulmonary

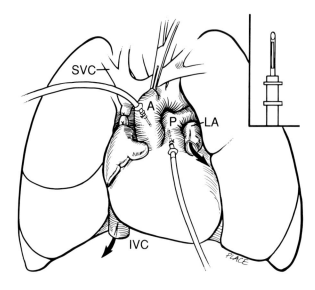

Figure 8–1. View via median sternotomy of heart-lung block ready for cardiac excision. Plegia lines are in place.

ligaments are incised to the lower veins. The right and left pulmonary arteries are released from the main pulmonary artery bifurcation to the pulmonary hili. When the organ harvest teams are ready, the patient is heparinized systemically. Prostaglandin E_1, (500μ g in 50 cc normal saline) is rapidly infused intravenously (Fig. 8–1). The superior vena cava is doubly ligated and divided. The inferior vena cava is transected. A high-volume Yankuer suction is inserted into the distal inferior vena cava to evacuate any hepatic perfusate. This step is appreciated by many liver transplant physicians. The tip of the left atrial appendage is transected before cross-clamping the aorta to minimize cardiac distention and decompress the left side of the heart. Two liters or so of Euro-Collins solution is infused in the pulmonary artery as the anesthesiologist continues to ventilate the lungs. Ventilation during the infusion of the pulmonoplegia provides even distribution of the preservative in the pulmonary artery vasculature. Simultaneously, infusion of cardioplegic solution in the ascending aorta is performed by the cardiac team. Ice saline slush should be placed generously over the heart and lungs. After completion of the pulmonoplegia and the cardioplegia, the heart may be excised leaving a small cuff of left atrium on the pulmonary veins (Fig. 8–2). This leaves plenty of left atrial tissue for the

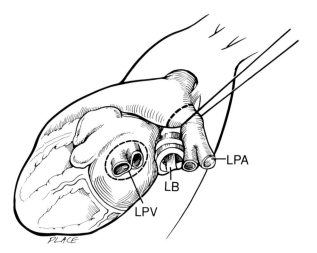

Figure 8–2. Appropriate lines of incision to allow separate lung harvest at time of cardiac excision.

cardiac surgeon to implant. The right and left pulmonary arteries are transected at their bifurcation. The heart is now removed in the usual fashion. At this point, cautery is used to divide mediastinal soft tissues to the level of the bronchus. **Care is taken to not devascularize the bronchus or clean it too vigorously.** The bronchus is doubly stapled and transected with the lung inflated. The lung(s) may then be completely excised and triply bagged, and subcarinal lymph nodes taken for tissue typing. This technique affords successful pulmonary ischemic times of up to 6 hours. Further experimentation with preservative solution should aid the protection afforded by the flush technique and further lengthen successful pulmonary ischemic times.

PULMONARY IMPLANTATION

Careful coordination of the recipient operation should be made with the procurement team. Time should be allowed for the successful induction of general anesthesia, placement of intracardiac and intra-arterial monitoring lines, positioning of the patient, and a thoracotomy with dissection of the hilar structures.

Anesthetic Considerations

A good thoracic anesthesiologist should be available. Single lung anesthesia has been obtained with the use of a standard endotracheal tube and a bronchial blocker on the left side or a double lumen tube for the right side. In the emphysema patient, we found that a bolus of colloid prevents poor cardiac filling with the advent of positive pressure anesthesia leading to a profound hypotension on induction and intubation. Additionally, low doses of dopamine in conjunction with several μ per kg per minute of nitroglycerin have aided cardiopulmonary stability during one-lung anesthesia during the time of pulmonary artery occlusion. Occasionally, a Siemens ventilator has allowed us to perform the operation without cardiopulmonary bypass on the otherwise very labile recipient.

Surgical Concerns

Once a patient is prepared for posterior lateral thoracotomy and broad spectrum antibiotics are given, the incision is performed in a generous fashion. In patients with predominantly emphysema, we have found the fifth interspace to afford excellent exposure, and for those with restrictive lung disease, the fourth interspace provides a better field. A retractor is placed and the lung deflated. The hilar structures are carefully dissected out, with care not to devascularize the bronchus as one encircles it and to open the pericardium anteriorly as close as possible to the pulmonary arteries and veins to maintain a large margin from the phrenic nerve. Electrocautery in this case may be used, but in decreased dose and with extreme care. The posterior veins are freed from the pericardium, and the bronchus is freed posteriorly as well. Inferior pulmonary ligaments are divided. A trial occlusion of the pulmonary artery may be performed. Should the patient be hemodynamically unstable with this, cardiopulmonary bypass will be necessary. The right chest allows easy placement of flexible cannulae in the atrium and aorta. In patients having a left thoracotomy, groin access is required. When a lung arrives, the patient is given 5000 units of heparin unless cardiopulmonary bypass is required, in which case full heparinization is performed. An angled vascular clamp works well on the pulmonary artery, placing it as close to the MPA as possible. A large Satinsky clamp can be placed across the left atrium as proximal to the pulmonary venous entrance as possible. The lung is then excised and hemostasis checked for. Bronchial arteries are either cauterized or clipped. On the left side, the bronchial blocker can be positioned with a DeBakey forceps by the surgeon in the mainstem. On the right side, a double lumen tube is already in place. The operation is technically facile. The pulmonary veins are sutured into place with a running 4-0 Prolene suture. The bronchial anastomosis is performed along the membranous portion with a running 4-0 Prolene suture; the cartilaginous portion allows telescoping the larger bronchus into the smaller one. The telescoping portion calls for secure figure-of-eight sutures to be placed around the cartilaginous rings of donor and recipient bronchus and removes tension from the membranous portion. Generally, the donor bronchus fits within the diseased and larger recipient bronchus. Occasionally, inspection before anastomosis reveals that the recipient bronchus would more easily overlap the donor bronchus, and in this case a "reverse" telescope is performed. Tying the figure-of-eight sutures naturally telescopes one ring inside the other (Fig. 8–3). In either case, **trim both donor and recipient bronchi as short as technically feasible to limit chance for ischemia.** With the bronchus intact, one may then start a running 4-0 Prolene pulmonary arterial closure. Before completing the artery anastomosis, the venous clamp is removed, allowing blood to "backperfuse" and vent through the nearly completed pulmonary artery anastomosis (Fig. 8–4). Partially air-freed in this manner, the anastomosis is cinched and tied, and the left atrium is needled along with the pulmonary veins to complete deairing. Hemostasis is checked for and achieved, and the lung is reinflated and placed immediately on PEEP. We close the incision with large PDS pericostal sutures and running Vicryl with skin staples. **Catgut sutures in the immunosuppressed patient have led to costal dehiscence and lung herniation.**

Posteroperative Management

Immediately after a procedure, patients are placed on mechanical ventilation using a Servo ventilator. Ventilator management is aimed at maintaining cardiac output while trying to ensure a relatively high mean airway pressure that will retard interstitial water accumulation. The newly implanted lung is susceptible to large amounts of interstitial water accumulation because of the phenomena of reperfusion injury, ischemic injury and possible hydrostatic changes. Ten millimeters of mercury PEEP with increased or even reversed inspiratory/expiratory ratios are often required for 36 to 72 hours. During this interval, paralysis, narcotics and vigorous diuresis are instituted. Pulmonary injury with resultant edema reaches a maximum of 8 to 12 hours postoperatively and then progressively improves. Recipients with some degree of underlying pulmonary hypertension develop tremendous ventilation perfusion mismatch and have increased hydrostatic pressures placed on the new lung, making them most difficult to manage. In all patients, aggressive pulmonary vasodilator therapy with nitroglycerin is pursued. Additionally, inotropic support with low doses of dopamine provides added hemodynamic stability and

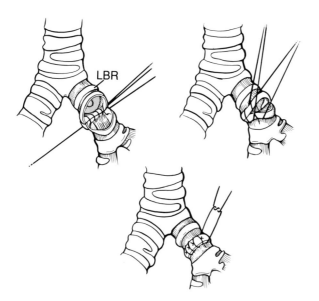

Figure 8–3. Telescoping anastomotic techniques. Trim donor and recipient bronchi short to limit ischemia. Figure-of-eight sutures around cartilaginous rings naturally promote telescoping effect when secured.

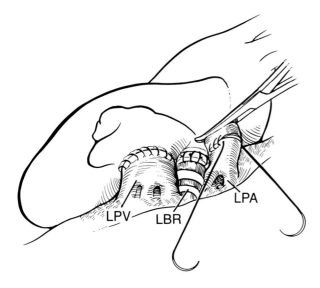

LPA

LPV LBR

Figure 8–4. Time for deairing. Remove venous clamp with native lung under gentle Valsalva pressure and the donor lung will retrograde air-free in several seconds.

diuresis. In severe cases of ventilation perfusion mismatch requiring high PEEP and high ventilatory pressures to maintain oxygenation, more potent inotropic and vasodilator therapy are required. In most patients with low pulmonary artery pressures, ample donor lung size and short ischemic times, postimplantation pulmonary edema is minimal and postoperative difficulty is rare.

Note: Our experience has been that attempts at extubation much before 48 hours postoperatively are met with frustration and morbidity.

Immunosuppressive Regimens

Lung transplantation is feasible today, as are all transplants, because of the advent of cyclosporine and triple drug immunotherapy. We have experimented with a variety of immunosuppressive regimens and currently use a cytolytic agent for the week after surgery in conjunction with triple drug immunotherapy. The perfect immunosuppressant regimen for lung transplants is not available, nor is the perfect regimen for other transplants currently. Each transplant patient is different and brings a different set of concerns, and it is my feeling that immunosuppression should probably be very carefully tailored to each individual recipient based on age, renal function, the number of antigens which cross match if any, and intangibles that we have not yet sorted out.

As pulmonary transplant patients are followed, one must be eternally vigilant of possible rejection or infection episodes. My own experience with daily pulse oximetry and bedside spirometry in the follow-up of a transplant patient has been positive. These aids only tell you when you have a problem, not what type it is. Pulmonary transplantation can be achieved successfully only through a team effort with the help of many fine transplant coordinators; a competent secretarial staff; and interested and dedicated colleagues in pulmonary medicine, cardiology, infectious diseases, and surgery.

RESULTS

Using these techniques and methods, we now have pulmonary transplantation being performed with actuarial survivals worldwide around 70% 2 years after transplant. In our own program, the intraoperative and early postoperative mortality has been zero in over 70 lung transplantations. The problem arises with the long-term follow-up of these patients because they continue to be prone to rejection episodes, allergic pulmonary reactions, long-term chronic rejection which takes the form of bronchiolitis obliterans, and finally, infectious processes that seem to be very difficult to totally eradicate once they are started.

Although it seems that the anastomotic problems have been solved, the problems of immunosuppression, rejection, and infection remain a challenge for those in the field. The postoperative management of a lung transplant easily correlates the amount of work generated by ten routine thoracotomies. Lung transplantation is the most time-consuming, yet rewarding, procedure that I have encountered to date.

9

Thorascopic Procedures

Homer S. Arnold

Thorascopic procedures have become the most popular subject in thoracic surgery. Thoracoscopy is not new. The Coryllos thoracoscope was used widely in the 1930s and 1940s. Its primary use was in lysing adhesions in patients with tuberculosis in whom artificial pneumothorax was to be used as a form of therapy. It also had a limited use in diagnosis.

The recent mushrooming of thoracoscopy has been, in part, the result of the availability of superior optics, the addition of video assistance, and the production of a wide variety of instruments that can be employed through additional ports.

The availability of the double-lumen endotracheal tube has also enabled the anesthesiologist to partially or completely collapse the lung, facilitating vision and operative procedures.

The procedure has been extended to perform a wide variety of operations, some of which seem to be nothing more than attempting to do, with difficulty and unnecessary risk, procedures more simply and safely done by conventional approaches.

The feature of a very short hospital stay makes thoracoscopy an attractive choice from the cost aspect. Unfortunately, it has become for some a fad and for some an opportunity for monetary return when a more major procedure might not be acceptable.

The procedure has been extended by some surgeons to include lobectomy and pneumonectomy, which seems to me to be unwise. Also, some have opted for local excision of primary lung cancer when the patient's condition and the stage of the disease make the patient a prime candidate for a curative resection. The evidence seems clear to the point that local excision leads to a greater incidence of local recurrence and is not an adequate operation for cancer.

Some surgeons perform a major pulmonary resection by means of the thoracoscope, requiring considerable expenditure of time and money. Then, at the end of the procedure, they make a thoracotomy incision to remove the specimen. This seems to be begging the issue and casts serious questions as to their motivation.

Since this manuscript first went to press, there has been and continues to be a constant, rapid improvement in instrumentation and electronics. Nonvalve ports and no-port techniques are evolving.

A definite feature of the thoracoscopic procedures is that training and experience under supervision are both necessary for safe, uncomplicated operations to be accomplished. This is not a field for self-teaching. Many good courses of instruction, given by recognized institutions, are available, and those choosing to utilize thorascopy should take advantage of these. (Ed.)

ANESTHETIC CONSIDERATIONS

Local Infiltration

It is possible to perform thoracoscopy under local anesthetic infiltration at the port site, using 10 to 15 mL of 1% lidocaine.

Advantages

1. Minimum equipment and instruments required.
2. The opening in the chest wall is adequate and tolerated well.
3. Spontaneous ventilation is possible without assistance.

Disadvantages

1. The awake patient may be apprehensive and may not cooperate adequately.
2. Some pain and discomfort are present.
3. The operating time is limited by the duration of the anesthetic agent and is short and insufficient in procedures requiring more than 30 minutes.

Indications

1. Diagnosis of pleural disease and pleural biopsy.
2. Visual diagnosis of intrathoracic trauma in patients in whom the extent of injury is not apparent.

Regional Anesthesia

The location of ports is plotted, and then from three to ten intercostal nerves are blocked intercostally, using 5 to 8 mL of 1% lidocaine injected into the center of the intercostal space. The anesthetic may be supplemented by the use of narcotic and neuroleptic agents given intravenously.

Advantages

1. Pain control is better than local anesthesia, and the patient is more sedated and quieter.
2. The open thorax is well tolerated.
3. Spontaneous ventilation is generally unimpaired.

Disadvantages

1. The technique is time-consuming and the presence of an anesthesiologist is required.
2. The patient may hypoventilate, with partial lung collapse and sedation and therefore require ventilatory assistance, which in turn may require general anesthesia.
3. The duration of the anesthetic agent, about 45 minutes, limits this technique to short diagnostic procedures.

Indications

1. Relatively short diagnostic examinations are the primary indications when visual inspection only is planned.
2. Small pleural or lung biopsies may be done.

General Anesthesia

1. General anesthesia without muscle relaxants and preserving spontaneous ventilation may occasionally be chosen when the patient is small or when a double-lumen tube cannot be used. The patient must not be a poor risk.
2. General anesthesia with the use of a muscle relaxant:
   A. A single-lumen tube is used with open thorax. This would be most useful in drainage and débridement in a patient with empyema.
   B. A single-lumen endotracheal tube is used in conjunction with a closed thorax and utilized CO_2 insufflation to collapse the lung. This is the approach in a small patient and in any situation where a double-lumen tube cannot be used.

C. A double-lumen tube is used in association with an open thorax. The majority of cases fall into this group.

D. A double-lumen tube is inserted and a closed thorax is used with CO_2 insufflation to collapse the lung. This technique is applicable when there is advanced emphysema with or without bullus formation. The inelasticity of the diseased lung, which results in noncollapse, is overcome with CO_2 insufflation.

Advantages

1. The patient is asleep.
2. There is no pain.
3. The thorax may remain open or closed.

Disadvantages

1. An anesthesiologist and full equipment for ventilation are required.
2. Tracheal intubation is necessary.
3. Special equipment of high technology level is required.
4. The expense to the patient is much greater.

Indications

These techniques can be used for all operative procedures.

Note

Intercostal block by way of one of the ports using marcaine and local infiltration of lidocaine will result in much less pain postoperatively.

TECHNICAL POINTS AND EXPERIENCE LESSONS

These are generally applicable to most operative procedures and facilitate thorascopic operations.

1. The surgeon must insist that the placement of the double-lumen tube is correct by using a fiberoptic tracheoscope or bronchoscope. Deflation of the lung may be difficult, and hypoventilation is an added risk.
2. The sites of ports to be used are marked on the chest wall before the surgical drapes are placed (Figs. 9–1 and 9–2). The plan for the procedure must be made at this time so that the position of surgeon, assistant, and video screen can be established.
3. The incisions should be small initially so that the pleural space can be kept closed in case the surgeon decides to use CO_2 insufflation. Each opening must be directed toward the site where the planned procedure is to be done. This ensures that the video camera will be able to see the area of surgery and that the instrument will be used properly.
4. The video screen should be facing the operator with the port placed to aim in that direction. The camera should keep the same orientation to the floor also.
5. Two display screens are useful, one on either side of the table.
6. Remember that if suction is used, the lung will expand unless there is sufficient opening in the chest wall to permit air to enter or unless CO_2 insufflation is used.
7. The surgeon should always have sufficient assistance so that the camera and retractors can be held without the necessity of changing hands (Fig. 9–3). The circulating nurse must be experienced in the management of video equipment.

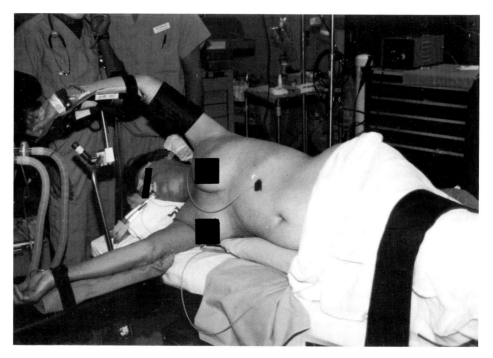

Figure 9–1.   Position of the patient after induction of anesthesia and insertion of the double-lumen tube, and before marking of port sites. Note the arm position.

8. When the surgeon has limited experience, it may be wise to work with a general surgeon who is experienced in laparoscopic procedures.
9. Practice using a training device, and assist in laparoscopic procedures to gain additional experience. Spend sufficient time to become familiar with the use of video equipment before actual use. Figures 9–4 and 9–5 show the instrument tray and fiberoptic scope, respectively.
10. Obtain an operative permit preoperatively for open thoracotomy in the event that a complication may arise or if the procedure cannot be completed as planned, to avoid having to terminate the procedure or proceed without a permit.
11. The chest tubes should always be inserted through a separate small tunneled incision. The port openings do not seal well when the tubes are removed.
12. When the visualization is poor, stop and correct the problem, checking the camera, videoscope, all connections, and any other source of problems. Do not proceed when vision of the operative field is poor.
13. At the end of the operative procedure, check carefully for pulmonary air leaks and do not terminate the operation with an air leak if it can be closed.
14. There is some postoperative pain during the first 24 hours arising from the pleura and incisions. Adequate analgesics are required. The pain should improve during the second day.

OPERATIVE PROCEDURE: MANAGEMENT OF PLEURAL EFFUSION

Patient Selection

The patient is usually referred, and is known to have a primary malignant lesion of the breast, gastrointestinal tract, or elsewhere, with a pleural effusion. The patient has usually

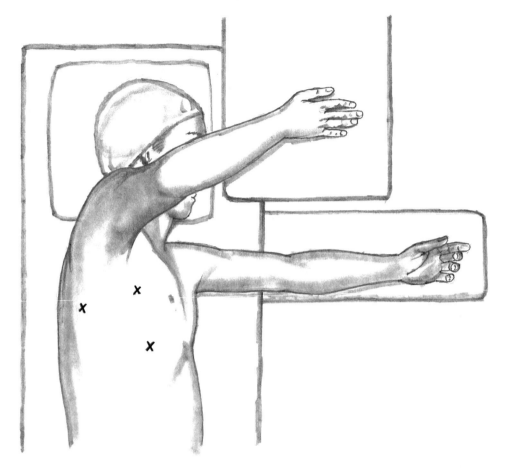

Figure 9–2. This diagram reiterates the position of the patient and shows the port sites marked before the skin preparation and draping.

had thoracentesis and a pleural needle biopsy, which may or may not have established the etiology of the effusion.

Preoperative Studies

The routine laboratory work that would normally be done for open thoracotomy should be done. A CT scan of the chest is necessary, seeking mediastinal adenopathy, a parenchymal lesion, or pleural nodules. The extent and localization of the effusion must be determined so that adequate operative visualization will be possible and complete drainage may be effected.

Anesthesia, Bronchoscopy

A general anesthetic using a muscle relaxant is necessary. The ECG/blood pressure and pulse oximeter are monitored.

Anesthesia is induced and a single-lumen endotracheal tube is placed. Bronchoscopy using a fiberoptic bronchoscope is then carried out to identify endotracheal disease. On completion of bronchoscopy, the single-lumen tube is removed and replaced with a double-lumen tube. The position of the tube is ascertained using a fiberoptic scope before placing the patient in position for operation.

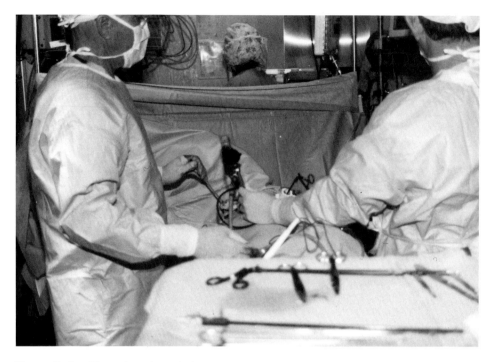

Figure 9–3. The orientation of the surgeon (left) and assistant to the operating ports is demonstrated. The videoscope screen is to the right at the head of the table. If two videoscopes are used, the second would be placed behind the surgeon and would better enable the assistant to stay oriented to the operative field.

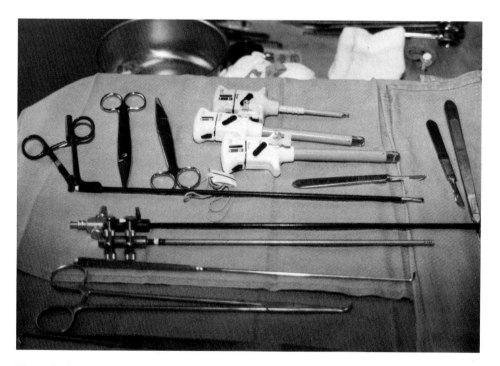

Figure 9–4. An instrument tray for thoracoscopy, with most instruments displayed except for the fibroscope.

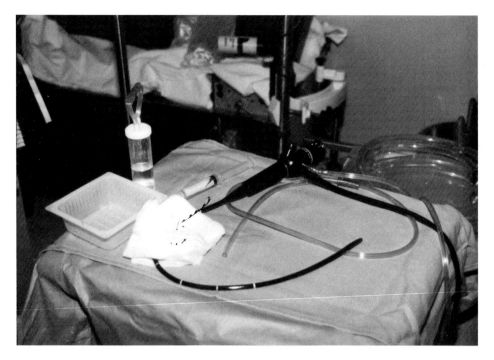

Figure 9–5.   Fiberoptic scope and its connecting cables to the videoscope.

Position

The patient should be placed in a full lateral position using an axillary roll to protect the axillary structures. The table is flexed. The sites of the ports to be used are identified and marked. The skin is then prepared and surgical draping for an open thoracotomy is done.

Procedure

The first incision is made over the region of the effusion as previously determined by CT scan, usually in the fifth or sixth interspace in the posterior line. A 10 mm port is inserted and the lung deflated. The contents of the space are aspirated and samples of the fluid are sent to the laboratory for cytologic study and culture.

The space is then inspected with the videoscope for evidence of neoplasm involving the pleura, lung, and mediastinum. An additional 5 or 10 mm ports are inserted which are used for suction tips, grasping forceps and biopsy forceps. This usually means three ports. One each in the anterior, mid, and posterior lines.

Assuming that a diagnosis of malignancy has not been established, biopsies are taken from suspicious areas and sent for frozen section examination.

Then, assuming that a diagnosis has now been made, the surgeon is faced with four choices of procedures to control the effusion:

1. **Chemical pleurodesis using 500 mg of Doxycycline mixed in a volume of 100 cc of water or saline.**
2. **Mechanical abrasion of the pleural surfaces with a dry sponge inserted through one of the ports, which has been enlarged.**
3. **Talc poudrage, 5 to 10 grams of talc in 100 cc of suspension.**
4. **Parietal pleurectomy.**

Each choice has a success rate of 60 to 80% except for pleurectomy, which is almost always successful.

The surgeon should now inspect each port and each biopsy site for bleeding and the lung for air leak. Electrocautery, hemoclips, or staples can be used. Suture is also possible.

Intercostal block, with video assistance, of several nerves in the operative area is now done using marcaine. A chest tube is inserted and properly placed under camera vision. The ports are closed and each site is infiltrated with marcaine.

The chest tube drainage begins to diminish and usually ceases in about 4 days, after which the chest tube is removed.

THORASCOPIC MANAGEMENT OF SPONTANEOUS PNEUMOTHORAX

Patient Selection

These patients are typically young individuals without evidence of lung disease and no history of trauma. An established air leak has been present for more than 48 hours. Patients with two or more episodes on the same side are candidates. At present, surgical treatment of remote and opposite side occurrence is open to discussion.

Preoperative Studies

Routine laboratory procedures and standard chest x-ray are done. CT examination has been recommended by some to identify blebs preoperatively, but I do not use it routinely in my practice.

The patient who has a chest tube in place should have the tube connected to a water seal system until after anesthesia has been induced and the patient turned into the lateral position.

Anesthesia, Bronchoscopy, and Double-Lumen Tube Replacement

A muscle relaxant is used and ECG and pulse oximeter are used for monitoring. Anesthesia is induced and a single-lumen endotracheal tube is inserted. Bronchoscopy is then done with a fiberoptic bronchoscope to search for endobronchial disease. On completion, the single-lumen tube is replaced with a double-lumen tube. The fiberoptic bronchoscope is used before and after positioning the patient.

Position

The patient is placed in the full lateral position, using an axillary roll. The table is flexed.

Procedure

Port sites are identified and marked and the skin of the chest is prepared and draped as for thoracotomy. A 10 mm port is introduced in the midaxillary line in the seventh or eighth interspace. The pleural space is inspected, and if adhesions are present, a 5 or 10 mm port is introduced in the anterior or posterior axillary line for retraction and lysis of all adhesions. This is done with electrocautery or blunt or sharp dissection.

The blebs and bronchopleural fistula are then identified, and saline irrigation and added ventilatory pressure are used to be certain of the air leak site. If the bleb and fistula are small, the bleb is elevated with grasping forceps encircled with an endoloop, and ligated. If it is a larger cyst, one port is enlarged to accommodate the stapling instrument. The area distal to the staple line may be left or excised. At this point, again using irrigation and ventilatory pressure, the site of the closure is inspected to be certain that there is no further leak. Additional staples, clips, or sutures may be required. The procedure is illustrated in Figure 9–6.

At this point, the surgeon must decide whether or not to do some form of pleurodesis. Cases should be individualized based on the pathologic findings and the surgeon's experience. Three choices are available:

1. Chemical—Doxycycline 500 mg in 100 cc of solution can be instilled and left in the pleural space.
2. Mechanical—The pleural space is abraded using a dry sponge on a sponge stick inserted in an enlarged port.
3. Talc poudrage.

The mechanical method is most often used.

The site of the resection and all port incisions are then inspected for bleeding and air leakage and appropriate corrective measures applied. Intercostal nerve blocks are done

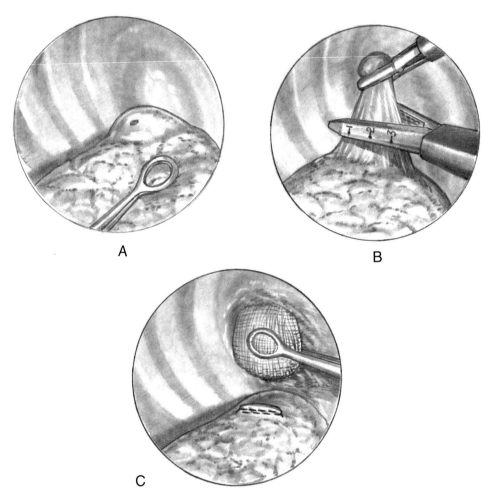

Figure 9–6. Spontaneous pneumothorax. *A,* The etiologic bleb or cyst is visualized through the videoscope. The point of rupture with its air leak is seen. This can be confirmed by submerging this area in irrigating solution and applying positive endotracheal pressure. *B,* The bleb has been grasped and elevated. *C,* The lung is being stapled proximal to the bleb. Staples or sutures do not hold well when applied to the thin-walled cyst. The area can be ligated as an alternative method.

using marcaine. This is done under videoscopic control through one of the ports. The chest tube is placed through a new incision and its position checked by videoscope.

The port sites are infiltrated with marcaine and then closed, suturing the musculature and subcutaneous tissue with absorbable material. The skin is then closed. The chest tube may again be checked with the scope for position.

Note

There has been a single failure with continuing air leak for 4 days. At operation, an electrocautery burn injury was the site of the leak rather than the original bleb and fistula. No infections have been seen.

THORASCOPIC MANAGEMENT OF BACTERIAL EMPYEMA

Patient Selection

Selection is usually from patients who have been under antibiotic therapy from 2 to 4 weeks and have had multiple thoracenteses. At this point, the pleural multiloculation is extensive and the pleural space contains considerable exudate and debris.

Preoperative Preparation

The extent of the empyema cavity and its location must be determined by CT examination or other means. CT is also useful in detecting mediastinal, parenchymal, or pleural nodules. The etiologic bacteria must be determined and sensitivity to various antibiotics ascertained.

Anesthesia, Bronchoscopy

General anesthesia with muscle relaxant with ECG and pulse oximeter monitoring.

After induction of anesthesia, a single-lumen endotracheal tube is inserted and bronchoscopy with a fiberoptic bronchoscope to exclude bronchial obstructive disease or other disease. The single-lumen tube is then replaced with a double-lumen tube and its position verified before and after positioning the patient.

Position

A full lateral position is used, employing an axillary roll and the table flexed.

Procedure

The port sites are determined and marked. The patient is then draped as for open thoracotomy. After reviewing films, make the first incision in the appropriate interspace in the posterior axillary line. A finger is inserted to verify that the empyema space is beneath the incision. Exudate is collected and forwarded to the laboratory for culture. A 10 mm port is inserted and the exudate is evacuated from the space and trabeculations broken down.

The video camera is inserted and the space inspected to search for neoplastic implants, size and extent of the space, evidence of parenchymal disease, and other pathologic processes. A second 10 mm port is inserted in the anterior axillary line in the interspace previously selected. The entry of the port into the pleural space is observed with the video camera.

Loculations are then completely broken up, using the suction tip and grasping forceps. The space is thereby fully developed and cleared of debris. The parietal pleural surface is debrided first, using grasping forceps or sponge forceps. The pleural coating of exudative membrane tends to keep the lung unexpanded and immobile.

After the parietal surface is as clear as possible, attention is turned to the visceral pleura. The surgeon must give particular attention to the fissures and must not be satisfied until the entire lung is mobilized. Some of the tissue removed should be submitted to the laboratory for pathologic study. Repeated profuse irrigation is used. Larger instruments should be considered, such as sponge forceps or a larger suction instrument, or sigmoidoscopy suction instrument, or whatever is necessary, if the débridement is difficult.

The videoscope should be withdrawn and moved from one port to another until the surgeon is fully satisfied that débridement of the space and the lung are complete, and with increased inflation the lung is shown to be fully expandable.

When the procedure is completed, the port sites and the entire operative field is carefully inspected for bleeding and saline solution is used to identify air leaks. Additional electrocautery, stapling, clips, or suturing may be required.

Marcaine is used to block several intercostal nerves under videoscopic control. The chest tube is inserted through a new incision and its intrapleural position verified with the videoscope. Operative sites are infiltrated with marcaine. The wounds are closed, using absorbable suture for the musculature and subcutaneous tissue. The skin is closed with suture, staples, or adhesive strips.

Postoperative Observation

The chest x-ray film may show considerable opacification for the first few days but shows progressive clearing. The patient may be febrile for the first 24 to 48 hours.

Antibiotic therapy is continued intravenously or orally. Wound healing without infection should be expected. Recurrence is a possibility and may suggest occult malignant or other disease.

EXCISIONAL BIOPSY OF PULMONARY NODULE

Patient Selection

These patients most often have a history of a prior malignancy and a pulmonary lesion discovered on follow-up chest x-ray. A CT scan has usually been done, and bronchoscopy and percutaneous thin needle biopsy have been attempted without a positive diagnosis. Also, patients of advanced age or with poor pulmonary function who are not suitable for a full thoracotomy may be subjects for thoracoscopic biopsy.

Preoperative Studies

A CT scan should be done if it has not already been performed. A careful study of the CT films must be done to localize the lesion exactly as to lobe, depth in the lung, and size. Pulmonary function studies may be indicated if respiratory status is unimpaired. Otherwise, routine laboratory procedures for anesthesia should be done.

Anesthesia, Bronchoscopy, and Double-Lumen Tube Placement

General anesthesia is induced and a single-lumen endotracheal tube is inserted. Bronchoscopy with a fiberoptic bronchoscope is performed to search for endobronchial disease. On completion, the bronchoscope is removed along with the single-lumen tube. A double-lumen tube is inserted and its position verified with a fiberscope before and after the patient is positioned.

Procedure

The sites of port placement are determined and marked. The chest is prepared and draped as for thoracotomy. A 10 mm port is inserted in the midaxillary line in the seventh or eighth interspace. A finger is introduced to be certain that no extensive adhesions are present and the pleural space is free. Pneumothorax is induced and the lung is allowed to collapse partially.

The entire pleural space and lung surface are inspected with the videoscope. A search is made for pathologic lesions not previously discovered by CT examination. A second port may be inserted at this time so that the lung may be retracted and adhesions divided, and to facilitate finding of the lesion.

The nodule is identified by video-vision if possible. If doubt exists, the port can be enlarged and a finger is inserted to palpate the nodule and lung. The lung should be allowed to become atelectatic as one means of delineating the nodule, particularly if it is subpleural. A ring or grasping forceps may grasp the lung to elevate it to the examining finger for better palpation.

A third port is established for entry of the stapling instrument. It should be far enough away from the lesion to allow application of the instrument. The stapling device or ligature carrier is positioned optimally for resection of the nodule. A large grasping instrument is used to pick up and elevate the nodule and place the adjacent lung in the stapling instrument. The lung is stapled and the lesion excised and removed. Figure 9–7 illustrates this procedure. A specimen removal pouch is recommended to prevent seeding of neoplastic cells into the chest wall.

A
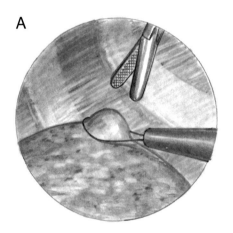

B
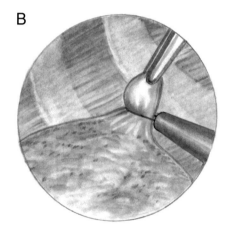

C
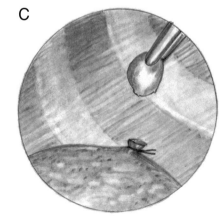

Figure 9–7. Excision of subpleural nodule. *A*, Subpleural nodule about 1 cm in diameter has been grasped and elevated above the lung surface. If the nodule is not clearly identified, a finger can be introduced through a port site to palpate the area. *B*, The area has been encircled with a ligature. After it is tied, the lesion is then excised.

The excision site is carefully inspected for bleeding and air leakage. Additional staples, cautery, or clips may be required. The ports are inspected and any bleeding points are controlled. A chest tube is placed through a new incision. The incisions are infiltrated with marcaine and closed with absorbable sutures for the muscle and subcutaneous tissue. The skin is closed with clips, sutures, or adhesive strips.

THORACOSCOPIC LUNG BIOPSY FOR DIFFUSE DISEASE

Patient Selection

Patients who are subjects for lung biopsy are usually referred by pulmonary internists. They have diffuse pulmonary interstitial disease and have usually already had extensive studies including bronchoscopy with transbronchial biopsy. A specific pathologic diagnosis has not been made. The question the surgeon is asked is usually, "Can you get a good biopsy?" The surgeon's answer is, almost invariably, "Yes."

Preoperative studies

Usually little is required. If a CT examination has not been done, it is necessary. On review, if there is evidence of hilar or mediastinal adenopathy, a cervical mediastinoscopy should be done before thoracoscopy. Otherwise, only routine studies are indicated as prerequisites for general anesthesia.

Pulmonary function may be marginal, and most patients have had no problems with thoracoscopy. Some patients with poor function studies may tolerate thoracoscopy with the addition of continuous partial airway pressure (CPAP) to the anesthesia ventilatory procedure.

Anesthesia, Bronchoscopy, and Double-Lumen Tube Placement

Monitoring should include ECG and pulse oximeter. A muscle relaxant is used.

General anesthesia is induced and a single-lumen endotracheal tube is introduced. Bronchoscopy with a fiberoptic bronchoscope is then performed to search for endobronchial obstruction, neoplasm, or other pathologic process. The single-lumen tube is replaced with a double-lumen tube, and its placement confirmed with a fiberscope before and after the patient is positioned.

Position

Full lateral, using an axillary roll with operating table flexed.

Procedure

Sites for port insertion are identified and marked. The patient is then prepared and draped for thoracotomy. A 10 mm port is placed, depending on the biopsy target area. It should be at some distance from the operating ports. The lung is deflated by opening the ipsilateral lumen of the double-lumen tube and opening the thorax.

The entire pleural space is inspected to identify unsuspected abnormalities and to define the area or areas of the lung to be biopsied. Additional ports are now introduced so that grasping forceps and stapling devices have good access to the designated site.

The area of the lung to be biopsied is grasped and elevated and the adjacent lung stapled. The biopsy specimen is then excised and sent to the laboratory. Studies requested may include permanent section, culture for acid-fast bacilli, culture for fungi, and any other indicated studies. If the specimen is too large to pass through the port, an endopouch can be used to extract the specimen.

The port incisions and the biopsy sites are carefully examined to detect bleeding or air leak. Immersion in saline solution and with increased ventilatory pressure must be the method of detecting air leakage. Electrocautery, restapling, clips, or sutures may be used to correct any problem identified.

Intercostal block of appropriate nerves is accomplished, with video assistance, via one of the ports. Then a chest tube is placed through a separate incision. The incisions are infiltrated with marcaine. The port incisions are closed, using absorbable material for the muscle and subcutaneous tissue. The skin is closed with sutures, staples, or adhesive strips.

Drainage may be expected for 24 to 48 hours, depending on the amount of fluid drainage and the duration of the air leak, if any.

Note

It has been possible to obtain a biopsy from the desired area and a pathologic diagnosis in all cases. No persistent bronchopleural fistulas have been seen beyond 48 hours. A single complication of empyema has been seen in a noninfected case.

THORASCOPIC CERVICODORSAL SYMPATHECTOMY

Patient Selection

The patients have vasomotor disturbances such as Reynaud's phenomenon, whether primary or secondary. Post-traumatic causalgic syndromes may also be managed by this procedure. Hyperhidrosis responds to this approach also.

Preoperative Studies

Studies in a vascular laboratory should be done to clearly identify the syndrome if possible. It is probably best to have performed at least three stellate blocks to be certain that vascular spasm is present, rather than vascular occlusive disease. Underlying collagen diseases must be diagnosed. It is doubtful that a surgical procedure is indicated in lupus erythematosus or scleroderma. Other routine laboratory procedures are accomplished.

Anesthesia and Double-Lumen Tube Placement

The patient is anesthetized and a double-lumen tube is inserted. Its position is verified by a fiberscope before and after positioning the patient.

Position

A full lateral position is used with the arm extended. An axillary roll is used and the table is flexed.

Procedure

The port sites are determined and marked. The patient is then prepared and draped as for thoracotomy. The port incisions are made and hemostasis is produced by electrocautery. Two ports are placed and the area of the sympathetic chain is visualized. With the scissors, the pleura is incised vertically overlying the chain, which can be seen through the intact pleura. A grasping forceps is used to grasp the ganglion and apply traction. Dissection is used to free up as much of the chain as the surgeon wishes to resect. Branches are clipped and divided as they are seen. Proximal and distal clips are applied to the main trunk superiorly and inferiorly. The structure is then excised and removed from the thorax. Figure 9–8 illustrates this procedure.

The site of resection is visualized repeatedly over several minutes to identify bleeding points. It is easy to injure intercostal arteries and veins as they may course over the chain. They may require clip, suture, or electrocautery.

A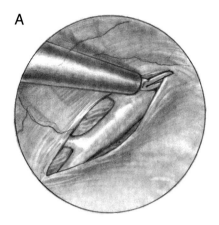

B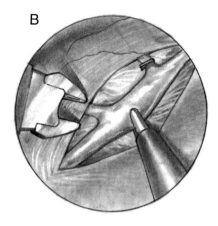

C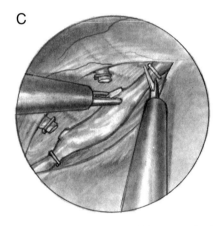

Figure 9–8. Cervical sympathectomy. *A,* The area of the sympathetic chain and stellate ganglion are being exposed by incising the parietal pleura. *B,* The ganglion has been grasped and placed under tension. Hemoclips are being applied to the branches from the ganglion. *C,* The sympathetic trunk has now had clips applied superiorly and inferiorly. The surgeon is now cutting the chain just above the inferior hemoclip.

Ports are inspected for bleeding. The chest tube is inserted and placed properly under videocontrol. Marcaine is injected to produce an intercostal block, also under video control. Port sites are infiltrated with marcaine.

The incisions are closed using absorbable suture for the musculature and subcutaneous tissue. The skin may be closed by sutures, staples, or adhesive strips.

COMPLICATIONS OF VIDEO-ASSISTED THORACOSCOPIC SURGICAL PROCEDURES

A lengthy list of major and minor complications has reported by others and experienced by the author. This emphasizes the fact that this form of thoracic surgery is major surgery and that the surgeon must use all precautions and care to avoid morbidity and the poor result that may ensue. These are listed by location:

Chest Wall

1. Hemorrhage from port site injury to an intercostal vessel or to other vessels in the wound.
2. Wound infection from internal or external sources.
3. Subcutaneous emphysema from a bronchopleura fistula or nonfunctioning chest tube.
4. Rib fractures.
5. Tumor seeding of operative wounds or tube tract.
6. Prolonged postoperative pain, usually intercostal neuralgia.

Pleura

1. Hemorrhage from operative site (lung, pleura, or mediastinum) or injury to a major vessel.
2. Empyema from operative contamination or dissemination from an abscess or localized infection in the lung.
3. Pneumothorax secondary to persistent air leak or nonfunctioning chest tube.
4. Recurrent empyema caused by inadequate drainage or improper tube placement.
5. Pleural tumor seeding from biopsy of a neoplasm of the lung or lymph node.

Pulmonary

1. Perforation or tear of the lung by:
   a. Trochar
   b. Excessive traction
   c. Inappropriate or poor biopsy technique
2. Air embolism
   a. Insufflation pressure in the presence of an open vessel
   b. Needle biopsy
3. Hemorrhage
   a. Parenchymal, from excisional procedures
   b. Pleural
   c. Injury to a pulmonary vessel
4. Bronchopleural fistula
   a. Site of operative invasion
   b. Missed leak (pneumothorax) at time of intervention
5. Re-expansion pulmonary edema
6. Atelectasis
   a. Operated side
   b. Contralateral side

10

Mediastinum

THYMECTOMY FOR MYASTHENIA GRAVIS

Indications

This has been an area of controversy for many years. The role of the thymus in myasthenia gravis is poorly understood; however, approximately 75% of patients manifest improvement following thymectomy, and approximately 30% sustain a permanent remission. Those in whom thymectomy is performed soon after diagnosis have better results than those operated on months to years following onset of symptoms. At present, most thoracic surgeons believe that thymectomy should be performed as soon as possible after muscular weakness appears. Myasthenia is more likely to improve when thymectomy is performed if there is no tumor present. Patients with thymomas may improve, but are less likely to.

Preoperative Preparation

Most patients with myasthenia gravis have been taking several drugs, which presents problems for the operative and postoperative periods.

Anticholinesterase agents are almost universally used. Patients should be weaned from these agents preoperatively. Plasmapheresis should be carried out preoperatively and assists in discontinuing anticholinesterase agents. Most patients are taking corticosteroids, and although it may not be possible to discontinue these drugs, the dosage levels can be reduced. Preoperative sedation should be minimal, and atropine should be avoided. Muscle relaxants should also be avoided.

The patient with respiratory insufficiency should be intubated while awake, using a nasotracheal tube. Prolonged postoperative ventilation is necessary in many of these patients.

Choice of Incision

The completeness of removal of the thymus tissue is a critical feature. Certainly a cervical incision can be used, but a large percentage of patients have some thymus tissue left behind. A partial sternotomy likewise produces poor exposure. A full median sternotomy is the incision of choice, and even then a cervical incision may be necessary to remove cervical thymus tissue. Cosmetic considerations should not play a significant role in choice of incisions; rather, adequacy of exposure should be the dominant concern.

Position

Supine.

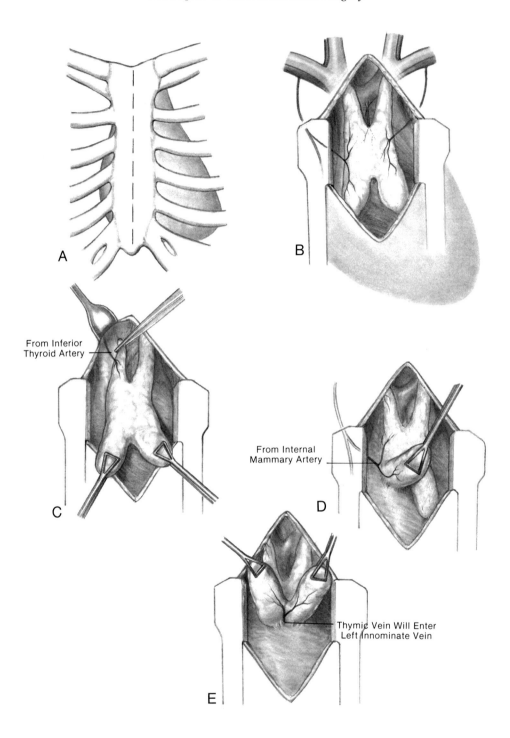

Figure 10–1. Thymectomy for myasthenia gravis. *A*, Median sternotomy is preferable to cervical approach. *B*, Exposure of thymus; note blood supply from the internal mammary artery. *C*, Additional blood supply is derived from the inferior thyroid artery. *D, E*, Sharp dissection is used, always being careful not to injure the left innominate vein. Thymic tissue should be excised totally.

Procedure (Fig. 10-1)

A median sternotomy incision is made and a retractor placed. The dissection is begun at the lower pole of either lobe of the thymus gland. A combination of blunt and sharp dissection is used to free the thymus from the pericardium and pleura. The thymic tissue usually dissects easily and cleanly. Should the dissection be difficult or should there be dense adherence to the pericardium, pleura, or any other structure, it is probable that a malignant tumor is present. The opposite lower pole is then dissected free and both lobes are elevated. As the dissection plane approaches the innominate vein, one to three thymic veins are encountered entering the innominate vein inferiorly or anteriorly. These should be doubly ligated and transected. The gland is deflected superiorly and laterally, and the dissection is carried into the thoracic inlet area. Typically, the upper pole extends well into the cervical area, becoming progressively smaller and containing less glandular tissue, terminating usually as a fibrous cord, the thyrothymic ligament. This may be ligated and severed when it is grossly apparent that there is no glandular tissue in the ligament at the level of division.

The arterial supply is derived principally from branches of the internal mammary arteries and usually poses no surgical problem.

The anterior mediastinum of some patients contains a large amount of adipose tissue surrounding the thymus. It may be difficult to identify the thymus with certainty; therefore, it is necessary to remove all of the adipose tissue in the anterior mediastinal area.

Thymic tissue may be detached from the anatomic thymus gland and be found at almost any point in the mediastinum, even as high as the superior pole of the thyroid gland.

Care must be taken to identify and protect both phrenic nerves during the dissection. The recurrent laryngeal nerves are not usually in jeopardy in this surgical field.

The pleural spaces should not be opened, but if an opening is made inadvertently, it should be enlarged and the pleural space drained by carefully placed tubes.

The field is carefully examined for remaining thymus tissue, for lymphatic fistulas, and for hemostasis.

The wound is then closed.

Note

Patients with prior respiratory distress may require prolonged intubation and occasionally tracheostomy for ventilatory assistance and control of secretions. The tracheostomy stoma should be placed above the thyroid isthmus, and the sternotomy incision should not extend to the suprasternal notch in an effort to keep the two fields separate.

MEDIASTINAL TUMORS

The variety of mediastinal tumor in origin, location, and size is almost endless, and a comprehensive surgical description for each variety is impossible. Therefore, only three surgical procedures are discussed here: resection of a posterior mediastinal neurogenic tumor, resection of an anterior mediastinal teratoma, and resection of a bronchogenic cyst. These represent three separate entities and perhaps serve as prototypes for resections of other neoplasms. Thymectomy has already been described as it is performed for myasthenia gravis, but the technique for resection of a thymoma, although essentially the same, has modifications determined by the pathologic process.

Figure 10-2 indicates the typical locations of the most common mediastinal masses.

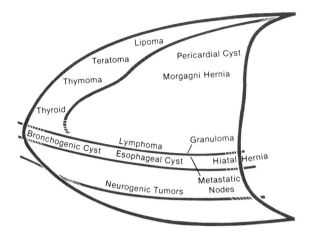

Figure 10-2. Location of mediastinal tumors.

RESECTION OF POSTERIOR MEDIASTINAL NEUROGENIC TUMOR

Indications

The most common posterior mediastinal tumors are neurogenic tumors. Several types occur, including neurilemmoma, ganglioneuroma, neuroblastoma, and phenochromocytoma. Determination of the exact type may be difficult and is not usually possible preoperatively. Many of the benign lesions have malignant potential, particularly ganglioneuroma.

The extension through the intervertebral foramen into the dural canal that commonly occurs makes the surgical approach more complicated. Some advise preoperative myelography. I prefer to include a neurosurgeon on the operating team so that the intraspinal extension, if present, may be managed without having to do a separate posterior laminectomy. This is usually not a difficult approach to the lesion. (Prior CT scan or lateral tomogram will establish involvement of the dural canal.)

Incision

Posterolateral thoracotomy.

Procedure (Fig. 10-3)

An incision is made and the pleural space opened through the fifth or sixth interspace, depending on the site of the neoplasm. After exposure has been obtained, the lung is retracted anteriorly and away from the area of the tumor. The neoplasm is inspected and evaluated for evidence of pleural, rib, and vertebral involvement. The relationship of the tumor to the sympathetic chain is determined.

The pleura is incised on the lateral surface and the tumor is freed laterally, superiorly, inferiorly, and finally medially. The most intimate involvement is to either an intercostal nerve or the sympathetic chain. Few sequelae result from sacrificing either. The gross appearance is often diagnostic in neurilemmoma and ganglioneuroma. The posterior dissection should be approached alternately from medial and lateral sides. The vascular supply is from intercostal vessels and should not pose a problem. As the area of the intervertebral foramen is approached, increasing care should be taken in the dissection to do this under direct vision, avoiding excessive traction and gently freeing the tumor. Involvement of the intervertebral foramen should have been diagnosed prior to surgery. If there is extension of the tumor through the foramen into the spinal canal, the

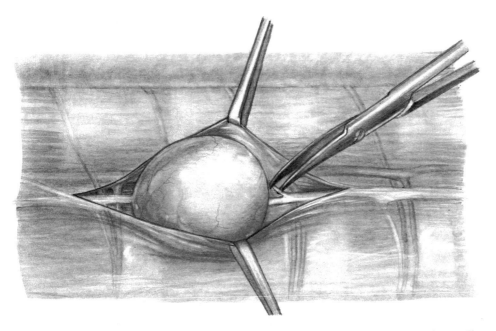

Figure 10–3. Technique of resection of neurogenic tumor of the posterior mediastinum. The pleura is opened and dissected away from the tumor. The tumor arises from an intercostal nerve or from the sympathetic chain. It may extend into the intervertebral foramen and require laminectomy for complete excision. Blood supply is from the intercostal vessels.

neurosurgeon should take over the procedure and perform a laminectomy so that the entire lesion may be removed intact without damage to the spinal cord.

There is usually no involvement of the lung or of the aorta unless the lesion is malignant and invasive outside its capsule.

Upon completion of removal, the area must be carefully inspected to be certain that hemostasis is complete. Also, the area of the intervertebral foramen must be examined for cerebrospinal fluid leakage. Any leakage must be controlled. Several methods are available. A simple one is to detach a single intercostal muscle anteriorly, dissect it free, and, with its posterior arterial and venous supply intact, suture it onto the area of the leak, closing it completely.

A single drainage tube is placed and the chest is closed.

RESECTION OF BRONCHOGENIC CYST (FIG. 10–4)

The nomenclature of cysts involving the bronchus, trachea, and esophagus is somewhat confusing. Cysts may be identical in location, size, and other features but be lined with either some form of gastrointestinal mucosa or a type of respiratory epithelium. The enteric cyst, bronchogenic cyst, and gastrointestinal reduplication cyst are actually similar lesions, because the trachea and esophagus are of common origin. Terminology can be based on the character of the lining epithelium. Most cysts occur in the mediastinum closely associated with the trachea, the esophagus, or both. The lesion may occur at any vertical level. Generally, bronchogenic cysts contain other elements of the tracheobronchial structure and may be more related to the trachea and bronchus than to the esophagus.

Position

Lateral.

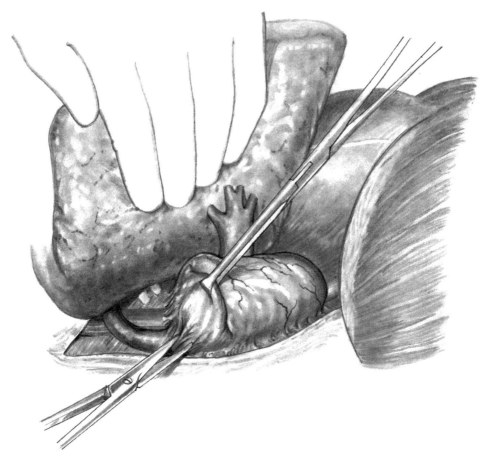

Figure 10–4. This illustration depicts a bronchogenic cyst in the mediastinum overlying the trachea and esophagus at the carinal area. Dissection is tedious and carefully done to avoid injury to either trachea or esophagus. The cyst may share a common muscular wall with either or both. Blunt dissection may be hazardous. View is from a right posterolateral thoracotomy. It is possible to produce an injury to the trachea or esophagus that is not grossly apparent. Using position pressure with the pleural space partially filled with saline will exclude tracheal injury. If esophageal injury is identified or strongly suspected, oversew the area and cover with pedicled pleura or muscle.

Incision

Posterolateral.

Procedure

An incision is made and the pleural space is opened through an appropriate interspace. The lung is partially collapsed and retracted anteriorly, exposing the cyst. Unless there has been erosion into the lung or the cyst has been infected, there are few if any adhesions. The pleura is opened either anteriorly or posteriorly, and the pleural incision carried transversely above and below the cyst. Dissection of the mass from its bed is usually begun inferiorly, retracting the cyst superiorly and laterally with the hand. The pleura can be left attached to the cyst in an effort to prevent opening the cyst. All surfaces except the medial one are freed. Bronchogenic cysts may have little blood supply or be extremely vascular. Dissection is generally easily accomplished unless the cyst either is infected or has been infected earlier. An active infection present at the time of surgery may destroy tissue planes and result in a difficult, bloody procedure.

It is usually possible to avoid entering the cyst, and unless an active infection is present, there is little consequence to inadvertently spilling the contents of the cyst.

The medial surface of the cyst is dissected free of the esophagus or trachea, whichever is closely involved with the cyst. The musculature of the cyst wall and either the esophagus or trachea may be common, and dissection results in opening either the cyst or the other structure. Great care must be taken to avoid opening either. Should an opening result, the resection of the cyst is completed, and then the esophageal wall is repaired using 4-0 Dexon or Vicryl reinforced with a second row of interrupted silk sutures. The trachea is best closed with 4-0 dexon or Vicryl as simple interrupted sutures. Presence of an air-fluid level on the x-ray film means that the cyst has eroded into the lung, tracheobronchial tree, or esophagus and that it is infected.

The blood supply is from local intercostal, esophageal, or bronchial arteries, and the venous drainage is to the azygos system.

If the cyst has recently been infected or is now infected, there will be marked edema and induration about the cyst, making dissection more difficult and hazardous. On occasion, it is easier to enter the cyst to be better able to find a dissection plane, and it may be wiser to leave a small portion of the wall of the cyst rather than risk damage to a neighboring structure.

Hemostasis is carefully secured. The pleural space is partially filled with saline solution to be certain that an air leak is not present. A single chest tube is inserted; if there is any persistent air leak from lung parenchyma, two tubes should be used.

The incision is then closed.

RESECTION OF TERATOMA OF MEDIASTINUM (FIG. 10–5)

In the past, a distinction has been made between dermoid cysts and teratomas based on an assumption that the dermoid cyst contained only ectodermal tissue, whereas the teratoma contained all three germinal cell layers: ectoderm, endoderm, and mesoderm. This is not realistic because both teratomas and dermoid cysts usually contain components of all cell layers. Almost any type of tissue may be found. Endocrine secretion may occur, and complications such as perforation can be the result of secretion of gastric elements. The malignant potential is relatively high. Teratomas most often occur in the anterior mediastinum, rarely posteriorly, and may be of almost any size. Presentation may be from compression of the trachea or bronchi or erosion into neighboring structures.

Position

Right lateral or supine.

Incision

A right thoractomy may be used. I prefer to use a median sternotomy. This description will assume that a sternotomy approach is used.

Procedure

A median sternotomy incision is made and a sternal retractor is placed. Relatively wide exposure is necessary if the tumor is large. The tumor, more often than not, presents to the right side. After initial inspection and evaluation, dissection is begun along the left side of the tumor, seeking a comfortable dissection plane. Unless the tumor is malignant and invasive, dissection is not difficult. Blood supply, while variable, usually arises in the superior mediastinum, principally from the internal mammary and pericardial vessels. The surgeon must constantly be aware of the position of the aorta, pulmonary artery, left innominate vein, and superior vena cava. It may be wise to remove an area of pericardium if there is no clear plane of dissection or if the tumor appears to be malignant. Invasion

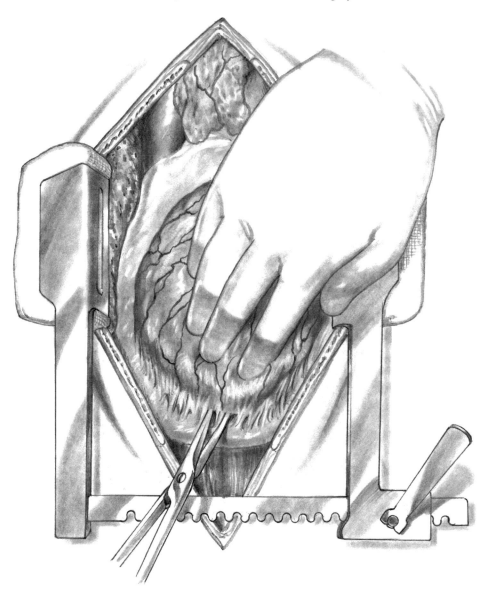

Figure 10–5. Resection of mediastinal teratoma. A view of beginning dissection of a large teratomatous lesion lying in the anterior mediastinum. Scissors are being used to dissect the tumor from the pericardium while the assistant's hand elevates the lesion. Most of the vascular supply will enter the tumor superiorly near the midline. If the tumor is malignant and invasive, dissection may be impossible and resection of the pericardium or adjacent lung may be required.

of pericardium, aorta, pulmonary artery, and lung may all occur. Careful examination, experience, and judgment are required to decide how extensive the resection is to be and at what risk. Certainly, an extensive resection in which tumor is left is not a wise choice. Pericardial resection poses no problem except for the phrenic nerve.

A malignant lesion may prove to be nonresectable. Whether removing as much of the tumor as possible as a debulking procedure is helpful or not is debatable, but probably it is not advisable.

A careful search for bleeding points should be made. Also, a careful inspection for lymphatic fistulas must be made. Control of both by suture and hemoclip is necessary. Electrocautery control of a lymphatic fistula is not advised.

A cystic lesion (dermoid cyst) may remain isolated or may erode into adjacent lung and establish a bronchial fistula with its lumen. These cysts may also become infected and enlarge rapidly, obstructing the trachea and displacing other structures. Involved lung may be resected transegmentally with the TA 90 or TA 55 stapling devices. Involvement of hilar structures is rare, but in some cases may require lobectomy.

Note

Cystic lesions of the mediastinum, including the teratomas, are uncommon in infancy, but when they do occur, they may produce severe respiratory obstruction by compression of the trachea or bronchus, necessitating urgent treatment. Intubation with the infant awake before anesthetic induction is a key point.

11

Pleura and Chest Wall

CHEST TUBE INSERTION FOR MALIGNANT EFFUSION

Many, but not all, pleural effusions that are massive are caused by malignant neoplasm metastasized to the pleura. It is often necessary to introduce a chest tube for drainage and for instillation of various agents to terminate fluid secretion. Whether related to malignancy or not, a significant mortality rate has been associated with this procedure, and in any major center, death or severe vascular collapse still occurs with unnecessary frequency.

The mechanism of respiratory distress, hypotension, and cardiac arrest following rapid drainage of fluid from the pleural space is poorly understood; several explanations have been advanced. Probably acute mediastinal shift is basic to most of these problems.

The following procedure is a didactic one, which may be unnecessary for many patients; however, no major sequelae are likely to occur if these guidelines are followed.

Salient Points

1. Use the basic technique as described elsewhere under *Chest Tube Insertion*.
2. Choose a surgical environment for tube insertion.
3. A small chest tube, No. 22 or No. 24, is usually adequate.
4. It is not critical that the tube be placed as dependently as for an empyema drainage, but by means of good chest films the surgeon should ascertain that the pleural space is free and that the effusion is not a loculated or a localized one. The sixth or seventh interspace in the posterior axillary line should be adequate.
5. Clamp the tube before insertion so that there will be no drainage of fluid until the tube is secured and the bottle connections are made.
6. Let 300 to 400 mL of fluid drain out and reclamp the tube.
7. Wait 5 to 10 min, let an additional amount drain, and reclamp the tube.
8. Stop immediately if the patient complains of dyspnea or pain, or if there is a marked change in vital signs.
9. Transfer the patient to the room or ward with the tube clamped and wait 20 to 30 min; then allow an additional 300 mL of fluid to drain, reclamp, and repeat at 10- to 15-minute intervals. If acute dyspnea or hypotension occurs, clamp the tube.
10. Do not leave the patient unattended at any time during this period.
11. If severe pain, marked respiratory distress, or hypotension is unrelenting, order a chest x-ray film immediately. Should the patient appear to be getting worse, disconnect the tube and allow air to enter the pleural space for about 10 seconds to re-establish the mediastinal position.

12. Do not apply suction until the x-ray shows the lung to be expanded, no mediastinal shift, and the patient is hemodynamically stable. Suction adds little to management of this problem.

Various agents such as quinacrine hydrochloride (Atabrine) and tetracycline may be instilled into the space, but this should be done before all fluid has been removed. The chest tube should remain clamped for 18 to 24 hours after instillation unless the patient has discomfort or x-ray shows rapid fluid reaccumulation.

EMPYEMA

Diagnosis and Management

Basic Considerations

Pleural fluid may accumulate for many reasons, so that accurate diagnosis of its cause is imperative. Brief mention of several examples will be made because etiology may modify the medical and surgical approach.

Pleural Tuberculosis. There are three general types: serous effusion, pure tuberculous empyema, and mixed tuberculous empyema.

1. Serous effusion. Tubercle bacilli may be difficult or impossible to recover. This has been thought by many to represent an allergic response of the pleura to the infection. However, with C-T examination, a parenchymal lesion not seen on the standard film is often seen and, with more sophisticated laboratory methods tubercle bacilli are usually identified. It requires no drainage or any surgical consideration.

2. Pure tuberculous empyema. This is produced when tuberculosis involves the pleura, which may be identifiable by pleural biopsy, and in which the pleural fluid contains tubercle bacilli (mycobacteria). This variety generally requires no surgical therapy, and inopportune chest tube drainage may serve only to secondarily infect the pleural space.

3. Mixed tuberculous empyema. Rupture of a tuberculous cavity into the pleural space will produce a pyopneumothorax wherein the pleural space is infected with *Mycobacterium tuberculosis* and with pyogenic bacteria. Surgical drainage is required and may be followed by more major procedures, such as decortication, resection, or thoracoplasty.

Mixed Anaerobic-Aerobic Empyema (Putrid Empyema). A primary or aspiration lung abscess may, without warning, rupture into the pleura. The immediate result is usually a tension pyopneumothorax. This is a catastrophic event, which requires immediate diagnosis, aggressive antibiotic therapy, and immediate surgical drainage.

The organisms are the flora of the mouth and teeth and include staphylococci, streptococci (microaerophilic), fusiform bacilli, spirochetes, and several gram-negative bacteria. This is a symbiotic infection.

The patient may not only have respiratory distress but also present with a picture of septic shock.

Thoracentesis is to be avoided, as is closed chest tube insertion. Both only help to spread the necrotizing cellulitis to the chest wall.

Immediate rib resection drainage is mandatory, preferably relying on clinical diagnosis only. By immediate is meant within the hour; even a delay of 2 to 3 hours may be fatal.

Staphylococcal Empyema. This entity has been seen principally in young children as a complication of staphylococcal pneumonia. Recently, in drug abusers, staphylococcal pneumonia has been noted as a complication of endocarditis and following mycotic emboli from infected areas elsewhere.

A characteristic feature of staphylococcal pneumonia is the formation of multiple pneumatoceles, which are prone to sudden rupture into the pleural space, resulting in tension pyopneumothorax. Empyema without pneumothorax may also occur. Individuals with pneumatoceles should be placed in an environment where constant observation is possible and where the facilities for chest tube insertion are always at hand.

Streptococcal Empyema. This is a relatively rare occurrence and usually complicates a major viral pneumonitis, such as influenza. The pleural fluid is usually very thin and produced rapidly. Early drainage is usually required. Open drainage is not necessary as a rule, and a simple chest tube in an appropriate intercostal space is usually sufficient.

Klebsiella, Pseudomonas, *Escherichia coli* Empyema. The gram-negative empyemas usually represent extensions from an area of pneumonitis, which is, in turn, the result of aspiration. These are most likely to be seen in elderly patients, in those on ventilators for extended periods, in those who are drug abusers or alcoholics, and in others with immunosuppression. More recently, Aerobacter and Proteus species have been included. Most are nosocomial infections. The prognosis has been generally poor. Other types of organisms may cause empyema, including fungi, but these make up a small percentage of pleural infections and will not be discussed here.

Empyema Management

This section is written briefly to emphasize key points.

When to Drain

1. **When any pleural effusion from which bacteria can be recovered is present.**
2. **When aspirate is frankly purulent.**
3. **When complete lung expansion is not obtained and maintained after thoracentesis.**
4. **When an air-fluid level is present, indicating a bronchopleural fistula.**

When Not to Drain

1. **When criteria for drainage are not present.**
2. **Tuberculous effusion not infected with pyogenic bacilli.**

Where to Drain (Fig. 11–1)

1. **Determine the anatomy of the empyema space. That is, determine its location, shape, volume, and most dependent level.**

Method

1. **Do a thoracentesis and inject 30 cc of air and 2 to 3 cc of iodized oil (Lipiodol) or oily propyliodone (Dionosil) into the cavity. Make posteroanterior, lateral, and decubitus films with "Bucky technique" or use a grid cassette and overexpose 10 kV.**
2. **Do not guess.**
3. **Drain at most dependent site; however, very rarely should a tube be placed lower than the ninth interspace.**

Intercostal Tube Drainage (See also Chest Tube Insertion, Chap. 4.)

1. **The procedure may be performed under local or general anesthesia.**
2. **Critically ill patients may require intercostal tube insertion in bed if tension pyopneumothorax is present. Revise in the operating room later.**
3. **Turn the patient into lateral position and strap in position.**
4. **Identify the rib and site to be drained.**
5. **Aspirate the area selected with a 10 mL syringe and No. 19 needle. If pus is obtained, move down one interspace; repeat the aspiration. Select the lowest space at which pus can be obtained. Make a 2 to 3 cm incision. Dissect bluntly with a hemostat until the pleural space is entered. Enlarge the opening and**

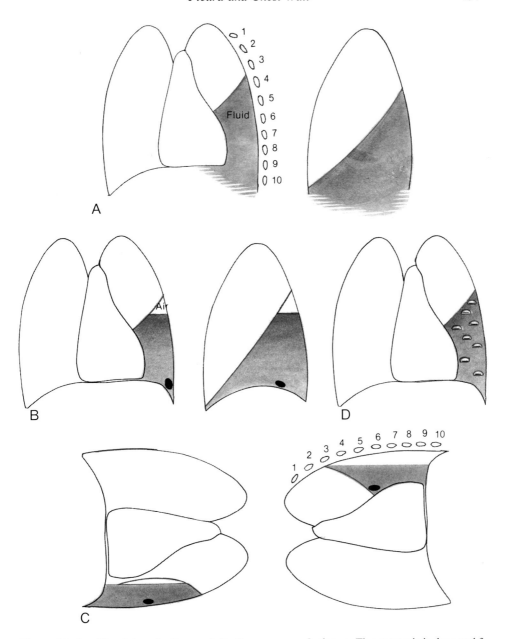

Figure 11–1. **The determination and site for empyema drainage.** Thoracentesis is done and 3 mL of heavy contrast material (Lipiodol, Dionosil) is instilled along with 50 cc of air. Films are made in the posteroanterior, lateral, and both lateral decubitus positions. The resultant films will show whether the space is unilocular or multiloculated *(D)* and the anatomic extent of the space in all planes. Dependent drainage is then easily accomplished.

explore the space with the finger. If the space is filled with fibrinous debris or is multiloculated, stop and convert to a rib resection. Otherwise, introduce a tube. Use the tube with the open end and only one side hole. Place the tube with the side hole just inside the pleura. Suture in place and connect to the chest suction system.

Rib Resection Drainage of Empyema

Position

Usually lateral. However, the condition of the patient may preclude a lateral position, and a supine or semilateral position may be necessary.

Anesthesia

Intercostal block and local infiltration or general anesthesia.

Procedure (Fig. 11–2)

For this discussion, it is assumed that studies have shown the most dependent part of the cavity to be posterolateral, at the level of the ninth rib. After positioning the patient, the skin is prepared and draped. A vertical incision is made, about 3 inches in length, centered over the ninth rib. The muscle is incised vertically and hemostasis is established.

At this point, a 10 mL syringe armed with a No. 18 needle is inserted into the eighth intercostal space. If the empyema space is entered, the needle is then inserted into the ninth interspace. No pus should be obtained if preoperative studies were interpreted correctly. Should the space be entered again, a lower space is then tapped as before. The selection of the rib to be resected is then finalized.

An incision is made in the periosteum with the electrocautery about 5 cm in length, and a transverse incision is made at either end. A periosteal elevator is used to remove the periosteum from the rib; a rib shear is used to cut the rib and remove it. The intercostal bundle is isolated, ligated proximally and distally, and resected.

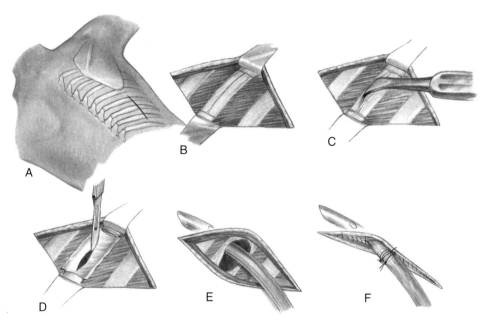

Figure 11–2.   Rib resection drainage of empyema. *A,* A vertical incision permits removal of the proper rib and gives access to additional ribs if necessary. *B, C,* The rib is resected subperiosteally, and the pleural space is opened through the periosteal bed *(D). E, F,* Tube insertion and wound closure following complete evacuation and irrigation of the empyema cavity and of fibrinous debris; also any loculations in the interlocular space are destroyed. The tube is inserted a short distance into the empyema cavity and has only the end hole and one side hole. The skin of the wound should be left open to prevent infection.

is guided through the periosteal bed and into the space. The incision is extended and the space is opened widely so that the exudate can be suctioned. A sponge forceps and repeated irrigation are used to remove fibrinous debris from the space. The space may be multiloculated and, if it is, it must be converted to a single space.

A finger should be used to explore the space to ascertain that the drainage site is dependent. If an error has been made, the drainage tube may be inserted through a lower intercostal space or an additional segment of rib resected.

A large (i.e., No. 32 or No. 36 French) tube with a single end opening and one side opening is placed so that the side hole is about 2.5 cm inside the cavity. The tube is sutured to the skin with heavy silk sutures, then connected to a water seal suction system.

The wound is partially closed using absorbable sutures for the musculature and the subcutaneous tissues. The skin is left open. A dressing is then applied.

Management of Empyema Tubes

1. Keep the tube open, with no dependent loops.
2. Measure drainage daily.
3. A bronchopleural fistula, if spontaneous and not a fistula surgically related to a bronchial stump, will probably close during the first week.
4. Obtain an x-ray film immediately postoperatively to check the tube position and degree of expansion and thickness of the pleural peel.
5. Obtain an x-ray film about every 3 days for the same reasons.
6. After the lung appears expanded for 2 to 3 days, discontinue suction and obtain chest films; if the lung expansion is maintained, leave only on water seal.
7. Measure the volume of the cavity by turning the patient to the lateral position and instill saline solution into the tube, measuring the volume used. Repeat this procedure every 3 to 4 days.
8. When the volume has diminished to less than 10 to 15 cc, perform a sinogram with diatrizoate sodium (Hypaque) to confirm that the space is obliterated.
9. Change and clean or replace the tube weekly and shorten by 2 cm each time. When the tract is extrathoracic, replace with a smaller tube (i.e., No. 18) and continue as before. Remove the tube when its length is less than 5 cm.
10. The chest tube may be converted to open drainage to permit ambulation or discharge at any time after lung expansion is maintained without water seal. Cut off the tube and secure it with a safety pin and strips of adhesive. The need to change dressing frequently will be determined by the quantity of drainage.

Reasons for Chronicity of an Empyema Space (Fig. 11–3)

1. The drainage site is not dependent.
2. The drainage tube is too far into the pleural space.
3. The tube placed is too low and occluded by the diaphragm.
4. The tube is too small. Never use a smaller size than No. 28, usually larger except in children.
5. Foreign material, such as fibrinous debris or blood clots, in the pleural space that has not been removed.
6. A bronchopleural fistula.
7. Specific infection, such as tuberculosis or fungal infection.
8. The pleural peel is too thick, indicating that either drainage was done too late or decortication should have been performed instead.
9. There is underlying disease, such as carcinoma, mesothelioma, or specific infection with parenchymal destruction.

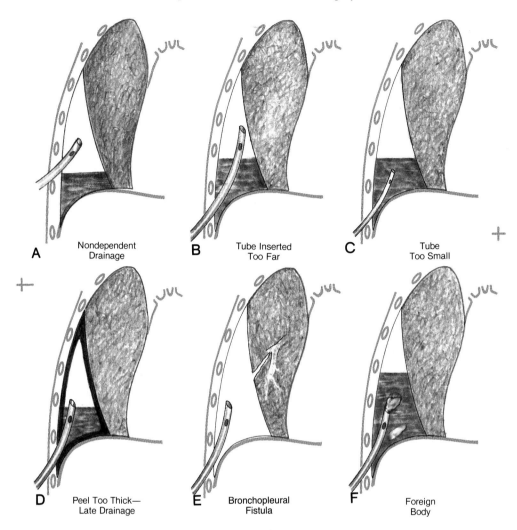

Figure 11–3. Reasons for failure of empyema drainage are several, and all represent failures in proper technique. Preoperative evaluation, planning, and technical adequacy should prevent any of these common failures.

Experience Lessons

1. **Perform drainage early and *correctly*.**
2. **Never do a thoracentesis on a patient with empyema resulting from rupture of a primary (aspiration, putrid) lung abscess, and never use closed intercostal tube drainage for this problem.**
3. **When an empyema caused by infection by mixed anaerobic organisms is drained by rib resection, close the muscle only; then pack the wound open and make no attempt at closure.**
4. **Wound infection can be prevented by leaving the skin and subcutaneous tissues open.**

Note

Technique of pleural decortication is discussed in the chapter on *Trauma*.

Closure of Postpneumonectomy Bronchial Fistula Following Pneumonectomy With Omental Graft (Fig. 11–4)

Position

Lateral.

Incision

Posterolateral thoracotomy.

Procedure

The incision is made by reopening the previous incision. Hemostasis is almost entirely by electrocautery if the surgeon stays in the old incision. The pleural space is opened. Additional rib resection is unnecessary unless a thoracoplasty is planned.

A second incision is made in the midline of the abdomen midway between the xiphoid process and the umbilicus. The incision should be long enough to provide adequate exposure. Usually a 10 to 15 cm incision is sufficient. The omentum is delivered and its length is estimated by laying it over the chest wall to the area of suture. It may be necessary to divide a portion of the omentum laterally to obtain additional length of the graft. The incision is retracted superiorly and a 5 cm incision is made in the diaphragm. After obtaining hemostasis, the omental graft is delivered into the thorax through an opening in the anterior area of the diaphragm. The opening should be large enough that vascular supply of the omentum is not compromised.

The area of the fistula is visualized and a decision made as to whether an attempt should be made to mobilize the bronchial stump and reclose it. This may be practical if the procedure is being done less than one month after the original operation. A fistula of several months' duration will be so embedded in scar tissue as to make dissection difficult and hazardous.

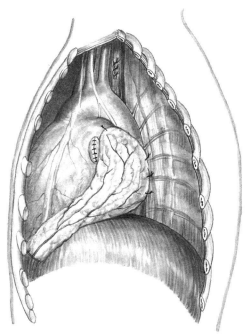

Figure 11–4.   Omental graft to close a bronchopleural fistula. This drawing demonstrates the anterior diaphragmatic opening through which the mobilized greater omentum is brought into the thorax to be sutured over the bronchial fistula.

The bronchus in the first instance is resutured using steel wire or prolene suture material. PDL may also be selected. The omentum is then sutured to the closed bronchus with interrupted nonabsorbable sutures. (Fig. 11–4). Closure of the fistula by direct suture may not be technically possible in some patients, and the graft will be used as primary closure.

After testing the closure with applied pressure of 30 to 40 mm of water pressure, the chest is closed. Pericostal sutures are preferred. The residual pleural space should be filled with dilute neomycin solution as described elsewhere.

The surgeon may elect to perform a thoracoplasty to obliterate the pleural space, as an alternative or myoplasty may be chosen.

Muscle Transplant To Obliterate a Chronic Empyema Cavity (Figs. 11–5, 11–6)

Recently muscle transplant (Fig. 11–5) has been popularized as an alternative to fill and obliterate a chronic empyema space. Any or multiple extracostal muscles may be mobilized, detached at one extremity, and placed in the pleural space, preserving the arterial supply of each muscle.

The advantage is that the unsatisfactory cosmetic result of thoracoplasty is avoided. However, the detachment of the principal muscles of the shoulder impairs shoulder motion and arm strength depending on the extent of the muscle transplanted.

Position

Lateral.

Incision

Posterolateral.

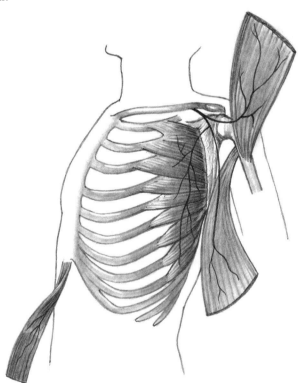

Figure 11–5. This drawing illustrates the principle of developing a vascularized muscle graft for intrathoracic transplantation. The rectus abdominis, pectoralis major, and latissimus dorsi and their blood supply are shown.

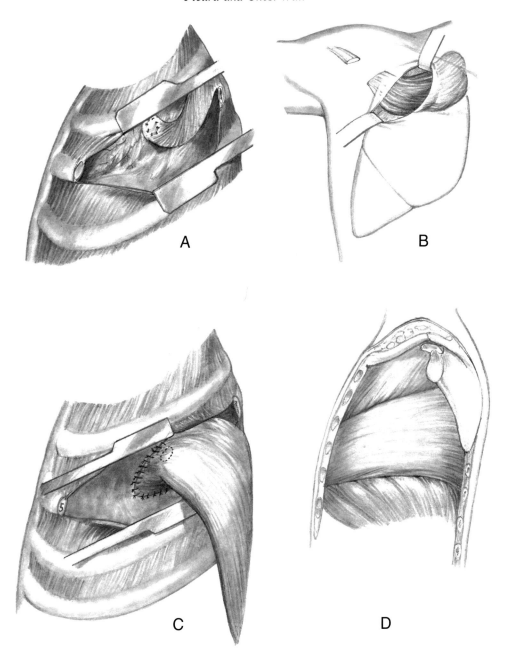

Figure 11–6. Diagram to emphasize the vascular base for muscle grafts used to close a postpneumonectomy fistula or to fill the postpneumonectomy pleural space.

A, Technique of using an intercostal muscle bundle to suture over a bronchopleural fistula.

B, Technique of using the pectoralis major for closure of a fistula.

C, Technique of using the latissimus dorsi for the same purpose.

D, A diagrammatic portrayal of using multiple pedicled muscle flaps to fill and obliterate a postpneumonectomy empyema space.

Procedure

A curved parascapular incision is made overlying the empyema space. No muscle transaction is done. A decision must be made as to which and how many muscles are to be transplanted.

In the case of the latissimus dorsi, it is mobilized and transected near its insertion into the humerus. Once it is mobile the site of entry into the pleural space is skeletonized and an 8 to 10 cm length of rib is resected and the empyema space is entered. The opening may be enlarged if necessary by resection of a second rib (Fig. 11–6A). The muscle is then gently placed in the empyema space and sutured in place with absorbable sutures. Suture of an area into and over a bronchopleural fistula may also be accomplished using prolene sutures.

The serratus anterior muscle may also be used, but its use will cause scapular deformity.

The pectoralis major (Fig. 11–6B) may also be used, but its use will require an anterior or anterolateral approach. As with the latissimus dorsi (Fig. 11–6C), the muscle is severed near its insertion into the humerus and an adequate opening is made by rib resection. The muscle is placed in the pleural space above, or either over or under a latissimus dorsi transplant, and sutured into place.

All of the above muscles and the rectus abdominus can be used at the same time to literally fill the residual pleural space. Some rib resection may be required in addition (Fig. 11–6D).

The skin incision is closed with adequate drainage by sump or Penrose drains.

Note

This procedure, like the Schedé thoracoplasty, should not be attempted early but deferred until the volume of the empyema cavity has been reduced in size to a relatively narrow space by contraction of the chest wall and diaphragm and by shifting of the mediastinum to the diseased side. If the procedure is attempted early, when the hemithorax is essentially normal in volume, the transplanted musculature will not even begin to fill and obliterate the space. This principle cannot be overemphasized because any attempt to obliterate the pleural space early will result in an unnecessary major procedure and will almost certainly fail.

Eloesser Empyema Drainage Procedure

Indications

This procedure establishes a permanent, skin-lined drainage of a chronic empyema space. It is used chiefly when the patient's age or general condition precludes a more major procedure, such as decortication, resection, or thoracoplasty. The space being drained is one that will not be apt to close spontaneously.

Advantages

1. **Requires no tube.**
2. **Little surgical care is required postoperatively.**
3. **A simple daily dressing change is the only care needed.**

Disadvantages

1. **A permanent, cosmetically displeasing opening is present.**
2. **Odor is occasionally a problem.**

Position

Full lateral position.

Procedure (Fig. 11–7)

The technique described under *Empyema Management* is used to determine the size, shape, location, and lowest point of drainage once this drainage site is identified; it is suitably marked. The patient is turned into the full lateral position. Exploratory thoracentesis is done to confirm which rib is to be resected by identifying the lowest point at which pus or air can be aspirated. Frequently, a previously placed chest tube is present. If so, and if its position is adequate, the tube is removed and this point becomes the lowest point in the center of the incision.

A U-shaped incision is made with the tip of the incision about 2 cm below the rib to be resected. The base of the incision lies superiorly and should be about 5 cm wide. The vertical limbs should be about 8 cm in length. The skin is reflected and a vertical incision is made in the latissimus dorsi muscle. The incised muscle is retracted, exposing the rib, which is resected extraperiosteally. The pleural space is entered through the base of the resected rib. The intercostal vessels and nerves of the resected rib are isolated, ligated proximally and distally, and resected.

The underlying thickened pleura is excised widely. The cautery is most useful for this procedure. The intercostal muscle superior to the resected rib is also excised. The skin flap is turned into the incision to determine if it is long enough to reach the intercostal space above the next unresected rib. An additional rib may be resected if necessary.

A nonabsorbable suture is then passed through the tip of the skin flap as a horizontal mattress suture. Each end of the suture is then attached to a large (4 to 5 cm) cutting needle, which is passed through the opening in the chest wall and then out through the interspace above the unresected rib and through the skin, leaving a bridge of skin about 1 cm between the two ends. The suture is then tied with minimal tension, thus bringing the skin flap into the pleural space and up the inner chest wall about 4 cm. The lower portion of the wound below the flap is partially closed with simple skin sutures.

The pleural space is manually debrided of as much debris as possible and irrigated. The wound is dressed with petrolatum gauze. The suture should remain for about 2 weeks before removal.

Note

The base of the skin flap may be oriented posteriorly if this appears to be better.

Claggett Procedure (Fig. 11–8)

Indication

Postoperative empyema without bronchopleural fistula following pneumonectomy.

Position

Supine or lateral.

Anesthesia

Local or general.

Procedure

An anterolateral site is selected to conform to the most dependent part of the pleural space as determined by radiograph. The anterior extremity of the original incision is usually satisfactory. A 6 to 8 cm incision is made in the old incision or a new incision may be made. The extracostal musculature is incised and the underlying rib exposed. A 5-cm length of the rib is removed. The pleural space is opened widely. All pleural fluid is aspirated and all fibrinous debris is suctioned or manually removed. The pleural space is

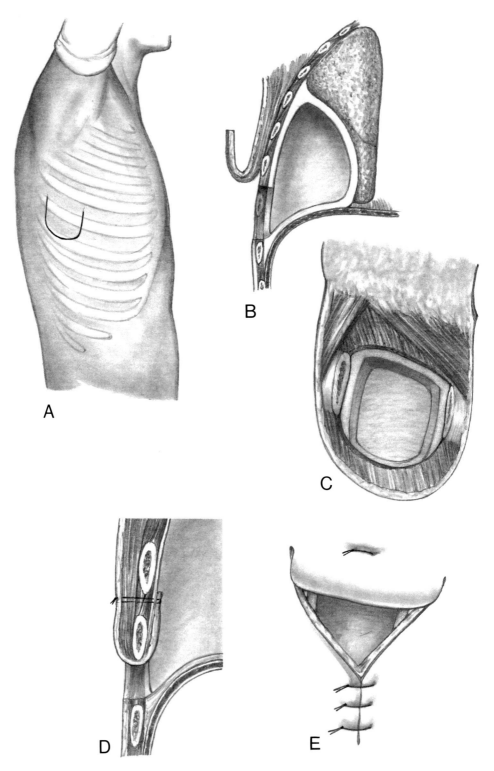

Figure 11–7. Eloesser flap. *A*, The position of the U-shaped flap should be over the rib preselected to be resected for dependent drainage. *B*, A section of rib is removed after the myocutaneous flap is developed. The parietal peel must be removed. *C*, View the flap elevated, the rib resected, and the empyema cavity exposed. *D*, The technique of turning the flap into the empyema cavity and suturing through the full thickness of the chest wall to secure it in place. *E*, The flap is in position and the lower portion of the wound is closed to narrow the area that will become a granulating wound.

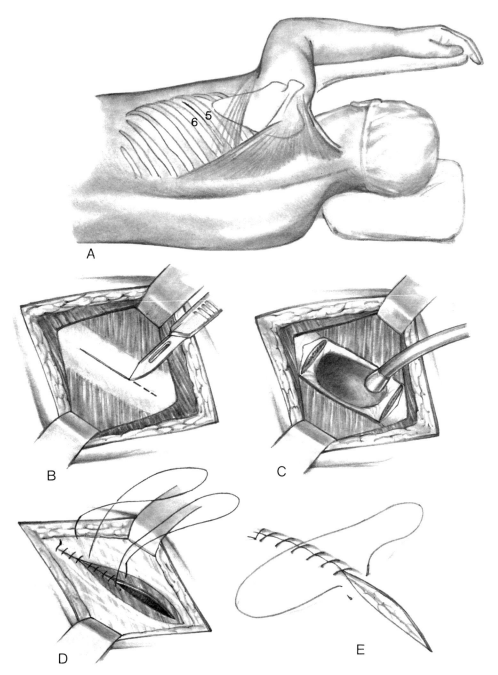

Figure 11–8. The Claggett method of pleural drainage following pneumonectomy. *A,* The incision is made near the lower end of the original incision. *B* and *C,* A small piece of rib is excised, and the pleura is opened. The pleural space is evacuated by suction and debridement. *D* and *E,* Six weeks later, the wound edges are excised. The pneumonectomy space is filled with 0.25% neomycin solution, and the wound is closed. (From Hood, R. M., et al.: Surgical Diseases of the Pleura and Chest Wall. Philadelphia, W. B. Saunders Company, 1986, p. 168. Used by permission.)

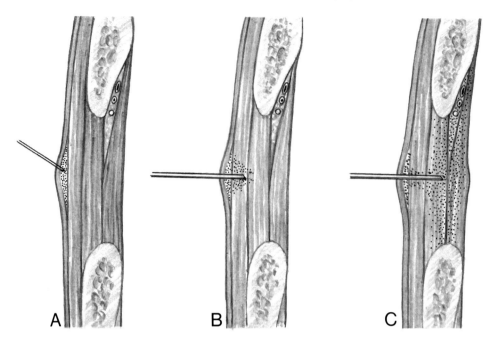

Figure 11–9. *A–C,* Techniques of local anesthesia to the chest wall before needle biopsy or thoracentesis. Adequate anesthesia should be produced and the procedure should be painless.

irrigated repeatedly with large volumes of saline. An irrigation solution of 0.25% neomycin may be used. The wound is then left open.

Six weeks later, the wound edges and all granulating surfaces are excised. The pleural space is irrigated with neomycin solution. The pleural space is then filled with 0.25% neomycin solution and the wound closed primarily without drainage.

Note

This procedure is successful about 50% of the time in sterilizing the pneumonectomy space. If it fails, the procedure may be repeated.

THORACENTESIS

This topic is discussed in greater detail elsewhere in this textbook (see chapter on *Trauma*).

INTERCOSTAL NERVE BLOCK (FIG. 11–9)

Intercostal nerve block using local anesthetic agents can be of significant benefit to the trauma patient with excessive pain from rib fractures and for relief from postoperative incisional pain. Unfortunately, poor technique has often resulted in further pain and unnecessary complications.

Anatomy of the Intercostal Space

Both an external intercostal muscle layer and an internal intercostal muscle layer are present. The intercostal nerve and vessels lie between these layers. Anterior to the angle of the rib, the neurovascular bundle is protected by the inferior margin of the rib above.

Posterior to the angle of the rib, there is no internal intercostal muscle, so that the nerve and vessels are essentially lying on the parietal pleura; consequently pneumothorax is more likely to result if the block is attempted in this area. The intercostal artery tends to lie in the center part of the intercostal space posterior to the rib angle and therefore is more vulnerable to injury here than it is farther anteriorly. An anatomic variant, the extension of the dural sheath laterally along the intercostal nerve for 2 to 4 cm, makes intradural injection of the anesthetic agent a possibility if the site of injection is too medial. These features determine, in part, the technique of anesthetic block.

Position

Lateral position.

Anesthesia

One per cent lidocaine (Xylocaine).

Procedure

The patient is placed in the lateral position and the intercostal nerves to be blocked are determined. The site of block should be at the rib angle or anterior to this point. Ribs are counted and sites are marked. A 10 mL syringe containing 1% lidocaine with a No. 25 to No. 27 needle is used to make an intradermal injection, producing a wheal of about 1 cm in diameter over each rib.

The small needle is replaced with a No. 20, 4 cm long needle, which is inserted into the anesthetized skin. The needle is advanced slowly, injecting a small amount of anesthetic until the rib is touched. The needle is "walked" off the inferior margin of the rib and advanced about 0.5 cm. No attempt is made to touch or locate the intercostal nerve. After aspiration, to be certain that no vascular structure is entered, 5 mL of anesthetic agent is injected without moving the needle further into the intercostal space. The needle is not maneuvered during injection.

This process is repeated with each intercostal space until the desired number of nerves have been anesthetized. About 10 minutes are required for maximum anesthesia. A band of anesthesia should extend from a point 5 cm anterior to the injection site to the midline anteriorly.

The duration of anesthesia may be prolonged by using epinephrine in the anesthetic solution or by using a longer-acting agent, such as bupivacaine (Marcaine).

The patient should be kept in a supine position for about 10 minutes because of the possibility of nausea or syncope secondary to hypotension. If dyspnea or chest pain results, physical examination or chest x-ray is mandatory to be certain that pneumothorax has not occurred.

Notes

1. **Do not inject at a site medial to the rib angle.**
2. **Do not try to touch the intercostal nerve with the needle.**
3. **Be aware of the complications of total spinal block and pneumothorax.**

PLEURAL NEEDLE BIOPSY

Position

Sitting or supine.

Anesthesia

Local, lidocaine.

Procedure

The site of thoracentesis and biopsy is selected. A skin wheal is produced using a No. 25 needle with 1% lidocaine. Subcutaneous, muscular, and intercostal infiltration with lidocaine is accomplished. A No. 18 needle is introduced into the pleural space to establish that fluid is present and a proper site has been selected.

A 2 to 3 mm skin incision is made with a No. 11 blade (Fig. 11–10). The Abrams needle is inserted into the pleural space. It is opened to be certain that it is in the space. The obturator is withdrawn slightly, and the biopsy blade is retracted against the pleura and the cutting sleeve is closed. This biopsy site can be lateral or inferior but not superior, for fear of injuring the intercostal vessels. The instrument is withdrawn and the biopsy specimen is removed. Second or third biopsy specimens may be removed through the same tract. Reinsertion of the instrument is necessary.

After the removal of tissue for biopsy is complete, the remainder of the pleural fluid may be removed after attaching a stopcock to the needle.

The patient should be carefully observed for about one hour for evidence of bleeding or pneumothorax.

OPEN PLEURAL BIOPSY (FIG. 11–11)

Indication

This procedure is useful when repeated needle biopsy specimens have been negative and there is an obliterated pleural space that will not permit needle biopsy without lung injury. Also, a larger pathologic specimen is obtained by this technique.

Position

Lateral or supine.

Anesthesia

General or local with intercostal block.

Technique

A 5 to 8 cm incision is made over a selected intercostal space. Hemostasis is obtained by electrocautery or ligatures. Electrocautery in an awake patient may stimulate muscle contracture and be less effective because the local anesthetic reduces conductivity of the tissues.

The intercostal muscle is incised and the parietal pleura exposed as widely as the incision permits. A circular area of pleura 1 to 2 cm. in diameter is excised. This should

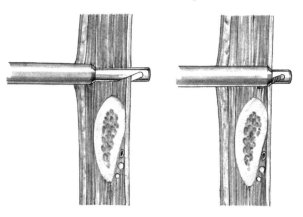

Figure 11–10. Technique of securing a biopsy specimen of the pleural lining by advancing the cutting cannula over the trochar tip. The biopsy forceps must not be turned superiorly to avoid injury to the intercostal vessels.

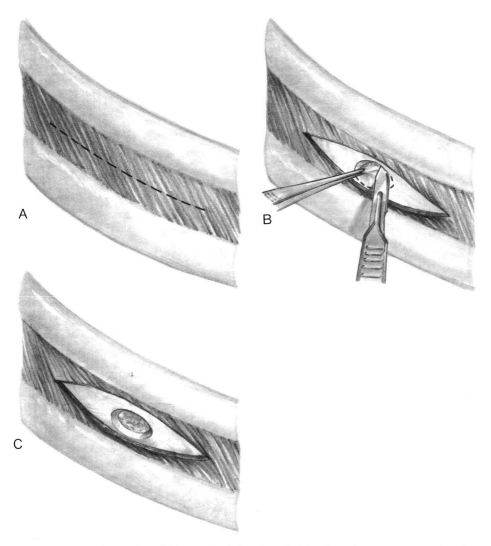

Figure 11–11. Open pleural biopsy. *A,* A 5 to 6 cm incision is made over an appropriate site. *B* and *C,* Through a small intercostal muscle incision, the parietal pleura is exposed, and a full-thickness disc is removed for biopsy. The surgeon must take care not to incise into adjacent, adherent lung.

be full thickness and accomplished with the scalpel rather than with electrocautery. The specimen may be divided for pathologic and bacteriologic purposes.

If the pleural space is entered and is free, a chest tube is inserted at a lower level. After hemostasis is complete, the extracostal musculature is closed with an absorbable suture and the skin and subcutaneous tissue closed. The chest tube may be removed later in the day or after 24 hours.

DRAINAGE OF SUBDIAPHRAGMATIC ABSCESS

Numerous methods have been advocated for the purpose of drainage of the subphrenic space. The most common method described in standard textbooks is that of draining posteriorly through the bed of the resected twelfth rib. Unless the abscess lies in this area, the abscess may be difficult to drain from this approach and the drainage tract will be unnecessarily long.

CT scanning has made it possible to localize a subphrenic collection accurately, making it possible to select the drainage site more accurately.

The technique described here is superior to the twelfth rib approach.

Procedure (Fig. 11–12)

By means of ultrasound, chest x-ray films, and CT scanning, the abscess is localized and the rib nearest to the collection is identified. A vertical incision 8 cm in length

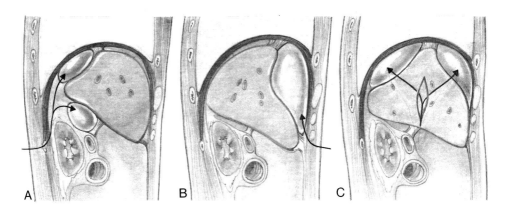

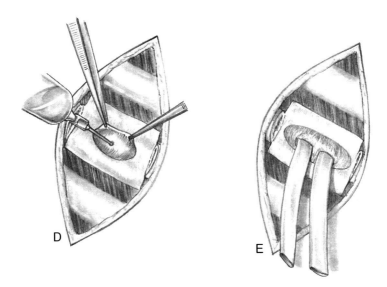

Figure 11–12. Drainage of subdiaphragmatic abscess.

A, The older method of draining a subphrenic abscess by means of a posterior incision with resection of the twelfth rib. The distance from the incision to the abscess is lengthy.

B, An anterior approach with the incision just below the costal margin. With this approach, injury to intraperitoneal structures is a risk.

C, Transthoracic approach through the periosteal bed of the resected sixth or seventh rib. Pleural synthesis must be present. This provides a simple, direct approach to most abscesses.

D, The technique of entering the abscess after carefully determining that the pleural surface is adherent to the diaphragm.

E, Appropriate drains are placed.

is made overlying this rib and the abscess. The musculature is incised and the rib cage exposed.

A 5 cm segment of rib is resected subperiosteally. The intercostal bundle is excised, and the parietal pleura is incised. Should the parietal pleura not be fused to the diaphragm, it should be sutured to the diaphragm with a continuous absorbable suture. The wound is then packed with gauze. Forty-eight to 72 hours later, after pleural adhesions have been ensured, the wound is reapproached.

A 3-inch No. 16 to No. 18 needle is used to identify and enter the abscess cavity. The needle is left in place and the scalpel or cautery used to open the diaphragm and enter the subphrenic abscess cavity.

After the space is evacuated, it may be packed with gauze, or sump drains may be left in the cavity. The wound is left open.

The pleural space is usually obliterated prior to surgical drainage so that the 48- to 72-hour delay described earlier is usually unnecessary.

Note

A complication of subdiaphragmatic abscess is erosion through the diaphragm with the production of either an empyema or a bronchial fistula communicating with the cavity. An empyema requires drainage of both the empyema space and the abscess cavity, whereas the bronchial fistula requires only abscess drainage.

REPAIR OF PECTUS EXCAVATUM

Indications

There are, without doubt, a few patients who manifest cardiac or pulmonary dysfunction because of severe pectus excavatum. In the vast majority of patients, however, the repair is solely for cosmetic reasons. Therefore, the potential improvement in appearance must be weighed, as must the results the individual surgeon has been able to accomplish, against the risk and complications. It is usually possible to effect a 90% improvement in a symmetrical pectus excavatum when the operation is performed in patients between the ages of 2 and 5 years. The results for asymmetric defects and in older children or adults are far less satisfactory.

Position

Supine.

Procedure (Fig. 11–13)

Numerous variations may be used. The description given here is probably the procedure most commonly used by the majority of thoracic surgeons.

The skin is prepared and draped, and a vertical incision is made in the midline from the level of inward displacement of the sternum to a point opposite the xiphoid process. Hemostasis is produced by electrocautery. Dissection is begun by incising the pectoral muscles about 0.5 cm from their origin and then dissecting the muscle and skin together from the rib cage. Penetrating vessels from the internal mammary and intercostal arteries are cauterized. The dissection should extend to the costochondral junction. Only one side need be dissected at this point. A cautery is used to incise the perichondrium from the sternum to very near the costochondral junction, which should be left undisturbed to preserve the growth center. The incision is "T"ed at both ends. A Freer elevator is then used to strip the perichondrium from the costal cartilage; usually the fourth cartilage is chosen first. The surgeon must try to avoid injury to the internal mammary vessels and pleura. The cartilage is divided near the costochondral junction lateral and as close to the sternum as possible and removed. Hemostasis is again secured.

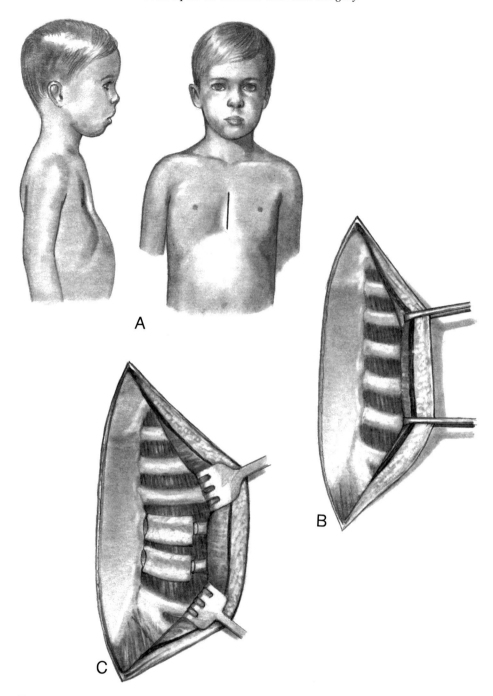

Figure 11–13. Pectus excavatum.

A, The incision is a short, vertical one. A transverse submammary incision produces a better cosmetic result in females.

B, The skin and pectoral musculature are reflected as a unit rather than separately.

C, Deformed costal cartilages are resected subperichondrially, usually beginning with the fourth.

Illustration continued on following page

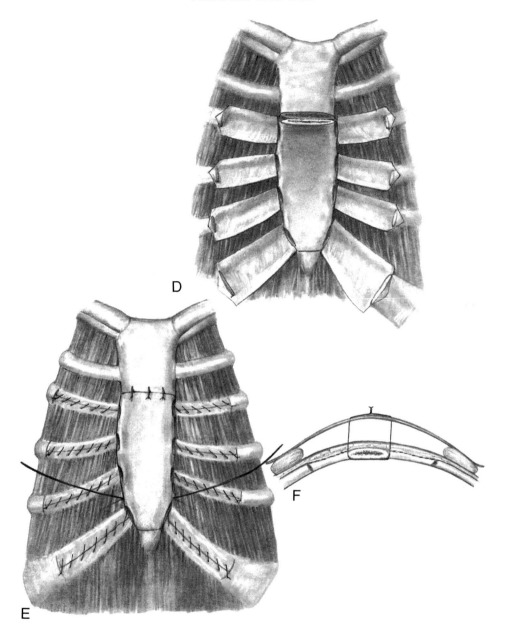

Figure 11–13. *Continued.*

D, The cartilage resection has been completed and transverse osteotomy of the sternum has been performed at the point of greatest angulation.

E, The perichondrium is closed with running 4-0 catgut or Dexon, and the osteotomy is closed with interrupted sutures of No. 28 steel wire. A No. 22 wire has been passed under the sternum and brought out lateral to the incision to be attached to an external support.

This process is repeated, removing only those cartilages involved in the deformity, usually the third through the sixth. The lower cartilage resections will require detachment of the rectus abdominis muscle.

The process of reflecting the myocutaneous flap and cartilage resection is repeated on the opposite side.

The sternum is exposed at the third costal cartilage or at the point of posterior deflection. A Stryker saw is used to transect the sternum completely. Older children or adults require a wedge osteotomy.

A heavy (No. 22) wire is then passed beneath the sternum, usually at the level of the fifth costal cartilage. There is a danger of injuring the mammary vessels and also of producing a pneumothorax if this is attempted from side to side. Preferably, beginning at the lower end of the sternum after resecting the xiphoid process, a substernal space is developed by finger dissection to the level desired, dissecting the pleura laterally. A wire can then be passed from the subxiphoid area to the external chest wall about 2.5 cm lateral to the sternal margin. The wire can be sharpened for passage through the skin by cutting it at an oblique angle; a No. 22 wire is usually adequate.

The transverse osteotomy is then closed by three sutures of No. 28 wires through the sternum and periosteum.

The perichondrium of each resected cartilage is closed with a continuous 4-0 absorbable suture. The pectoralis major muscle is resutured to its origin with 3-0 suture, either absorbable or nonabsorbable. The two muscles may be sewn together in the midline in the smaller child. The rectus fascia is reattached with similar sutures.

The subcutaneous tissue is closed with running 4-0 absorbable suture, catching the periosteum of the sternum to obliterate dead space. The skin is closed with a subcuticular suture of 4-0 or 5-0 absorbable material.

Any number of external support structures may be selected for attachment of the substernal wire. I prefer a wire spint padded on either end. The wire is brought to the support and the sternum is elevated to a slightly overcorrected position, and the ends are then twisted together.

Notes

1. **The technique of perichondrial stripping must be "learned" with each operation. The key is finding the proper space initially.**
2. **Some surgeons prefer not to use an external support. It is believed, however, that recurrence of the defect is more likely if it is not used.**
3. **The support may be removed as soon as the anterior chest wall is stable, usually 2 to 3 weeks in the 2 to 5 year old age group and 4 to 5 weeks in the older patient.**
4. **A variation, which I do not favor, is to resect the sternum, invert it, and sew it back into position.**
5. **An identical procedure may be used to correct pectus carinatum.**
6. **A variety of internal supports have been used to stabilize the sternum, but again it is felt that these give no better result than the technique described.**

CORRECTION OF PECTUS EXCAVATUM BY STERNAL REVERSAL

This procedure is an old procedure advocated by Ravitch and others for severe asymmetrical pectus excavatum. The procedure has been rarely used because (1) it is a more extensive procedure and (2) it uses the sternum as a free autograft. In smaller children, this should not pose a problem, but in older children the graft may not be successful and may necrose.

Position

Supine

Procedure (Fig. 11–14)

The incision is the same as that used for the usual pectus repair. Once complete exposure has been obtained, the sternum is transected at the point of deformity and the

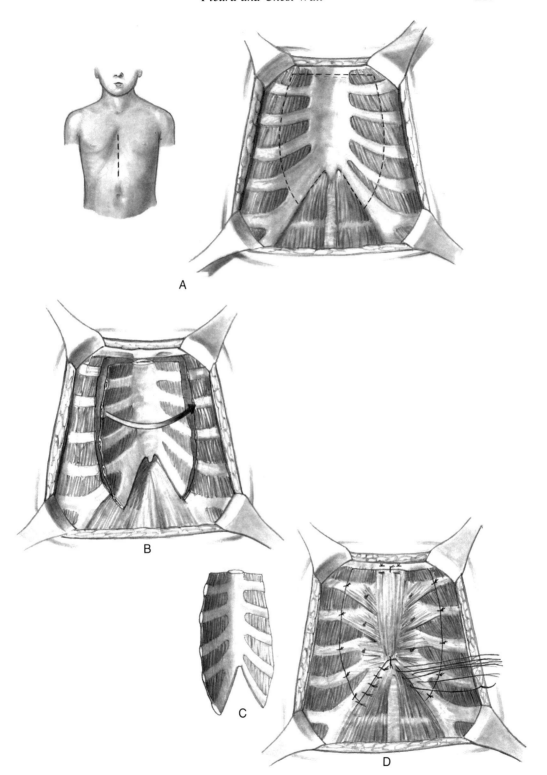

Figure 11–14.   Sternal reversal, pectus excavatum. *A*, Extent and lines of excision for sternal reversal.

B through *D*, Reimplantation of the inverted sternum. Chest tubes are not shown.

incision carried laterally and then inferiorly, as shown. Internal mammary arteries must be doubly ligated and each intercostal vessel ligated. The rectus abdominis is detached and the sternal plate freed by gentle blunt dissection, attempting not to open the pleura. The pleura will more than likely be opened, however. The plate is inverted. Three simple or horizontal mattress wire sutures are placed in the sternum and tied. Each costal cartilage is then sutured with a simple suture of nonabsorbable material. Chest tubes are placed if necessary through separate stab wounds. The pectoral musculature is then sutured to the sternum and sutured together in the midline if possible. The rectus muscles are reattached to the plate with multiple sutures.

A single sternal wire is placed beneath the sternum and brought out through the skin on either side of the incision at the fourth interspace level.

The wound is closed without wound drainage as previously described.

External support should be maintained until the sternum is stable, which may be longer than for the standard procedure.

RESECTION OF FIRST RIB OR CERVICAL RIB

Indication

Thoracic outlet syndrome.

Note

This procedure devised by Roos has gained great popularity. The first rib is the key to the outlet syndrome and, regardless of the anatomic cause, its resection and that of a cervical rib, if present, will relieve the patient's symptoms. The procedure has been carried out far too often, more recently even for pain syndromes related to trauma. The procedure is acquiring a bad name for this reason. When reserved for the relatively uncommon thoracic outlet syndrome, which is clearly established, it is a useful operation.

Position

Full lateral or slightly turned toward the back. The arm should be prepared fully and covered with a stockinette.

Procedure (Fig. 11–15)

A transverse incision 3 inches in length is made at the lower margin of the axillary hair. The incision is carried down to the chest wall, resisting the tendency to dissect superiorly too early. The lateral margins of the pectoralis major and latissimus dorsi muscles determine the anterior and posterior limits of the surgical field.

An assistant then grasps the arm, elevating it with moderate force, opening the axillary space. Blunt dissection will expose the upper three ribs. The cautery is used to detach the origin of the serratus anterior muscle from the second rib. The intercostobrachial nerve, arising from the second intercostal nerve, will be seen and should be preserved if possible.

The remainder of attachments of the scalenus medius and scalenus anterior muscles are then divided with sharp dissection. The exposure thus gained should expose the first rib well. Two Deaver retractors will be useful in gaining full exposure.

The first rib is then stripped free of its attachments. Most surgeons remove the rib subperiosteally, but it is better to remove the rib extraperiosteally to prevent bone regeneration in the area. The scalene tubercle of the first rib is a reliable guide to the location of the adjacent subclavian vein and the subclavian artery. Periodically, the arm traction should be relaxed for several minutes. The rib is then removed. A Bethune rib shear is used to cut the rib as far posteriorly as possible. Traction and torsion may be used to break the costochondral junction anteriorly, or the rib may be cut at that level. The remainder of the rib posteriorly is then removed with a Sauerbruch rongeur. Smaller rongeurs are difficult to use and control. The rib should be resected to the level of the transverse process. A common practice of cutting the rib in its midportion, then removing

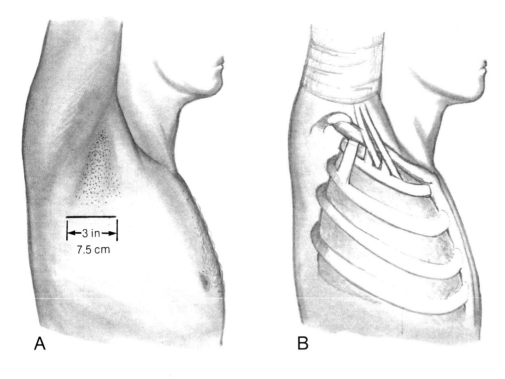

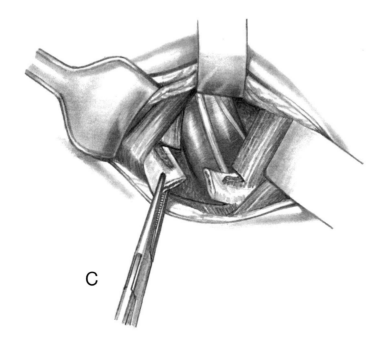

Figure 11–15. First rib resection for thoracic outlet syndrome.

A, The site of a 3-inch transverse incision at the hairline in the axilla.

B, The arm has been elevated and retractors placed, bringing the first rib into view and showing its relationship to vascular, neural, and muscular structures.

C, The rib has been transected and is being removed. Scalene musculature is divided. The rib resection should be extraperiosteal.

it piecemeal, is time-consuming and actually more hazardous. Hemostasis is produced with the cautery, and the wound is closed. Only the subcutaneous tissues and skin require closure. A Jackson-Pratt or similar type of drain may be left in place via a stab wound for 24 hours.

A chest x-ray should be made before the patient leaves the operating room to detect pneumothorax. A chest tube may be required if the pleural opening is large. Some surgeons prefer to put in a catheter through the wound and remove it at the end of the procedure.

Warning

Stretch injuries to the brachial plexus may occur, and care must be taken not to retract too heavily on the arm.

Should an injury to the subclavian artery or vein occur, it probably will not be controllable through this exposure, and bleeding should be controlled by packing while the patient is turned into the supine position; the area of bleeding is then approached by a cervical incision and clavicular resection. Control of the artery may be obtained on the left by opening the pleura through the third or fourth interspace through the original operative incision and clamping of the subclavian artery near the aorta. Even so, the patient must be approached through the cervical incision for repair.

PRERESECTION OR TAILORING THORACOPLASTY

Indications

Thoracoplasty, during earlier days, had its major indication for collapse of the tuberculous cavity. Today, its only usefulness lies in reducing the volume of the pleural space preceding or following resection and in obliterating chronic empyema spaces.

Resection of more parenchyma than one lobe, such as upper lobectomy plus superior segmentectomy, creates a difficult problem for the remaining lung to fill the pleural space. Previous parenchymal or pleural disease in a remaining lobe may prevent its expansion to an adequate size.

Ideally, the surgeon should anticipate the problem and add thoracoplasty to the procedure preoperatively or concomitantly. The principles that evolved many years ago for operative management are still valid, even though the procedure is performed for another purpose.

Position

Lateral.

Procedure (Fig. 11-16)

This discussion assumes that the procedure is being done as an isolated operation, although it may be associated with resection. A curved parascapular incision is made, extending superiorly to the upper scapular margin. The incision should be midway between the medial border of the scapula and the spinous process. A more lateral incision is liable to injure the accessory nerve. The latissimus dorsi and the lower 3 inches of the trapezius and the rhomboid muscles are severed. Then the serratus anterior muscle is divided as far distally as possible.

The exposure may be facilitated by stripping the periosteum from the superior surface of the fifth rib and placing one blade of a rib spreader against the rib and the other beneath the scapula. The subscapular space may then be exposed with minimal effort. The attachments of the serratus anterior muscle to the second and third ribs are divided as close to the rib as possible using the electrocautery. An effort is made to identify and preserve the intercostobrachial nerve arising from the second intercostal nerve.

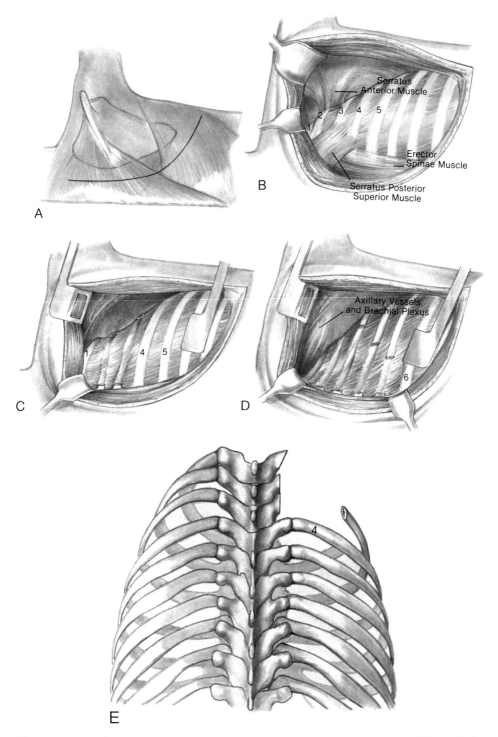

Figure 11–16. Extrapleural thoracoplasty. *A*, The patient is in the lateral position, and the extent of the skin and extracostal muscle incisions is indicated. *B*, The extent of exposure gained by this approach. *C*, The second and third ribs are resected, but the first rib is still intact. *D*, The extent of collapse following resection of five ribs in an effort to produce a uniform collapse anteriorly and posteriorly. *E*, Progressively less anterior rib is resected after complete resection of the first three ribs. *E*, The "squaring off" obtained by resecting posterior parts of the lower rib.

The extent of rib resection should be predetermined from the chest x-ray and from the resection planned. Usually three or four ribs are resected. Some surgeons prefer to leave the first rib intact; however, should an empyema space later result, its management may be made more difficult.

Resection is begun by stripping the periosteum from the third rib, leaving its anterior one third intact. The Haight and Alexander periosteal elevators are well designed for this procedure. The Doyan elevator is not a good instrument and usually leaves periosteum on the rib and injures the intercostal muscles. The rib is cut posteriorly within 1 to 2 cm of the tip of the transverse process. The Bethune rib shear is the most suitable instrument for rib resection. The anterior transection should be 3 to 4 cm lateral to the costochondral junction.

The second rib is removed in a similar manner except that it is removed totally. The insertion of the scalenus medius muscle must be severed. The first rib is approached by first severing the attachments of the scalenus anterior muscle to the rib. The inferior or lateral edge of the rib is then stripped. Next, the superior surface of the rib is cleared of periosteum. Lastly, the inferior surface is stripped. The superior or medial edge is then approached with the finger above, and the periosteal elevator is applied firmly to the rib edge. The scalene tubercle is a guide to the location of the subclavian vein and must be cleared carefully. Once the rib is free, it is cut posteriorly and then grasped with a bone-holding forceps and retracted inferiorly and medially while the anterior extent of the rib is cleared. Usually the rib fractures at the costochondral junction and does not require cutting.

A decision can be made at this point as to whether the fourth rib should be resected. If it should, only the posterior half need be resected. Attention is then directed to the remaining rib and transverse process posteriorly. The sacrospinalis muscle is detached and retracted, and the elevator is used to clear the medial surface. Attachments of the sacrospinalis muscle to the transverse process must be cut with the Mayo scissors. The elevator is used to complete the exposure of the rib and process. A Sauerbruch rongeur is then used to first resect the rib and then the process flush with the lamina. The first rib is resected to the tip of the process and the process is left intact.

Hemostasis is then secured with electrocautery, and the incision is closed without drainage.

Notes

1. **Use of the periosteal elevator requires considerable force, which must be controlled to prevent slippage and injury to the lung or subclavian vessels.**
2. **The tip of the rib shear is always directed superiorly and advanced only as far as the rib edge.**
3. **The rongeur is placed with the cutting edge in an anterior-posterior plane so that the lamina will prevent entering the spinal canal and injuring the cord.**
4. **Good hemostasis is necessary to prevent formation of a subscapular space hematoma and secondary infection.**

SCHEDÉ THORACOPLASTY

Indications

1. To obliterate an empyema cavity following pneumonectomy.
2. To manage an empyema cavity when the lung cannot be decorticated and expanded because of advanced parenchymal disease.
3. To close an empyema space in a patient whose general medical status does not permit extrapleural pneumonectomy or in a patient with a localized empyema space in whom decortication is not possible.

Schedé thoracoplasty is deforming, cosmetically undesirable, and, to a degree, disabling. The primary object is to close a chronic empyema space and allow complete healing without drainage. The surgeon must weigh the physical deformity against the disability and the threat of chronic empyema. The patient must be fully informed of the expected result and physical appearance following this procedure. This type of surgery is not often required, but when it is indicated, there is no other procedure or recourse, and the surgeon should not be reluctant to recommend this operation.

Preoperative evaluation must be exacting, and preparation should bring the patient to optimal condition. Many of these unfortunate patients are undernourished, sometimes

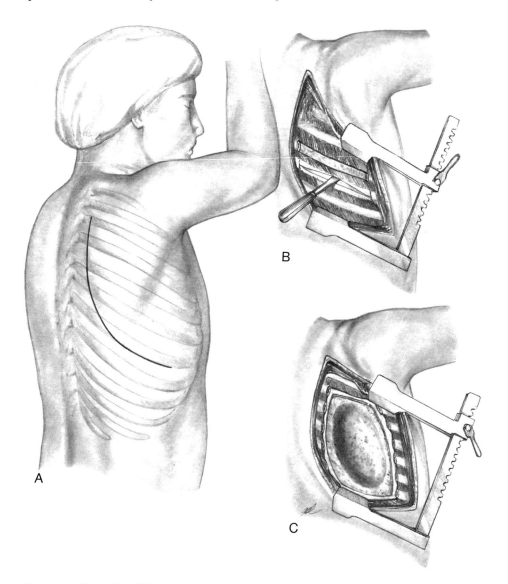

Figure 11–17. Schedé thoracoplasty.

A, Position of the usual incision, which is carried much higher posteriorly than is a thoracotomy incision.

B, C, Rib resection is begun. The ribs may be resected as shown in *B,* or the chest wall may be removed as a plaque by progressively cutting intercostal muscle and ribs *(C).* The rib resection must extend to the point at which there is no "overhang," and the thickened parietal pleura excised to completely unroof the space.

even cachectic. Control of infection, transfusion, and even a period of enteral or parenteral alimentation are necessary components of the preoperative period. To embark on this procedure without having instituted these measures is usually disastrous.

Position

Full lateral.

Procedure (Fig. 11–17)

This description proceeds on the basis that the problem is a postpneumonectomy empyema. Empyemas of lesser size require modification to adapt to the problem at hand.

The incision should begin at the level of the superior margin of the scapula, midway between the spinous process and the medial border of the scapula. It then sweeps inferiorly and anteriorly, passing about 6 cm below the tip of the scapula and ending in the midaxillary line about 5 to 6 cm below the nipple in the male or in the inframammary fold in the female. The electrocautery is necessary in making this incision and throughout the procedure; otherwise blood loss may be excessive.

The extracostal musculature is incised. Hemostasis is accomplished after the entire incision has been made. A rib, usually the sixth, is resected subperiosteally. This may occasionally be difficult because of the triangular thickening and irregularity acquired by ribs overlying an empyema of long duration. Also, contraction of the chest wall with narrowing of the intercostal space makes the rib section difficult. The rib may be resected by incising the intercostal muscle with the cautery as close to the rib as possible. The cautery is then used to cut through the periosteal bed and thickened parietal empyema wall into the empyema cavity. A second rib, usually the next lower one, is resected, and again the periosteal bed is incised. This now leaves the intercostal muscle as a "ribbon" attached at both ends.

The space can now be explored to determine its extent and to make an accurate appraisal of the extent of the chest wall resection needed to completely unroof the empyema cavity. Successive ribs are removed, and the posterior periosteum and empyema wall are incised. The thickness and rigidity of the pleural peel must be managed by excising the empyema wall from each intercostal muscle bundle with the scalpel or preferably with the cutting current of the electrocautery. Excision of this peel leaves the intercostal muscle as a thin, pliable, vascularized ribbon of muscle, which is able to fall in and partially fill the cavity.

Successive ribs are resected until the entire cavity is completely unroofed. There must be no overhang of chest wall, but the cavity should be completely saucerized, leaving the walls sloping outward. Each rib must be resected several centimeters beyond the edge of the cavity.

The surgeon must then return to each rib posteriorly, resecting the remainder of the rib as far as the transverse process, after which the transverse process and rib are resected to within 1 to 1.5 cm of the lamina of the vertebra. The transverse process of the first rib and the rib medial to the process are not resected. Rib disarticulation is undesirable and actually enlarges and deepens the empyema cavity posteriorly. The length of rib resection anteriorly is determined entirely by the extent of the cavity. Occasionally the first rib may be left intact if the empyema space does not extend to that level.

After the rib resection is completed and the parietal peel has been removed from each intercostal muscle, these are allowed to fall into the cavity. Hemostasis is then made as certain as possible. Three or four large Penrose drains are brought out at different levels from the upper to the most dependent portion of the space and wound. They are sutured to the skin edges securely. The wound is then closed in layers with absorbable sutures, leaving the skin open but closely approximated with subcutaneous absorbable sutures.

Occasionally, a bronchopleural fistula may be present. The fistula will be seen clearly on completion of the chest wall resection. Closure of the fistula is best accomplished by detaching one of the intercostal muscles anteriorly and suturing it securely into the fistulous opening after scarifying the area about the fistula. The rhomboideus major muscle or even the latissimus dorsi muscle may be used for this purpose.

Postoperative Management

There is rather profuse drainage for the first 48 hours, gradually diminishing over several weeks.

The drains should be removed one at a time, beginning with the most superior drain at 1 week, with the most dependent drain being withdrawn slowly no sooner than 6 to 9 weeks after the procedure. Wound infection is uncommon despite the contaminated field unless the skin is closed. Early ambulation and arm and shoulder physical therapy should be begun. Extended physical therapy is necessary to prevent severe scoliosis.

Notes

1. **The leaving of intercostal groups to partially fill the space is a modification from the original procedure that may, at times, be practical. At the least, it preserves the intercostal nerves and prevents undesirable anesthesia. The thickened empyema wall must be resected from each intercostal muscle if this structure is to be left.**
2. **The standard procedure is to excise the chest wall en bloc, leaving only extracostal tissues to fill the space. Some patients will already have had an unsuccessful extrapleural thoracoplasty. This situation necessitates resecting the entire chest wall en bloc because of the extensive regenerated bone. There is more extensive blood loss and generally more technical difficulty. The use of the electrocautery is almost a necessity if excessive blood loss is to be avoided. The surgeon should take care when using the cautery near the vertebrae lest heat be transmitted to the spinal cord.**

12

Esophageal Procedures

CORRECTION OF ESOPHAGEAL ATRESIA (WITH AND WITHOUT TRACHEOESOPHAGEAL FISTULA)

Preoperative evaluation of these infants must identify the type of atresia (Fig. 12–1) and location of the fistula if one is present. A careful evaluation of the patient's pulmonary status is vital, and aspiration pneumonia must be managed if it has occurred. The state of hydration and the electrolyte balance are also important and must be assessed. Timing of surgical intervention is critical; the disorder does not need urgent correction, and the patient's condition must be optimal. The presence of other coexisting defects must be determined and their significance evaluated.

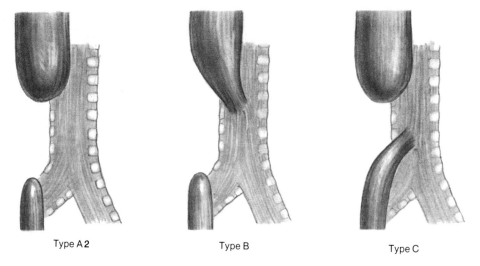

Type A 2   Type B   Type C

Figure 12–1. Esophageal atresia according to the Gross classification system. Types *A* and *C* make up approximately 95% of all defects, with type *C* predominant, producing approximately 85% of the abnormalities.

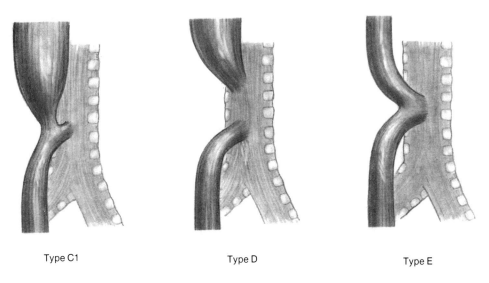

Type C1   Type D   Type E

Figure 12–1. *Continued.* A modification (type *C1*) is not common but does occur. Type *D* is extremely rare and the H-type fistula (type *E*) is also relatively rare.

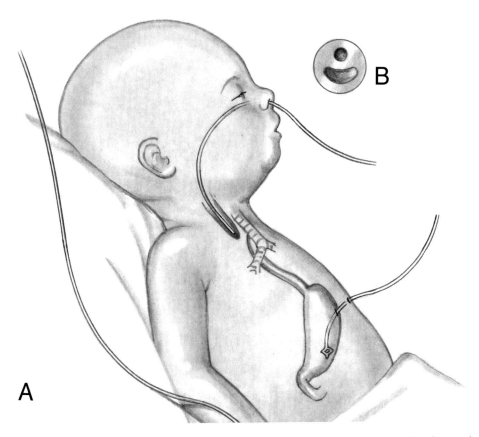

Figure 12–2. Diagram of preferred position of infant with esophageal fistula and tracheoesophageal fistula. The elevated position helps to prevent aspiration of gastric contents into the tracheobronchial tree. *B,* A double-lumen, sump type nasogastric tube (Fig. B) is placed in the blind upper esophageal segment to aspirate saliva and minimize aspiration.

Operative Procedures

Gross Type A: Esophageal Atresia Without Fistula.   This lesion makes up about 10 to 12% of defects. Primary repair is rarely possible. Recently techniques of stretching the upper segment by daily bougienage has made primary anastomosis possible in some patients. Generally, this lesion is managed initially by bringing the upper segment out in the cervical area as a salivary fistula and establishing a gastrostomy. Transplantation of colon or jejunum is accomplished at a later time, usually around 18 months of age.

Gross Type C: Esophageal Atresia with a Blind Upper Segment and the Distal Segment Communicating Directly with the Trachea or Major Bronchus.   This type affects about 85% of patients with esophageal atresia. Selection of the surgical approach is based principally upon the size of the fistula and condition of the patient. Should the infant weigh under 2 kg, if there are serious other defects that are endangering the infant's life, such as a major cardiac lesion, or if the respiratory status is poor and cannot be improved, a rapidly performed extrapleural division or ligation of the fistula, combined with establishment of a cervical fistula and gastrostomy, may salvage the patient's life with a much lesser risk; reconstruction, however, is deferred until the child is 18 months old or older (Fig. 12–2).

A child weighing over 2 kg with no associated defects and in good condition, with minimal or no pulmonary infection, should be subjected to complete repair.

Position

Full right lateral.

Anesthesia

General, although it is possible to use local anesthesia with tracheal intubation and respiratory support.

Incision

Posterolateral. It is unnecessary to curve the incision, as is done in adults, but it should be made transversely. A lengthy incision is unnecessary.

Procedure (Fig. 12–3)

The incision is made and hemostasis is secured by electrocautery. The intercostal muscle of the fourth or fifth interspace is carefully incised, taking great care not to enter the pleural space. The extrapleural plane is developed using blunt dissection. The best instruments for this are cotton-tipped applicators, changed often. After extrapleural dissection is well begun, a rib retractor is placed. The azygos vein is a good guide in identifying the transition from the chest wall to the posterior mediastinum. The dissection should be carried medially until the trachea is clearly in the field.

The azygos vein is dissected free, doubly ligated, and transected. The proximal esophageal pouch is then identified. Its lowest extent should have been identified by the preoperative esophagogram. It may extend as low as the T4 level, but frequently it lies higher in the mediastinum. Dissection is begun to free as much length of the proximal pouch as possible, avoiding injury to the pouch. The anterior wall may be firmly fused to the posterior tracheal wall, and entry into the trachea must be studiously avoided. A 5-0 silk suture in the tip of the pouch provides traction without instrument trauma.

The distal esophagus is usually identified easily. It is dissected free about 1 cm below the tracheal bifurcation and encircled with a 4-0 silk suture for traction. The site of entry into the trachea is identified. The esophagus is transected transversely, leaving a cuff of about 2 mm on the trachea. This cuff is sutured with an interrupted or continuous 6-0 Prolene or silk suture. It is preferable to partially incise and suture simultaneously to minimize air leakage. The closure should be immersed in saline solution and checked for air leakage.

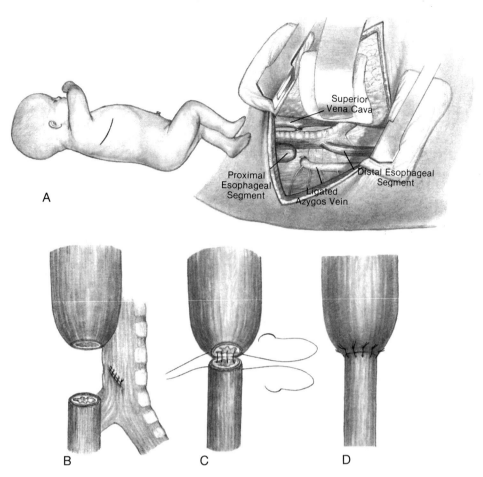

Figure 12–3. Esophageal atresia and repair of tracheoesophageal fistula of Gross type C.

A, The child is placed in the lateral position and a relatively small, almost transverse incision is made. The thoracic cavity is entered through the fourth intercostal space, and extrapleural dissection is accomplished with the mediastinal structures being exposed by retracting the lung anteriorly, the pleura remaining intact.

B, The azygos vein has been ligated and transected, exposing the proximal pouch and the distal fistula.

C, D, The fistula opening into the trachea is closed with fine Prolene sutures, and an opening is made in the proximal pouch. The anastomosis is small with a single row of interrupted Prolene or Tev-Dek sutures and may be reinforced after the method of Haight by a second row of sutures telescoping the proximal pouch down over the distal segment *(D).*

Measurement of the distance between the esophageal ends will indicate whether primary anastomosis can be accomplished without undue tension. A distance of more than 1.5 cm measured with no traction applied indicates that anastomosis will be hazardous and probably should not be attempted. It is unwise to try to gain length by mobilizing more than 1 to 2 cm of the lower segment for fear of devascularizing the segment.

An incision is made into the proximal pouch about 3 mm in length. Simple sutures of 6-0 Prolene or silk are used to anastomose the two segments, end to end. Sutures should include the full thickness of both ends. Some infants already have aspiration pneumonitis and are in such poor condition that immediate operation is contraindicated. The child should have a gastrotomy established and be placed in the position shown in Figure 12–3. Adequate hydration and nutrition can be maintained while antibiotic therapy is used. It is wiser to avoid infant formula and use only clear glucose solution so that fewer pulmonary problems are likely if aspiration should occur. The disproportionate size makes very careful placement of sutures necessary. Some have recommended using the full thickness of the lower segment and mucosa only on the proximal segment. This necessitates making a second row of sutures. No more than six to eight stitches are necessary. If there is adequate redundancy, a second layer of four to six stitches can be used to suture the proximal musculature downward over the original suture line after the method of Haight. Some surgeons prefer to introduce a No. 8 catheter through the anastomotic area to be used as a stent during the procedure.

It is preferable to interpose some mediastinal tissue between the tracheal closure and the anastomosis. A small Penrose drain or a simple strip of drain material is placed in the area and brought out posteriorly. The wound is then closed by approximating the ribs with two sutures of 2-0 Dexon, and the extracostal musculature is closed with continuous 4-0 Dexon. The skin is closed with subcuticular 5-0 chromic catgut or Dexon. A culture of the anastomotic area is taken before closure. If the pleura is inadvertently entered, a chest tube is necessary.

Gastrostomy should be established using a No. 8 or No. 10 mushroom catheter for feeding.

Critical Points

1. **Operate when patient's condition is optimal.**
2. **Use an extrapleural approach.**
3. **Do not attempt anastomosis under excess tension.**
4. **Prevent intraoperative hypothermia.**
5. **Avoid giving an excess of fluid and sodium intraoperatively and postoperatively.**
6. **The assistant should have a sandbag or similar mass about 5 to 6 inches high on which to rest hands during the procedure. This provides for constant exposure with minimal motion.**
7. **Interrupt the procedure frequently for lung re-expansion.**
8. **Early dilatation, i.e., at 14 to 21 days, with a filiform catheter and follower will prevent most strictures.**
9. **Contrary to the view of some pediatricians, fluids should be limited to 65 mL/kg/24 hours for the first 48 hours or until use of the gastrostomy is initiated, particularly in the premature infant.**
10. **Ventilatory support may be required, particularly in the premature infant and in those with preoperative aspiration pneumonitis.**

Infants who have esophageal atresia only, without tracheoesophageal fistula, pose a different problem. The two esophageal segments are usually separated to such a degree that primary anastomosis is not possible. Esophageal reconstruction using colon, stomach, or jejunal replacement is not feasible in the newborn and is best performed at about 18 months of age after considerable growth has occurred. The proximal esophageal blind segment is converted to a cervical esophagostomy, and a gastrostomy is established in the neonatal period. The stomach is not usually used because of its disproportionate size. Colon interposition has most often been used and is generally a successful and satisfactory graft. A full bowel preparation is used preoperatively.

ESOPHAGEAL RECONSTRUCTION WITH COLON INTERPOSITION (FIG. 12–4)

Anesthesia

General

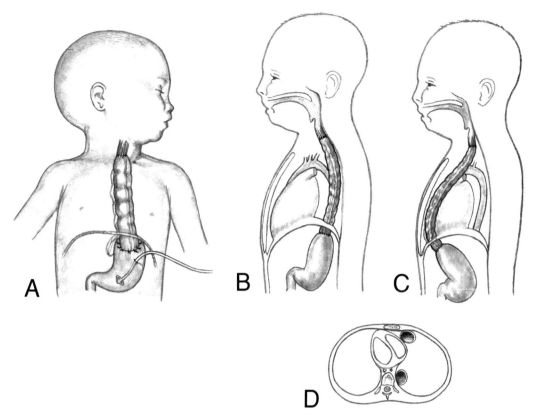

Figure 12–4.

A, Diagram of colon substitution for the thoracic esophagus in patients with insufficient esophageal length to permit primary repair.

B, The interposed colon may be placed in the posterior mediastinum in the anatomic plane of the esophagus.

C, Alternately, the colon may be placed in the anterior mediastinum in the substernal position. Either position is satisfactory and generally a matter of personal choice.

D, Diagram of cross-section of thorax showing the position of the colon in both positions.

Position

Supine

Procedure

A midline upper abdominal incision is made and the vasculature of the stomach and colon are evaluated. The right, transverse, or left colon may be selected based on the vascular pattern. I generally prefer the left colon. If the vascular arcade or marginal artery is intact and in full continuity, the graft may be based on the middle colic artery. If there is any doubt, the inferior mesenteric artery can be occluded with a vascular clamp for a period of 10 to 15 minutes, observing the appearance and color of the left colon.

Unless there is some concern, the inferior mesenteric artery branches are ligated and divided. The left colon is mobilized, being careful not to injure the mesentery or any mesenteric vessels. The transverse colon is transected, leaving the middle colic artery intact. The vascular supply is interrupted, preferably distal to its first branch. The left colon is transected at about the juncture with the rectosigmoid segment. Bowel clamps are left in place and the proximal transverse colon is anastomosed to the distal end of the left colon. A two-layered anastomosis is constructed by whatever technique the surgeon

232 of Techniques in General Thoracic Surgery

prefers. The defect in the mesocolon is closed to prevent herniation. The graft segment is then carried through the lesser omentum.

A decision is to be made at this time as to whether the graft is to be placed in the anterior or in the posterior mediastinum in the esophageal plane. The anterior technique will be described. A rake or Robinson retractor is used to elevate the sternum moderately. Using sharp dissection initially and then blunt finger dissection, the substernal plane is developed.

A second cervical incision is made along the sternocleidomastoid anterior edge and on either side of the cervical fistula. The deep cervical fascia is incised and the proximal esophagus detached from the skin edges and mobilized superiorly.

The substernal space is further developed with sharp and blind dissection until the two planes meet. The space is widened to a size that will accommodate the colon. The distal end of the colon is then advanced into the substernal space manually and very carefully. It is grasped with a Babcock clamp and delivered into the cervical area. Care must be taken not to produce volvulus in performing this part of procedure. The surgeon should then ascertain that the vascular supply arterial and venous are not under tension or obstructed in any way. A site is selected on the anterior wall of the stomach on the anterior surface at about the middle of the lesser curvature. It may have been necessary to take down the pre-existing gastrostomy during the preceding part of the operation. A longitudinal incision about 2 to 3 cm in length is made in the anterior stomach wall and a two-layer end-to-side anastomosis is constructed. A posterior row of mattress sutures is placed and tied. The mucosa is then sutured with continuous 4-0 or 3-0 Vicryl or Dexon suture material. The anterior mucosa is closed with the Cushing technique, an anterior row of interrupted Cushing sutures of non-absorbable material. The gastrostomy is then re-established.

Attention is then turned to the cervical area. If the color of the colon appears satisfactory, an end-to-end anastomosis is effected. A two-layer technique as described in this text is used. Upon completion, the colon is sutured to cervical fascia to prevent tension. The cervical incision is closed without drainage.

The peritoneum may be partly but not completely closed interiorly. Some prefer not to close it at all. The fascia is closed with nonabsorbable suture material and the subcutaneous tissue and skin are closed with the technique the surgeon prefers.

Notes

1. **If there is a serious question as to colon viability, the procedure may be aborted. If the procedure is completed, it is wise to reopen the cervical incision in 24 hours and inspect the bowel rather than risk mediastinitis.**
2. **Drainage only serves to infect the area and should not be used.**
3. **Postoperative dilatation may be done after the first week using Hurst-Malony dilatation with filiform dilators and followers.**

ESOPHAGEAL RECONSTRUCTION USING GREATER CURVATURE GASTRIC TUBE (FIG. 12–5)

Indications

This technique may be an alternative to colon interposition for esophageal reconstruction in infants with esophageal atresia. An indication would be when the vascular anatomy is not suitable for use of the colon.

Anesthesia

General.

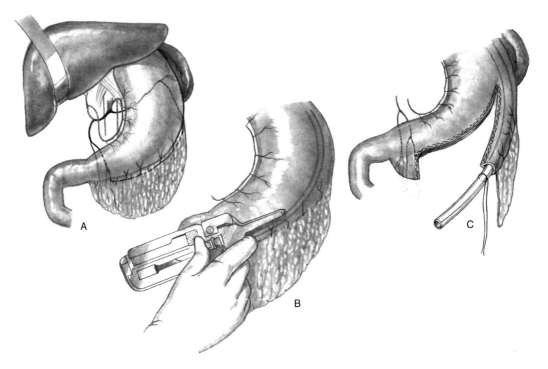

Figure 12–5.

A, Anatomic features of the stomach as related to creating a greater curvature tube for esophageal replacement.

B, Use of a G.I.A. stapling device to begin creation of the greater curvature tube. An indwelling dilator or catheter-size 40 to 42 in the adult and size 30 in the 18-month-old infant.

C, The completed tube. The staple line may be oversewn if desired, but many do not consider this necessary.

Position

Supine

Procedure

An upper midline laparotomy is made. The gastrocolic omentum is divided. The terminal splenic artery and the left gastroepiploic artery are inspected and evaluated because they will be the sole blood supply of the tube to be created. The right gastroepiploic artery is then identified, dissected free, doubly ligated, and divided.

From this point, either of two techniques can be used. One technique involves the use of the G.I.A. stapling device. A transverse incision is made across the stomach about 2 to 3 cm proximal to the pylorus. A 30 mm stapling instrument can be used for this incision. A catheter of size 18 to 26 French size is inserted into the stomach along the greater curvature to determine the size of the gastric tube. A G.I.A. stapling device is then used to create a staple line and incision parallel to the greater curvature. At least two and probably three applications of the instrument will be necessary to create a tube of at least 15 cm in length. Additional length can be produced if desired.

The alternative technique consists of making a transverse incision as previously described. Parallel anterior and posterior walls of the stomach about 2 cm from the greater curvature. The flap thus created is then closed again over a catheter to produce the greater curvature tube. A two-layer closure is used. The mucosal layer should be a continuous simple suture of 3-0 Dexon, Vicryl or catgut. The seromuscular suture line is then completed using interrupted nonabsorbable suture. The last 1 to 2 cm of the gastric suture line are left unsutured or sutured with interrupted sutures so that it can be adapted to the size of the cervical esophagus.

A second incision is made along the anterior border of the left sternocleidomastoid muscle. The proximal esophageal stomach is encircled by the incision. The proximal esophagus is dissected free and the distal lumen is trimmed to normal mucosa.

A substernal tunnel is then created by blunt finger dissection from the cervical area and the abdominal incision simultaneously. The gastric tube is then gently drawn through the tunnel into the cervical area, being careful not to twist the tube.

The size of the gastric opening is then tailored to the size of the esophagus and a two-layered anastomosis is constructed. A posterior row of interrupted muscular-seromuscular sutures are placed using a 4-0 nonabsorbable material. The posterior mucosa is sutured using a continuous simple suture of 3-0 or 4-0 absorbable material. An interrupted suture line of non-absorbable sutures is preferred by some surgeons. The anterior mucosa is closed with interrupted sutures and the muscular-seromuscular layer is completed with simple or mattress sutures.

A gastrostomy tube is placed in the gastric remnant and brought out through the abdominal wall.

The incisions are then closed by whatever technique the surgeon prefers. Gastrostomy feedings are begun in 2 to 3 days.

Note

An alternative technique can be used if one wishes to make esophagogastric anastomosis in the thorax. In this case, an incision is made in the diaphragm posterolateral to the hiatus. A left thoracotomy or thoracoabdominal incision is used. The tube is placed in the posterior mediastinum in the esophageal plane. This technique is applicable in patients with esophageal structure (lye) when the proximal esophagus can be preserved.

ESOPHAGOMYOTOMY (HELLER)

Indications

Relief of achalasia.

Contraindications

1. Fibrous stricture formation.
2. Previous dilatation with pneumatic or hydrostatic dilators.
3. Ulcerative esophagitis.

Position

Left lateral position.

Incision

Posterolateral thoracotomy.

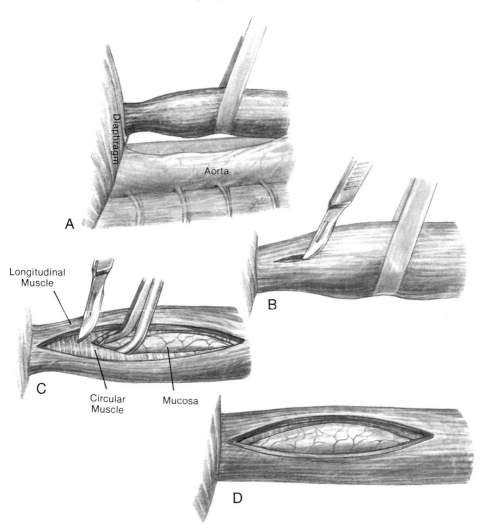

Figure 12–6. Esophagomyotomy (Heller procedure).

A, The distal esophagus has been mobilized. The area of muscle hypertrophy is noted in the terminal area.

B, The myotomy incision is made on the lateral aspect of the esophagus and extended superiorly for about 10 cm to the level of the inferior pulmonary vein. The incision is extended to the cardiac but not on to the stomach, as this extension usually results in perforation.

C, A blunt right angle clamp is used to separate the esophageal musculature and elevate it for incision.

D, The completed myotomy is shown with the myotomy wound left unrepaired. A Hurst-Maloney bougie may be placed in the esophagus to facilitate myotomy and make it safer.

Procedure (Fig. 12–6)

The seventh interspace is used to enter the pleural space. A Hurst-Maloney dilator, No. 40 to No. 44, is passed and left in the esophagus.

The mediastinal pleura is incised over the esophagus from the diaphragmatic esophageal hiatus to the inferior pulmonary vein. The esophagus is mobilized by sharp and blunt dissection. Care is taken not to injure either vagus nerve or to enter the opposite pleural space. The esophagus is encircled with a Penrose drain and elevated from the mediastinum.

The esophageal musculature is incised longitudinally beginning about 5 cm above the hiatus. The incision is gradually deepened and gently spread apart until the mucosa is seen to bulge into the wound. Then, using a right angle clamp, gently insert the clamp in the plane between the mucosa and the circular muscle, then centimeter by centimeter, incise and spread the musculature. Extend this incision to the level of the cardia but not on to the stomach; otherwise penetration into the lumen of the stomach is likely to occur. The myotomy should be extended superiorly to the level of the inferior pulmonary vein or higher if the musculature still appears to be hypertrophied.

Hemostasis is secured by careful application of the electrocautery. The Penrose drain is then removed. No attempt is made to close the mediastinal pleura, and the surgeon must be certain that no entry has been made into the esophageal lumen.

If the mucosa is opened inadvertently, it should be closed with catgut or other absorbable suture and covered by stomach or other tissue with interrupted sutures of silk in the overlying musculature.

A single drainage tube is left in the pleural space, and the chest is closed. The Hurst-Maloney dilator is removed (prior to closure).

Note

Postoperatively, esophageal reflux is almost invariably present, and an antireflux procedure may be done. Regurgitation and aspiration in the immediate postoperative period should be prevented by elevating the patient's head and by limiting intake until it is certain that intestinal activity is adequate and the patient is ambulatory.

RESECTION OF PHARYNGOESOPHAGEAL DIVERTICULUM

Indications

The three stages of Zenker's diverticulum, as described by Lahey, should be reviewed. The mere presence of a small, asymptomatic diverticulum is not an indication for operation. When the opening of the diverticulum is transverse and the sac is dependent, operation should be considered for the patient.

Procedure (Fig. 12–7)

The diverticulum may be approached via a longitudinal incision along the anterior border of the sternocleidomastoid muscle on either side, although the left is usually preferred. The deep cervical fascia is incised in the direction of the incision. The omohyoid muscle is divided, and the carotid vessels and vagus nerve are retracted laterally. The retroesophageal area is developed by blunt dissection. It may be necessary to ligate the middle thyroid vein in order to produce adequate exposure. The diverticulum is found in this area of dissection, just inferior to the cricoid cartilage. However, it is seldom as large as might be expected from the preoperative barium swallow.

The diverticulum is grasped with a Babcock forceps and freed from surrounding tissue. The diverticulum does not have a muscular coat but consists of mucosa and submucosa only. The muscular hiatus in the posterior esophageal wall should be freed from the neck of the sac and be clearly defined. After the dissection is complete, the sac may be stapled transversely with a TA 30 stapling instrument with 3.5 mm staples, or it may be excised and the mucosa closed with continuous 3-0 absorbable sutures. In either case, the surgeon must not exert undue traction at the time of stapling or excision lest too much mucosa be resected, producing a stricture postoperatively.

A 4-0 continuous Prolene or 4-0 interrupted silk suture is used to close the muscular wall of the esophagus transversely.

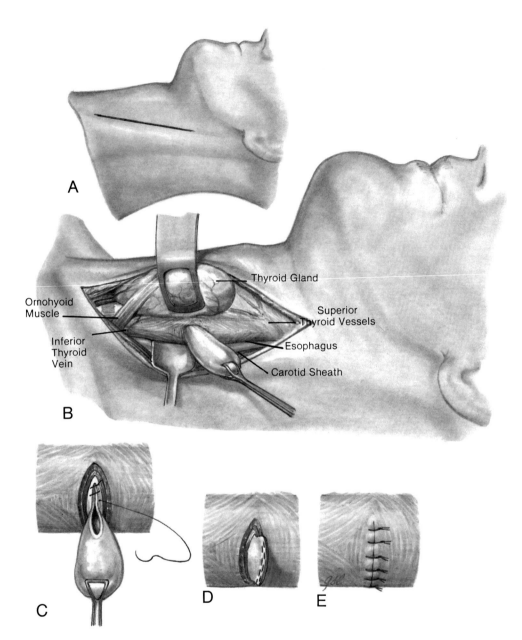

Figure 12–7. Pharyngoesophageal diverticulum.

A, The incision is made along the anterior border of the sternocleidomastoid muscle.

B, The exposure is demonstrated, and the diverticulum has been dissected free and mobilized.

C, The mucosa and diverticulum have been dissected, the neck of the diverticulum has been incised transversely, and the incision is being closed with a continuous 3-0 absorbable suture. Care is taken not to excise too much mucosa, which will produce a stricture.

D, An alternative method is to staple the neck of the diverticulum with a TA 30 stapling device in a transverse plane.

E, The esophageal musculature is approximated with interrupted nonabsorbable sutures.

A single Penrose or Jackson-Pratt drain is left in the retroesophageal space and brought out through a stab wound laterally.

The wound is closed with several interrupted sutures reapproximating the deep cervical fascia. The subcutaneous tissue is closed with continuous absorbable suture. The skin may be closed with a running subcuticular suture.

Note

Many patients with pharyngoesophageal diverticulum are aged and have severe cardiovascular disease. For these patients, the procedure may be done under local anesthesia.

PROCEDURES FOR ESOPHAGECTOMY

The following are operative procedures for partial or total esophagectomy, or esophagogastrectomy, for carcinoma. There is great disagreement in the surgical world at this time as to the medical and surgical approach to esophageal carcinoma. Some oncologists feel that results are so dismal that no effort at surgical resection is warranted, and prefer chemotherapy with or without radiation. Despite a poor 5-year survival for all cases, the survival rate for Stage I and II tumors is from 20 to 40% following curative resection. Some surgical groups feel that all surgical procedures should be considered as palliative only. Still others, particularly the Japanese, have devised more extensive procedures involving extensive lymphatic resection, and report better results than those in the United States.

This text is a technical manual, and its purpose is not to discuss or judge the merits of each procedure. I feel, in general, that preoperative cis-platinum is beneficial, followed by total esophagectomy, except for tumors of the gastroesophageal junction.

One comment about transhiatal esophagectomy, proposed by Orringer, is that it has been shown clearly that this procedure can be accomplished with a mortality-morbidity rate comparable to that of other forms of resection. However, I, along with several others, do not feel that this procedure has the necessary components of a definitive cancer operation. Further data and experience are required to determine whether or not this technique is a good cancer procedure for any stage of the disease. Certainly, for benign disease it probably will displace all other procedures.

RESECTION OF THE LOWER ESOPHAGUS WITH PROXIMAL GASTRECTOMY

Resection procedures involving the cardioesophageal junction can best be approached by a left posterolateral thoracotomy. Total gastrectomy can be approached similarly. One should not hesitate to extend the thoracotomy incision across the costal margin if additional exposure is necessary, although the majority of patients do not require more than a thoracotomy. This procedure is indicated for carcinoma of the cardia of the stomach or the lower one-third of the esophagus (Fig. 12–8A)

Position

Left lateral. The semilateral exposure renders the most critical part of the procedure, the esophagogastric anastomosis, the most difficult to see.

Procedure

A posterolateral thoracotomy incision is made, and the pleural space is entered through the seventh intercostal space. The lung is retracted superiorly. The diaphragm is incised

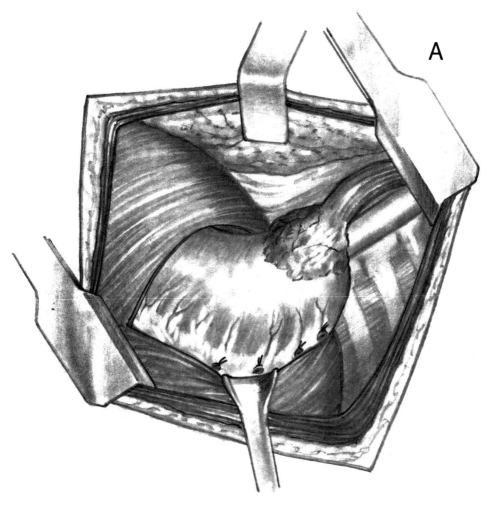

Figure 12–8.
A, View via left posterolateral thoracotomy with the patient in the lateral position. The diaphragm has been incised for 10 to 12 cm and the lower esophagus and proximal stomach have been mobilized. The tumor at the esophagogastric junction is seen.

in a semilunar curve, extending laterally from the hiatus and curving anteriorly to the costal margin at the anterior extremity of the chest wall incision. Hemostasis of the diaphragmatic incision is produced by suture ligature. The neoplasm is inspected at this point to determine mobility, involvement of the diaphragm, and extension into neighboring structures. The presence, size, and resectability of involved lymph nodes are then evaluated, including nodes along the splenic artery and into the splenic hilum. The liver is examined for evidence of metastatic disease.

The procedure is begun by mobilizing the esophagus above the lesion and then carrying the dissection inferiorly and laterally, freeing the region of the cardia posteriorly and detaching the fundus from the diaphragm. The short gastric vessels are then divided and ligated. The spleen may be removed if hilar nodes are involved or if the spleen itself is involved, but it should not be removed routinely. The greater curvature mobilization is

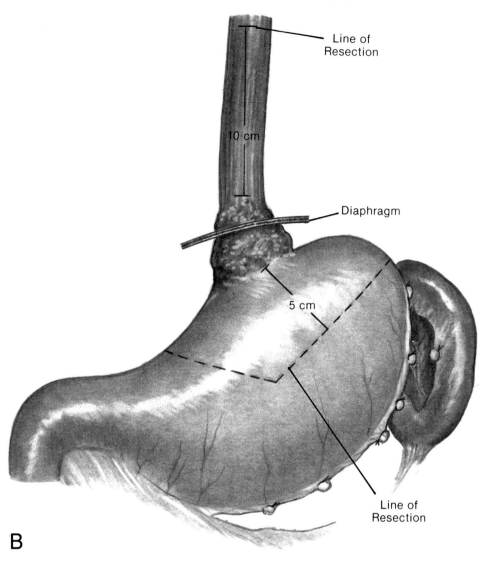

Figure 12–8. *Continued. B,* **Resection for carcinoma of the cardia.** It is wise to extend the gastric resection 5 cm from the margin of the tumor as seen grossly, and it is believed that the esophagus should be resected 10 cm above evidence of tumor. The lines of resection are outlined.

continued, clamping, dividing, and ligating the left gastroepiploic artery near its origin. The greater omentum is progressively detached from the greater curvature distal to the vascular arcade, which must be preserved. This line of division can usually be terminated about 5 to 8 cm from the pylorus.

The stomach is elevated and reflected medially, and the region of the cardia is further mobilized, carefully attempting to include any involved nodes in the specimen. The left gastric vessels are identified, doubly ligated, and divided. The stomach is then returned to its anatomic position and retracted laterally. The mobilization of the lesser curvature is completed with multiple ligatures and hemoclips.

A pyloromyotomy or pyloroplasty is accomplished; a myotomy is simpler and has proved to be adequate.

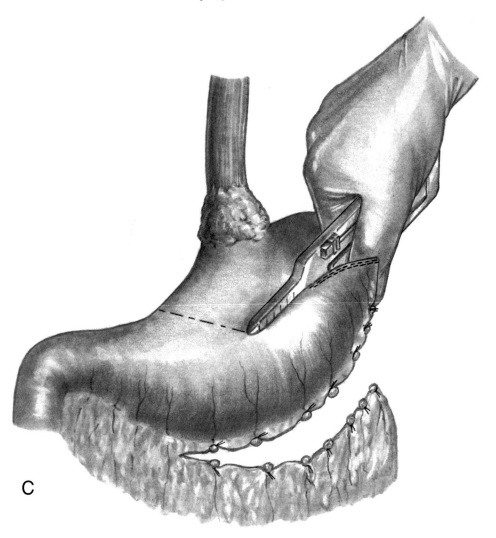

C

Figure 12–8. *Continued. C,* **Resection for carcinoma of the cardioesophageal junction.** The G.I.A. stapling instrument is being applied to the stomach along the line previously determined.

The gastric resection line is then determined (Fig. 12–8B). Usually this is begun superiorly, at the midportion of the fundus, then angled medially, removing about 50 to 60% of the lesser curvature. The G.I.A stapling instrument is used (Fig. 12–8C and D). At least three cartridges are necessary to complete the staple line. The resection should have at least a 5 cm clearance from visible neoplasm. I prefer to oversew the staple line with a running Lembert suture of Prolene or interrupted Lembert sutures of 4-0 silk.

The detached tumor-bearing portion of the stomach is elevated, and the esophagus is mobilized after incising the pulmonary ligament. The distance to the proposed resection line above obvious tumor must be 10 cm. The esophagus should not be mobilized much above the anastomotic site to minimize devascularization. The esophagus is then clamped with a right angle Sarot bronchus clamp about 1 cm below the anastomotic site, and the specimen is amputated distal to the clamp and removed.

The fundus of the stomach is brought into the thorax. A site on the anterior wall near

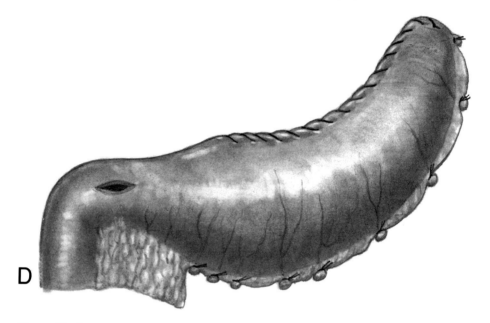

D

Figure 12–8. *Continued. D,* **Resection for carcinoma of the cardioesophageal junction.** The staple line has been oversewn with a running Lembert suture of 4-0 Prolene and the anastomotic site has been selected.

E

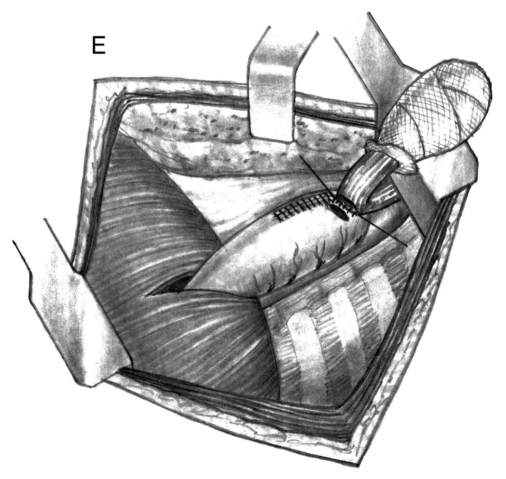

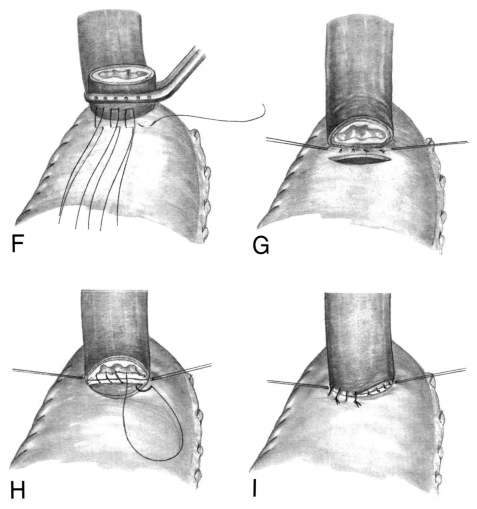

Figure 12–8. *Continued. F–I.* **Esophagogastrostomy.** This technique is useful whether the stomach is being anastomosed within the thorax or in the cervical area. The Sarot clamp shown would not be used for a cervical anastomosis.

F, A series of horizontal mattress or Cushing sutures is being applied to the posterior wall of the esophagus and the anterior wall of the stomach.

G, These sutures are tied and two are left, after which an opening is made into the stomach.

H, The posterior mucosal edges are closed with a continuous suture using 3-0 catgut or Dexon, and the anterior row is closed with interrupted sutures of the same material.

I, Horizontal mattress sutures are used to close the muscular wall of the esophagus to the gastric wall, as was done on the posterior wall. The anastomosis is shown in a nearly completed state. It is wise to attach the stomach to adjacent pleural structures to produce stability and to prevent tension on the suture line.

Figure 12–8. *Continued.*

E, The stomach and esophagus are again shown in situ. The esophagogastric anastomosis is being constructed. See F through I.

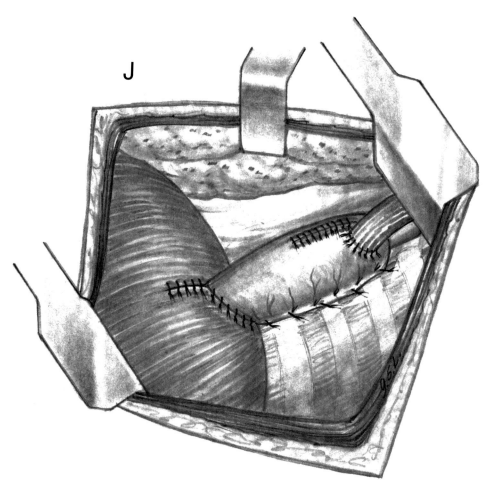

Figure 12–8. *Continued.*

J, Completed procedure. The esophagogastric anastomosis has been completed. The diaphragm has been closed with interrupted nonabsorbable sutures and the stomach fixed to the margin of the newly created hiatus with similar sutures. The stomach has been sutured to the chest wall with several interrupted sutures to prevent any traction on the anastomosis. Failure to close the diaphragm well may result in postoperative herniation of the small bowel.

the apex is selected (Fig. 12–8E through J). The clamped esophagus is angulated laterally, exposing the medial wall of the esophagus. A series of about five 4-0 silk horizontal (Cushing) sutures are placed in the stomach and esophageal walls. All sutures are placed before any are tied. The two end sutures are tagged and the others are cut. The esophagus is then reamputated just proximal to the Sarot clamp. A small (2 cm) incision is made in the stomach wall parallel to the previous suture line, about 6 to 8 mm away. The mucosal edges are then sutured together. Several techniques can be used. I prefer a simple continuous absorbable suture, including all layers, for the posterior wall and simple interrupted sutures anteriorly. A nasogastric tube is passed into the stomach before the anterior row is completed.

An anterior row of interrupted horizontal mattress sutures (Cushing) of 4-0 silk is then placed.

The diaphragm is repaired in two layers, as described elsewhere. The margin of the diaphragm is sutured to the stomach wall to prevent any change in position and to close the hiatus and prevent herniation of the bowel. Several sutures of silk are also used to attach the stomach to the mediastinal pleura to prevent any traction on the anastomosis.

The thoracotomy incision is then closed. A single chest tube is placed posteriorly with the tip near but not touching the anastomosis and the stomach.

This anastomosis can be easily made with the EEA stapling device, as described under Alternative Technique 1 and shown in Figure 12–9.

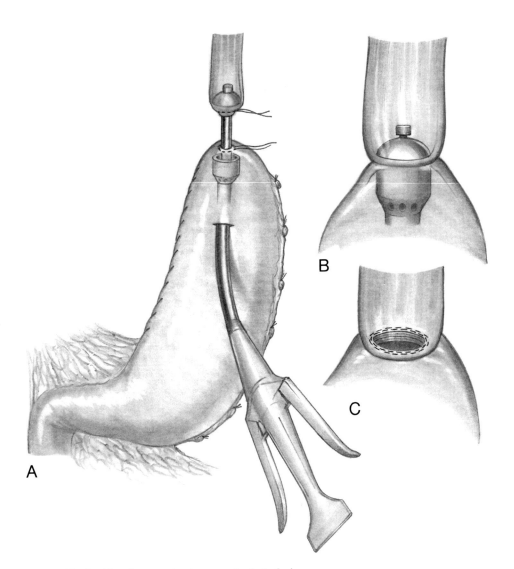

Figure 12–9. Esophagogastrostomy—staple technique.

A, The stomach has been mobilized. The tumor at the cardia in this instance has been resected, closed by stapling (G.I.A. instrument), and oversewn with continuous Lembert sutures. A gastrostomy opening is made in the anterior wall of the stomach. The EEA stapling instrument has been introduced and brought through the gastric wall at the site of anastomosis. The anvil is attached to the stapler and has been introduced into the proximal esophagus. Both the stomach and the esophagus have been closed tightly about the instruments with pursestring sutures.

B, The EEA device has been closed and staples fixed.

C, The instrument has been removed along with the "doughnut" of resected stomach and esophagus, both of which must be complete rings of tissue.

ESOPHAGECTOMY—SUBTOTAL (VIA RIGHT THORACOTOMY) (FIG. 12–10)

This procedure is best done in two stages during a single anesthesia session. I, among many others, have concluded that it is more expedient to perform the abdominal phase with the patient in the supine position and then turn the patient into a full right lateral position, redrape, and carry out a standard right posterolateral thoracotomy; this method also provides better exposure. Placing the patient in a semilateral position and attempting both laparotomy and thoracotomy, or using a thoracoabdominal incision and attempting to use two teams, results in poor exposure, prolonged operating time, and a higher morbidity rate.

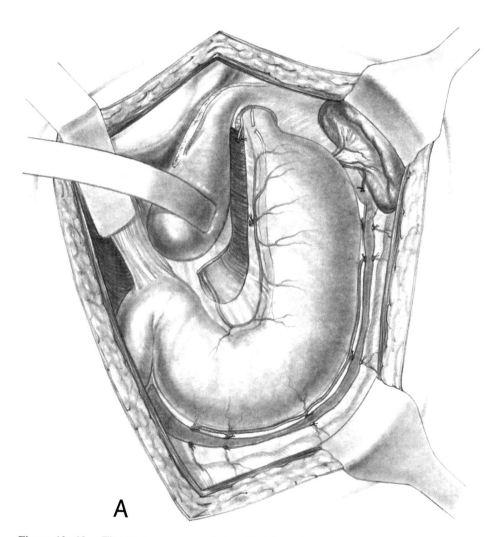

A

Figure 12–10. Thoracotomy approach to subtotal esophagectomy.
A, A view of the upper midline laparotomy showing the extent of mobilization of the stomach, which includes ligature and division of the left gastric artery, left gastroepiploic artery, and the short gastric arteries. The esophagogastric junction and the lower third of the esophagus should be completely mobilized. The drawing does not show the pyloroplasty, which is done before the incision is closed.

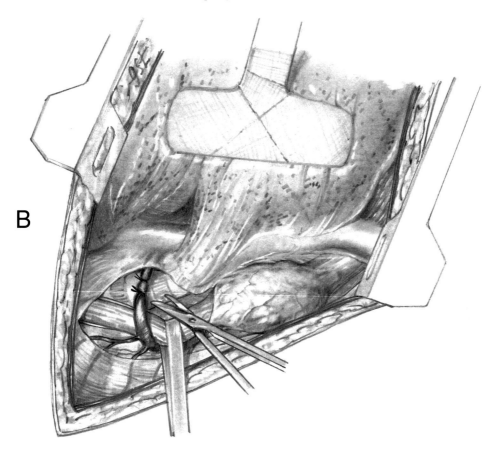

B

Figure 12–10. *Continued.*
B, This view is from the right posterolateral thoracotomy and demonstrates the incision through the mediastinal pleura and beginning mobilization of the esophagus proximal to the tumor.

This procedure may be modified, as described later; the surgeon may perform total esophagectomy or do a palliative cervical esophagogastrostomy, leaving the thoracic esophagus in situ.

Procedure (Fig. 12–10A through F)

The patient is placed in a supine position with the arms at the sides. A midline incision is made from the xiphoid process to a point 2.5 cm below the umbilicus. Hemostasis is produced by electrocautery.

Exploration of the abdomen is first carried out to determine if any pathologic processes unrelated to the primary problem are present. A careful exploration is then done to identify liver metastases and involvement of nodes around the celiac axis or along the lesser curvature that might preclude or modify the operation.

The dissection is begun by opening the gastrocolic omentum along the greater curvature in the antral region. The right gastroepiploic artery is identified and the line of dissection established about 2 to 3 cm distal to this vessel, which must be preserved. The omentum is severed between clamps, including no more than 2 to 3 cm of tissue each time. Ligation of each segment is accomplished using 2-0 nonabsorbable suture. This line of resection is carried distally to within 2 cm of the pylorus and then proximally, until the left gastroepiploic artery is identified, ligated, and transected.

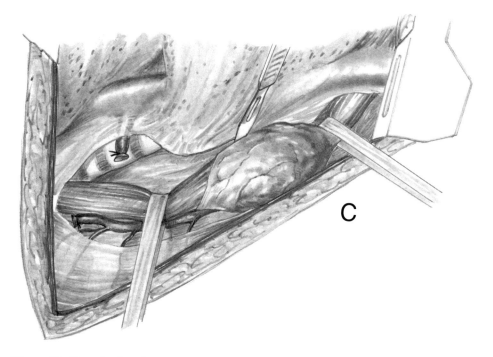

Figure 12–10. *Continued.*
C, This drawing depicts the completed esophageal mobilization including the area of neoplasm.

The avascular area is divided. Then the gastrosplenic omentum and the short gastric vessels are similarly ligated and divided. Great care must be taken not to injure the spleen or splenic vessels.

The stomach is retracted inferiorly and the lesser omental sac is entered superiorly to the right gastric artery. This omentum is divided between clamps and ligated. The left gastric artery and vein may be approached anteriorly, or the stomach may be elevated and displaced cephalad. The left gastric vessels are easily identified from this posterior approach. They should be doubly ligated separately but in continuity, with two proximal ligatures being employed. The vessels are then divided.

The stomach is then retracted inferiorly, and from the anterior approach the remainder of the lesser curvature is mobilized by dividing the gastrohepatic omentum between clamps. As the cardioesophageal junction is approached, the peritoneal reflection from the diaphragm is divided. After this the remaining tissue attaching the fundus to the inferior surface of the diaphragm is divided, and ligatures or hemoclips are used to secure branches of the phrenic artery lying in this area. Traction is applied to the stomach, and the distal esophagus is freed for 2 to 3 inches by blunt finger dissection. The surgeon must be certain that no peritoneal or omental attachments of the stomach remain.

A pyloromyotomy is then done. An incision about 2 cm in length is necessary. Care must be taken not to injure the duodenal mucosa at the distal end of the myotomy. Hemostasis is accomplished by electrocautery. The myotomy must be converted to a Heineke-Mikulitz pyloroplasty if the lumen is entered, or this type of pyloroplasty may be used if the surgeon prefers. Some surgeons have advocated not doing any form of pyloroplasty.

A careful inspection is then made to determine the adequacy of hemostasis.

The incision is closed by whatever technique the surgeon wishes. I prefer to close the peritoneum with a size 0 Dexon suture and to close the fascia with interrupted

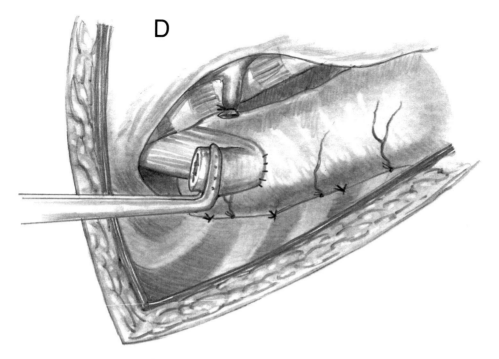

Figure 12–10. *Continued.*
D, The distal esophagus has been removed and the transected esophagus is held with a Sarot clamp while the posterior row of mattress sutures is being placed. Stay sutures are placed on both ends of the suture line. Only four or five sutures are needed.

figure-of-eight sutures of No. 28 (2-0) stainless steel wire. The wound is dressed and the drapes removed.

The patient is turned into the right lateral position, and the skin of the chest is prepared and draped. A standard right posterolateral thoracotomy incision is made. The lung is retracted anteriorly, and the mediastinal pleura is incised over the esophagus from a point about 8 cm above the azygos vein to the diaphragm. The azygos vein is doubly ligated and transected. Dissection is begun well above the neoplasm, usually in the region of the azygos vein, and the esophagus is mobilized and encircled with a Penrose drain. Blunt and sharp dissection is used to carefully mobilize the entire esophagus. There is usually a single fairly large esophageal vessel arising either from the aorta at about the sixth rib level or from the fifth or sixth intercostal artery, which must be identified and ligated.

The surgeon must dissect the area of neoplasm most carefully from adjacent structures, which include the bronchus or trachea, aorta, left atrium, and inferior pulmonary vein. Considerable experience and judgment may be required to decide resectability and when to abandon resection.

The diaphragmatic hiatus is freed from the esophagus, and gentle traction is used to deliver the stomach into the thorax. One must keep the lesser curvature oriented to the right side and avoid producing volvulus.

A G.I.A. stapling instrument is used to divide the stomach just inferior to the cardia. Should a larger extent of the lesser curvature of the stomach need to be resected, a TA 90 stapling instrument may be used. Oversewing the suture line with interrupted silk Lembert sutures or continuous 4-0 Prolene may be unnecessary, but I prefer it. A Sarot bronchial clamp is then applied to the proximal esophagus about 1 to 2 cm below the intended anastomotic line. The esophagus is transected distal to the clamp, and the specimen is removed. The Sarot clamp is elevated, exposing the left lateral wall of the esophagus. The

E

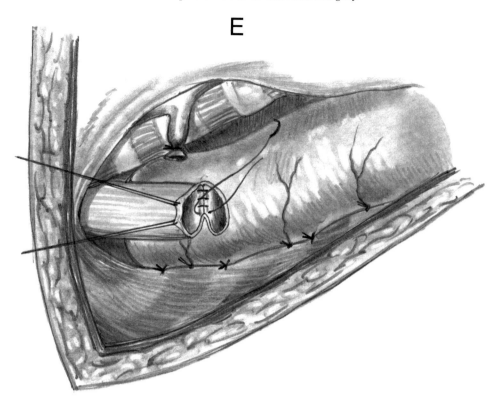

Figure 12–10. *Continued.*

E, The posterior row of sutures is completed and the esophagus again amputated. The mucosal suture is being placed. It is a continuous suture of absorbable material. A nasogastric tube is then passed through the anastomotic area as soon as the posterior suture line is completed. The anterior suture line is an interrupted Lembert suture with the knots tied intra.

fundus is delivered to this area and a site on the anterior gastric wall is selected. This anastomosis may be constructed of two layers of interrupted silk sutures, an inner layer of continuous catgut or Dexon, or a single layer of silk or Prolene interrupted sutures. The first method will be described.

A horizontal mattress (Cushing) type suture of 4-0 silk is used, beginning posteriorly. Each suture should be about 3 mm in width. All sutures are placed before any are tied. After the posterior row of silk sutures are in place, knots are tied. The suture at either end is tagged with a hemostat, and all others are cut.

The esophagus is completely transected proximal to the Sarot clamp. An incision is made into the stomach about 0.5 cm from the suture line. Care must be made not to make the opening too large. A 3-0 catgut or Dexon suture is used as a simple continuous suture, sewing the full thickness of the esophagus to the full thickness of the gastric wall. The suture is then tied and a sump-type nasogastric tube should be introduced from above, while the mucosal suture is still incomplete. The mucosa is closed with a continuous 3-0 catgut or Dexon suture or with simple interrupted sutures. Again, using interrupted Cushing sutures of 4-0 silk, the musculature is approximated on the anterior (actually lateral) aspect of the anastomosis.

The stomach is sutured to the mediastinal pleura and posterior chest wall in several areas to prevent motion or tension on the suture line, and the mediastinal pleura is sutured over the anastomosis for greater security.

A single chest tube is inserted with the tube lying posteriorly and the tip near the anastomosis.

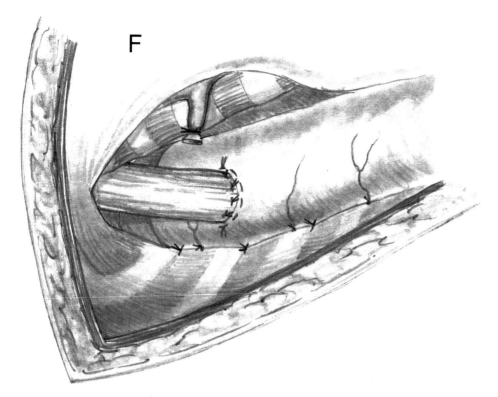

Figure 12–10. *Continued.*
F, Completed anastomosis using 4-0 interrupted mattress sutures as the anterior row. Several sutures have been placed to attach the stomach to the chest wall to prevent tension on the suture line.

Alternative Technique I

The esophagogastrostomy may be constructed with the EEA autosuturing stapling device (see Fig. 12–9). Large series are not available as yet, but reported series indicate a lesser incidence of anastomotic leaks but a slightly higher incidence of stricture compared with suture techniques. The curved, shorter disposable instrument is easier to use in the right side of the chest and has the advantage of being available in multiple sizes. The anastomosis will have to be established on the posterior wall of the fundus rather than anteriorly, as is usual with suture techniques.

A 2 to 3 cm opening is made into the anterior wall of the stomach 5 to 6 cm below the intended anastomosis site. A small stab wound is made through the stomach wall at the site of anastomosis and the anvil is then attached to the shaft of the stapler. A pursestring suture is placed about the circumference of the esophagus at its cut end, or the suture is placed with the supplied device. The anvil is then introduced into the esophagus and the pursestring suture firmly tied.

The stapler is then closed and fixed, after which the stapling instrument is partially opened and then removed. The anastomosis is inspected for any imperfection or leakage.

The wound in the stomach is then closed, and the remainder of the procedure is completed as described earlier.

Note

The surgeon should become thoroughly familiar with the principles and techniques of stapling devices before attempting to use them. When they are used

correctly, much operating time can be saved, and the quality of suture lines is at least as good as and probably better than that obtained with conventional techniques.

Alternative Technique II

Occasionally the neoplasm and involved esophagus may prove to be nonresectable after the laparotomy stage has been completed. There are at least four options at this point.

1. The entire procedure may be abandoned, leaving the patient in the preoperative state except for the mobilized stomach.
2. The stomach may be brought through the hiatus and the area of the cardia divided with the G.I.A. stapling instrument. The staple line is oversewn as described previously. The esophagus may be stapled well above the neoplasm

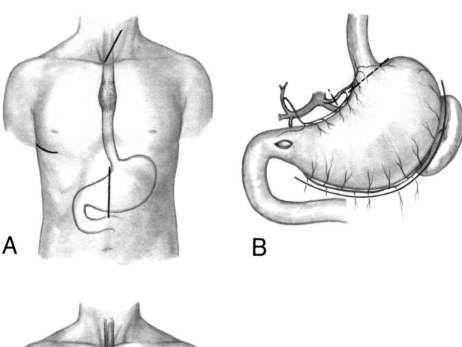

A   B

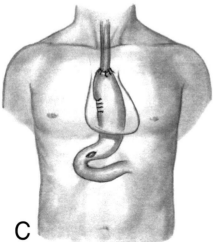

C

Figure 12–11. *A–C,* **Subtotal esophagectomy and thoracic esophagogastrostomy via laparotomy and right thoracotomy.** *A,* Incisions. *B,* Vascular anatomy of the stomach with preservation of the right gastroepiploic artery and right gastric artery as the blood supply for the transplanted stomach. (Note pyloromyotomy.) *C,* The completed resection and intrathoracic esophagogastrostomy in the posterior mediastinum.

Illustration continued on page 254

and an end-to-fundus anastomosis constructed, leaving the esophagus and neoplasm in situ.

3. The stomach may be brought up as described, and a side-to-side anastomosis performed above the neoplasm.

4. The cardia may be divided, after which the thoracotomy incision is closed and the patient turned back to the supine position. A cervical incision is made, and a substernal space is developed as described under *Total Thoracic Esophagectomy*. A cervical esophagogastrostomy is then constructed. This approach leaves the mediastinum accessible for extensive radiation. The esophagus becomes a blind pouch in the mediastinum. This procedure occasionally produces a mucocele, which in turn may be infected, resulting in drainage into the subphrenic area or into the mediastinum and pleural space.

TOTAL ESOPHAGECTOMY FOR CARCINOMA OR CORROSIVE INJURY OR STRICTURE

Indications

The choice of total resection versus subtotal resection may be dictated by the location or extent of the disease process or left to the surgeon. There are at least two reasons for performing a total resection. First, Ankiyama and others, who have extensive experience, are convinced that total removal of the esophagus is more likely to result in long-term survival. The second reason is based on the assumption that an anastomotic leak in the thorax is frequently a lethal complication, whereas an anastomotic leak when a cervical esophagogastrostomy has been done rarely produces fatal sepsis and can easily be drained and managed.

Position

Supine

Procedure (Fig. 12–11D to I)

The laparotomy phase of the procedure is the same as that described earlier in this chapter under *Esophagectomy—Subtotal (Via Right Thoracotomy)* and will not be repeated here. As soon as the gastric mobilization is complete and pyloromyotomy has been accomplished, the esophagus is transected across the cardia using the G.I.A. stapling instrument. The suture line may be oversewn with interrupted or continuous 4-0 silk or Prolene.

The laparotomy is covered temporarily with a drape. An incision is made along the anterior margin of the left sternocleidomastoid muscle, the head being turned to the right. The platysma muscle and the deep cervical fascia are incised. Anterior cervical veins are ligated and severed. The carotid sheath is gently retracted posteriorly after the pretracheal fascia is entered. The omohyoid, sternohyoid, and sternothyroid muscles are transected. Additional exposure may be gained by detaching the sternal head of the sternocleidomastoid muscle. The inferior thyroid vein is doubly ligated and transected, and the thyroid gland retracted medially. The recurrent laryngeal nerve should then be identified. The esophagus can now be seen clearly. The retroesophageal space is developed by blunt dissection and the esophagus carefully mobilized and encircled with a Penrose drain. The mobilization is extended well into the superior mediastinum. The TA 30 stapling instrument is then placed across the esophagus and the staple line placed as far distally as possible. The esophagus is transected on the proximal side of the instrument.

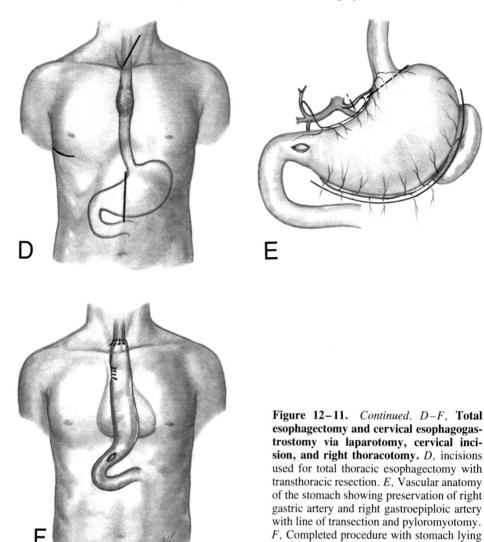

Figure 12–11. *Continued. D–F,* **Total esophagectomy and cervical esophagogastrostomy via laparotomy, cervical incision, and right thoracotomy.** *D,* incisions used for total thoracic esophagectomy with transthoracic resection. *E,* Vascular anatomy of the stomach showing preservation of right gastric artery and right gastroepiploic artery with line of transection and pyloromyotomy. *F,* Completed procedure with stomach lying in substernal position.

A substernal tunnel is developed by blunt dissection with the hand. The space must be wide enough to accommodate the stomach easily. This requires that the entire hand be used to develop the space. This requires careful monitoring because the compression of the heart will cause severe hypotension and the duration of manipulation must be intermittent and brief.

The thoracic inlet sometimes poses a problem, and it may be difficult to provide sufficient room. It may be necessary to resect a portion of the manubrium and the head of the clavicle. A blunt, double-action rongeur is adequate for this purpose.

The stomach is placed in the substernal space, being certain to keep the lesser curvature to the right. The fundus can be grasped with a Babcock clamp as it appears in the cervical area. Additional length may be secured by mobilizing the duodenum by the Kocher maneuver, although the limitation of mobility is determined chiefly by the right gastric artery. Enlargement of the liver may make it impossible for the stomach to be brought into the cervical area.

G

H

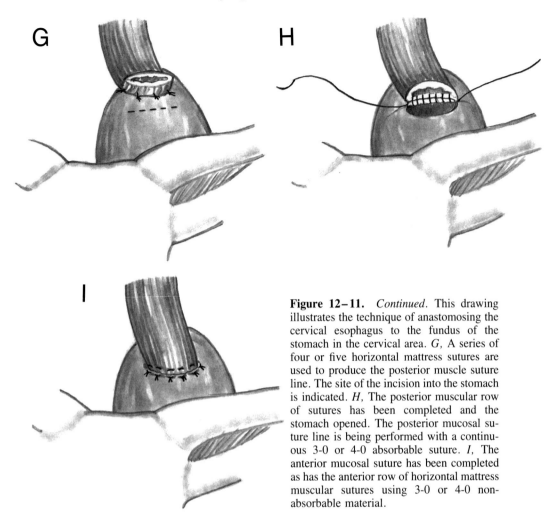

I

Figure 12–11. *Continued.* This drawing illustrates the technique of anastomosing the cervical esophagus to the fundus of the stomach in the cervical area. *G,* A series of four or five horizontal mattress sutures are used to produce the posterior muscle suture line. The site of the incision into the stomach is indicated. *H,* The posterior muscular row of sutures has been completed and the stomach opened. The posterior mucosal suture line is being performed with a continuous 3-0 or 4-0 absorbable suture. *I,* The anterior mucosal suture has been completed as has the anterior row of horizontal mattress muscular sutures using 3-0 or 4-0 non-absorbable material.

The technique of esophagogastrostomy is similar to that described under *Esophagectomy—Subtotal (Via Right Thoracotomy)* (see Fig. 12–8).

The cervical area is drained with Penrose or Jackson-Pratt drains that are brought out through a separate stab wound laterally. The wound is closed, leaving the anterior cervical muscles severed but repairing the sternocleidomastoid muscle with interrupted figure-of-eight nonabsorbable sutures. The deep cervical fascia is loosely closed with absorbable sutures and the subcutaneous tissue with continuous 3-0 absorbable sutures. The skin is closed with a subcuticular suture of 4-0 absorbable material.

The laparotomy incision is closed after reinspection for hemostasis and reassessment of the tension on the right gastric artery.

Following closure of the cervical and laparotomy wounds, the patient is turned into a right lateral position. A posterolateral incision is made, and the pleural space is entered through the fifth interspace. The pleura is incised vertically over the esophagus from the diaphragm to the apex of the pleural space. The azygos vein is doubly ligated and divided. Esophageal mobilization is begun well above the neoplasm, and a Penrose drain is placed around the esophagus to use for traction. A second area of mobilization is initiated well below the tumor. Blunt and sharp dissection are used to free the esophagus. A fairly large esophageal artery usually arises from the aorta or an adjacent intercostal artery at about the

T6 level. Great care must be used in dissecting the area of neoplasm from adjacent structures, such as the aorta, trachea, and left atrium. An overaggressive or careless approach may result in disaster. The esophagus should already be free at both extremities. Considerable time should be spent in ensuring hemostasis at this point. The pleura is left open.

Total esophagectomy for corrosive injury of the esophagus during the acute injury period is occasionally indicated. Before embarking upon this procedure, the surgeon must explore the stomach and small bowel carefully to be certain that there is no extensive injury to either that would make esophagectomy useless. Perforation and mediastinal soilage may also occur before the operative procedure is done.

A lengthy or total esophageal stricture may be an indication for operation. Usually the technical aspects of esophagectomy are not difficult, but occasionally there is extensive periesophageal inflammation and scarring, making dissection difficult and resulting in excessive blood loss.

One or two chest tubes are placed, and the incision is closed as discussed previously.

Note

Should the vascularity of the stomach be uncertain and viability in question, re-exploration of the cervical wound in 48 hours may prevent a major disaster.

ALTERNATIVE PROCEDURE USING COLON FOR RECONSTRUCTION

The stomach is preferred for reconstruction; however, prior gastric surgery or disease may make its use impossible. The risk of colon interposition is at least two times or more as compared with the stomach. A preoperative arteriogram should be done for study of the colonic blood supply. Right, transverse, and left colon all have been used, and some surgeons have preference for each. The right colon has more variable blood supply. Isoperistaltic or antiperistaltic reconstruction is also a matter of preference. The left colon antiperistaltic procedure will be described (Fig. 12–12A through C). The reconstruction may be delayed following esophagostomy and gastrostomy or even following esophagectomy, or it may be accomplished at one operative period. These decisions depend on the patient's nutritional status and general condition.

Procedure (Fig. 12–12)

The technique for esophagectomy via a right thoracotomy has already been described. A midline laparotomy incision is made. The colon is examined and its blood supply pattern confirmed. The branches of the inferior mesenteric artery are ligated and transected, and the middle colic artery is preserved. The colon is divided in the midtransverse area and at the junction of the descending and sigmoid colon, being certain that length is adequate. The colon and its vascular mesentery are passed posterior to the stomach and brought out anteriorly through the gastrohepatic omentum. The surgeon must be certain that (1) the colon is not twisted and (2) no undue tension is placed on the vascular pedicle. Venous occlusion is as damaging as arterial embarrassment.

The transverse colon is then anastomosed to the anterior wall of the stomach close to the lesser curvature, at about the juncture of the middle and lower thirds of the lesser curvature.

A substernal tunnel is prepared as described earlier, and the colon is gently passed to the cervical area. Either the previous incision has been reopened and the esophagus mobilized or incision described earlier is made and the esophagus mobilized, stapled, and transected. An end-to-end anastomosis in two layers is constructed using an inner continuous absorbable suture of 3-0 caliber and an outer row of interrupted silk, polyester or Prolene material. An end-to-end colocolostomy is then accomplished, restoring bowel continuity.

The blood supply of the colon is much more precarious than that of the stomach. Therefore, reexploration of a portion of the cervical wound 24 hours later may be wise if there is any doubt about viability.

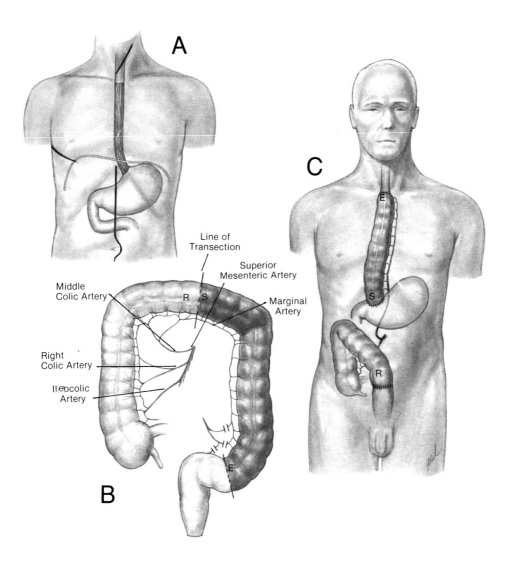

Figure 12–12. Total esophagectomy with colon reconstruction. *A*, The three incisions that are normally used and the extent of resection accomplished. *B*, The portion of the colon to be mobilized for placement and the lines of transection and vascular resection. The middle colic artery is the source of blood supply to the colon in this technique. *C*, The antiperistaltic type of anastomosis to the prepyloric region of the stomach and to the cervical esophagus. The transverse colon is reanastomosed to the rectosigmoid colon.

TRANSHIATAL ESOPHAGECTOMY (FIG. 12–13)

Position

Supine with head turned to right or left.

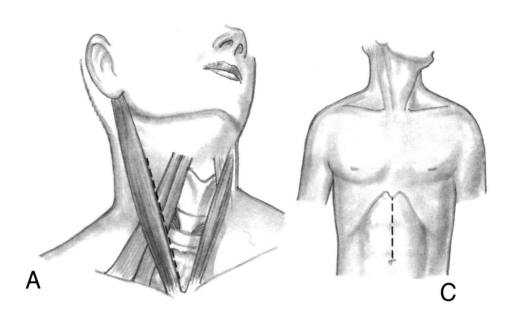

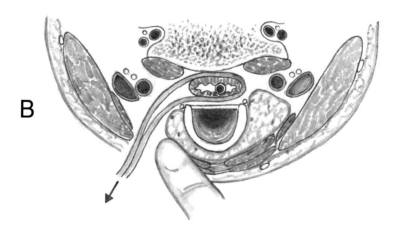

Figure 12–13. *A–C,* The basic technique of blunt dissection of the intrathoracic esophagus. The cardia and the lower third of the esophagus should be mobilized by blunt and sharp dissection under direct vision. The upper esophagus is also freed by blunt dissection, with care not to injure the membranous trachea or major bronchus and the recurrent laryngeal nerve.

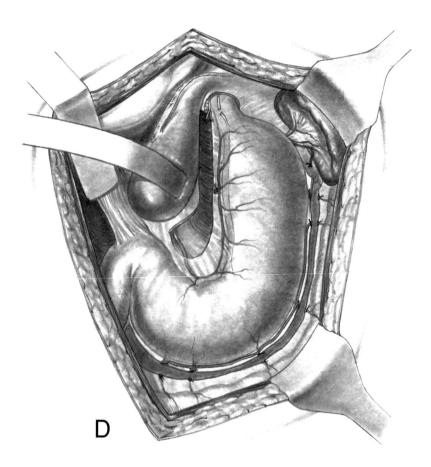

Figure 12–13. *Continued. D.* **Transhiatal esophagectomy.** The laparotomy field showing the fully mobilized and partially devascularized stomach. The right gastric and right gastroepiploic arteries are left intact and supply the entire stomach. Pylorotomy, which should be done, is not shown.

Anesthesia

General, preferably with double lumen intratracheal tube.

Procedure

A midline abdominal incision from the xiphoid process to below the umbilicus. The stomach is mobilized by dividing the gastrocolic mesenteric structures and leaving the omentum in the abdomen. The line of transection is just wide of the right gastroepiploic

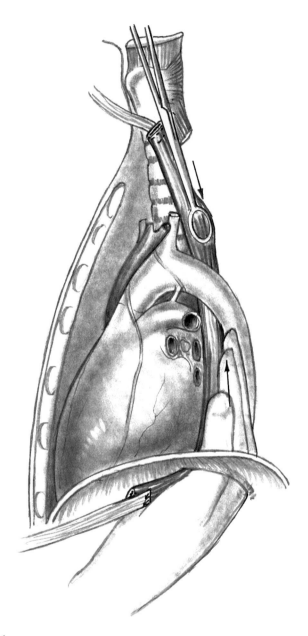

Figure 12–13. *Continued.*
  E, lateral view of the mediastinal dissection of the thoracic esophagus. The technique utilizes primarily the surgeon's hand for both the abdominal and cervical incisions.

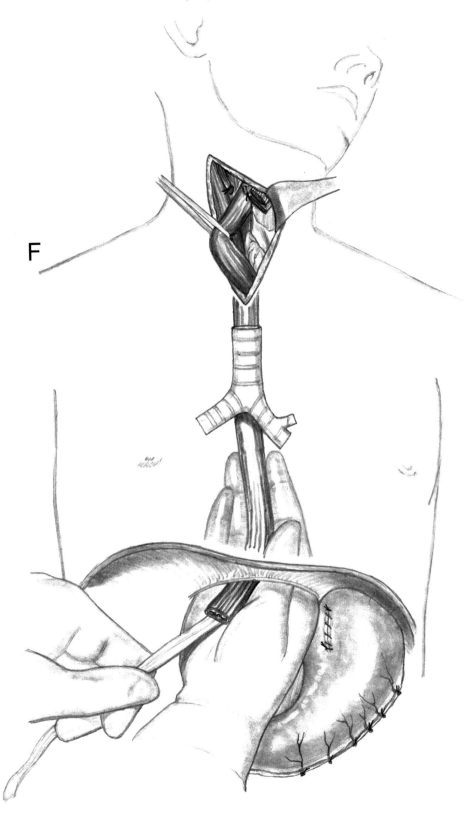

Figure 12–13. *Continued. F,* An anterior view illustrating the dissection again. The esophagus has been detached at the cardia after being stapled. The cervical esophagus has been mobilized.

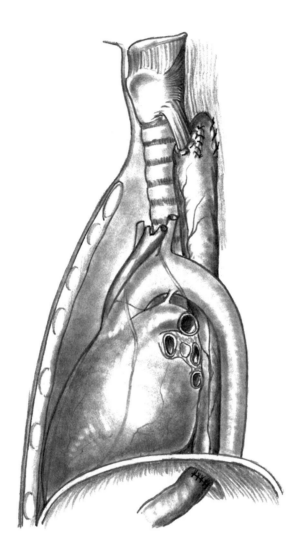

G

Figure 12–13. *Continued. G,* A lateral view diagram, shows the transplanted stomach lying in the esophageal plane posteriorly. The technique of esophagogastric anastomosis is demonstrated in Figure 12–11 G–I.

and left gastroepiploic arteries, taking care not to injure either and preserving this vascular arch. The left gastroepiploic artery is ligated and divided at its origin. The greater curvature is further mobilized by dividing the gastrolienal mesentery and ligating and dividing the short gastric arteries. The surgeon should take care not to include gastric wall in these ligatures. The stomach is then reflected superiorly and medially to expose the left gastric artery, which is doubly ligated and divided. The stomach is placed in its normal position and the lesser omentum is entered carefully, preserving the right gastric artery. The gastrohepatic mesentery is divided in multiple segments. Vessels of varying size from the left gastric artery to the left lobe of the liver are carefully ligated and divided. Varying amounts of this mesentery may be excised to remove lymphatic tissue if the surgeon desires. A strip of the lesser curvature can also be excised with the G.T.A. stapling device. The folds of peritoneum about the hiatus are divided and the phrenic vessels are identified, clipped, or ligated and divided.

This should leave the stomach fully mobilized. Additional mobility can be secured by performing a Kocher maneuver. The author has not found this necessary.

The remainder of the intra-abdominal esophagus is fully mobilized and a large Penrose drain is placed about the terminal esophagus to provide traction. The esophageal hiatus is enlarged by blunt stretching and can be incised laterally until the opening will admit the surgeon's entire right hand easily. Esophageal vessels to the lower one-third can be visualized and divided from the abdominal side. Heavy retraction, manually, or a mechanical retractor fixed to the table may be used to expose the hiatal area. The left lobe of the liver may also be mobilized by incising the triangular ligament.

At this point, the cervical procedure is begun. An incision is made along the anterior border of the sternocleidomastoid muscle on either side. The deep cervical fascia is incised and the visceral compartment entered. The esophagus is visualized and mobilized posteriorly with blunt dissection. An esophageal tube or dilator should be placed in the esophagus to facilitate dissection. The tracheoesophageal groove is entered and developed to the point that it can be encircled with a Penrose drain. Retraction of the thyroid is necessary, and one should avoid the use of metal retractors to protect the recurrent laryngeal nerve. The esophagus is then mobilized inferiorly. As far as possible, use primarily blunt finger dissection. One of the complications has been injury to the membranous wall of the trachea, so that gentleness is important.

The lower and middle thirds of the esophagus are mobilized transhiatally by finger dissection keeping as close as possible to the esophagus. Again, when the carinal area is reached, the anterior dissection must be carried out carefully to avoid injury to the membranous, posterior wall of the lower trachea and main bronchi. The presence of the surgeon's hand can compress the left atrium and inferior vena cava, causing severe hypotension from low output. The blood pressure should be carefully monitored and the hand may have to be removed often to restore and maintain adequate cardiac output.

When the esophagus has been completely mobilized, the distal esophagus can be transected with the G.T.A. stapler and the gastric staple line oversewn. The distal esophagus is sutured to a Penrose drain and then extracted from the thorax. The Penrose drain is sutured to the anterior wall of the fundus of the stomach. With gentle traction from the cervical incision and guidance with the hand, the stomach is advanced to the cervical area through the posterior mediastinum. Axial alignment of the stomach must be maintained so that volvulus does not inadvertently occur.

A two-layered esophagogastrostomy is then performed using the technique previously described and illustrated in Figure 12–11G through I. The stomach is sutured to the anterior spinal ligament at several points. A nasogastric tube is introduced into the stomach just before closure of the anterior row of sutures.

I prefer to establish a pyloromyotomy before the stomach is delivered into the thorax. Some recommend that a feeding jejunostomy tube be placed before the abdominal wound is closed.

LARYNGOESOPHAGECTOMY WITHOUT THORACOTOMY (FIG. 12–14)

Indications

This procedure is indicated for carcinoma of the cervical esophagus with laryngeal involvement as conversely occasionally for advanced carcinoma of the larynx with pharyngeal involvement. It is my opinion that the older Wookey procedure is probably no longer a valid approach.

Anesthesia

General

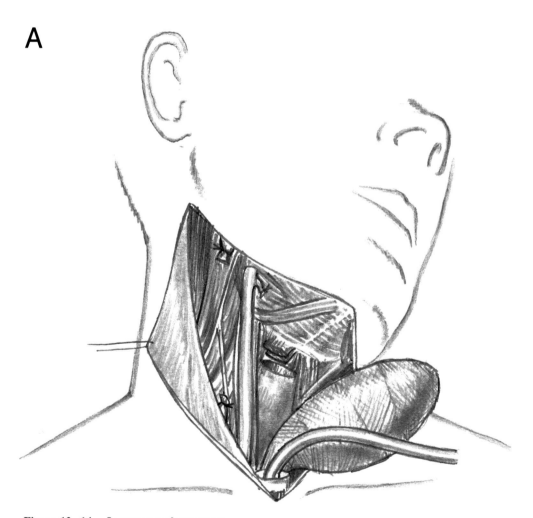

Figure 12–14. Laryngoesophagectomy.
A, A view of the completed neck dissection. The hypopharynx and trachea have been transected. The tumor-bearing larynx and esophagus are wrapped and lying to the left of the operation field.

Position

Supine

Operation

This procedure is best done by two teams, which are multidisciplinary. A general surgeon and an otolaryngologist or plastic surgeon who are regularly performing head and neck surgery should officiate for the cervical procedure. It may be wisest to begin the cervical procedure first to be certain that the lesion is resectable before proceeding with the abdominal phase.

The cervical incision can be transverse, bilateral, or Y-shaped. After hemostasis has been produced, exploration is carried out to the point that the full extent of the tumor and any extension are determined and resectability established, and that lymph node involvement does not prohibit an attempt at a curative procedure. The surgeon, by preference, may choose to perform a standard neck dissection first. Preserving one internal jugular vein seems wise. After the neck dissection is completed or carried to the extent that en bloc removal of the larynx and esophagus remain, the trachea is transected after the endotracheal tube has been withdrawn. A new endotracheal tube is inserted into the distal trachea.

The hypopharynx is transected above the neoplasm level. The specimen is then wrapped in a rubber or plastic container, leaving the distal esophagus intact for the moment.

The second phase requires an upper midline laparotomy. The technique of gastric mobilization is the same as that described in the immediately preceding procedure, *Transhiatal Esophagectomy,* and will not be repeated here. Gastric mobilization must be as complete as possible because of the additional length to be bridged by the stomach. Pyloroplasty is optional, although I feel that it is necessary.

The mobilization of the normal thoracic esophagus is then initiated from the cervical area and via the diaphragmatic hiatus chiefly by careful blunt dissection. Care must be taken to avoid pleural entry and injury to the membranous trachea and major bronchi. Experience will result in less complications and greater safety. When mobilization is complete, the stomach is slowly advanced into the posterior mediastinum by gentle traction and with assistance from below. After the stomach is delivered into the cervical area, the esophagus is divided at the cardia using a G.I.A. stapling device. The stapled area may be oversewn if desired but is not necessary. The entire specimen is then removed from the operative field.

The highest point of the fundus of the stomach is then incised widely enough to anastomose to the hypopharynx. This technique, except for size, is the same previously described. The stomach should be sutured at several points to the prevertebral fascia to prevent traction on the anastomosis.

Permanent tracheostomy should then be produced; it varies depending on the incision used for the cervical part of the procedure.

266

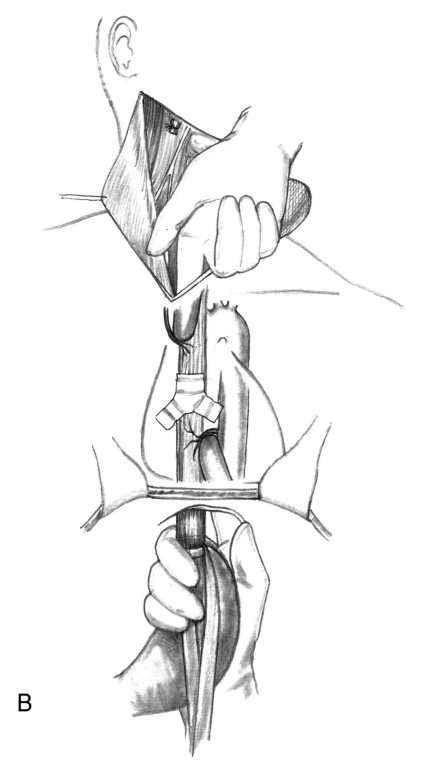

Figure 12–14. *Continued.*

  B, The blunt mobilization of the thoracic esophagus is being done from the cervical area and simultaneously from the abdomen. The lower third of the esophagus can be mobilized by blunt and sharp dissection from the abdominal side. The stomach has been previously mobilized as described and shown in previous text and drawings.

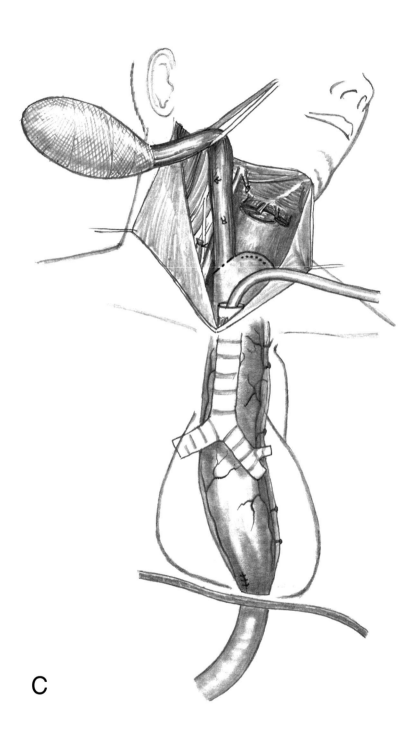

Figure 12–14. *Continued.*
  C, The thoracic esophagus and stomach have been drawn up into the cervical area. A G.I.A. stapling device should be used to close and divide the cardia. The endotracheal tube is shown in the distal trachea.

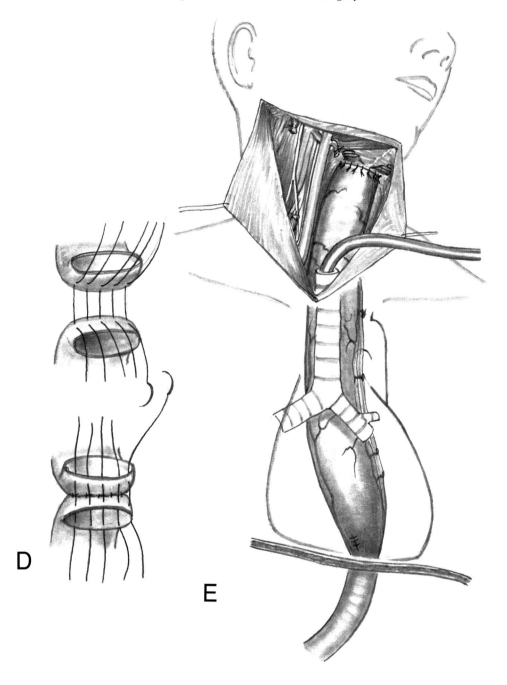

Figure 12–14. *Continued.*

D, The technique of anastomosing the stomach to the hypopharynx. Except for the larger diameter of the anastomosis, the technique is the same as that used for the anastomosis of the cervical esophagus to the stomach.

E, Completed procedure with the fundus of the stomach anastomosed to the hypopharynx. The stomach should be sutured to the prevertebral fascia to relieve tension (not shown). The permanent tracheostomy stoma has not been established.

Antireflux Procedures

For many years, a multiplicity of surgical procedures has been performed with the aim of correcting esophageal hiatal hernia, esophageal reflux and parahiatal hernia. Emphasis on repairing the hernia was emphasized earlier, before sufficient knowledge of the physiologic function of the esophagogastric junction. The Allison procedure was characteristic of this surgical approach.

More recently, emphasis on reducing or obliterating reflux has resulted in three procedures. The Nissen procedure has been most popular, but late complications and failure have been disappointing. Similarly, the Belsey procedure has been used extensively, but has proved less than perfect and has a higher rate of operative and postoperative problems. The Hill procedure has been less popular, but in the hands of Hill has had a commendable statistical record. It seems, from a theoretical and anatomic viewpoint, to more nearly restore the normal relationship of the structures in and about the gastroesophageal junction.

The reader is reminded that esophageal reflux is best managed medically if possible. The typical esophageal hiatal hernia without reflux is not an indication for surgery. The large parahiatal hernia should be repaired. Also, when advanced stricture formation has occurred, no procedure including resection is likely to prove altogether successful.

It should be emphasized that hiatal hernia repair without an adequate antireflux procedure is generally futile. Furthermore, in the absence of reflux, incarceration, or gastric ulceration in the herniated stomach, hiatal hernia repair is not indicated.

The Belsey procedure accomplishes the same result as the fundoplication, but thoracotomy is required. Published results of most long-term studies indicate a slightly higher percentage of unsatisfactory results and a higher morbidity rate.

There are a number of unpleasant sequelae to any form of reflux procedure; one should not advise such a procedure unless there is a clear failure of medical management.

NISSEN FUNDOPLICATION

This procedure has emerged as the most satisfactory one for the control of gastroesophageal reflux. Usually it is performed by laparotomy rather than thoracotomy. A variant is the Collis-Nissen procedure, which should be done transthoracically. The procedure may also be done transthoracically if there is adequate reason for thoracotomy apart from the Nissen procedure.

Procedure

A laparotomy is performed for exposure of the upper abdomen. After visceral exploration, suitable exposure of the cardiac area and fundus is obtained. The peritoneum over the cardia is incised and, by blunt and sharp dissection, the distal esophagus is mobilized and encircled with a Penrose drain for traction. The fundus is detached from its peritoneal attachments to the diaphragm and mobilized.

A Hurst-Maloney dilator, No. 52 to No. 56, is passed orally and guided into the stomach; it is left in place while the remainder of the procedure is accomplished. Often a stricture must be dilated acutely with several dilators before one of this size can be passed.

The fundus is then passed posteriorly to the esophagus and wrapped anteriorly around it, until it touches the remaining stomach. Occasionally it may be necessary to divide several short gastric vessels to carry out a 360-degree wrap. Silk sutures, 3-0, are placed in the stomach, the esophagus, and the fundus. Several should be placed before any are tied. The total width of the wrap should be about 2-3 cm. The sutures are tied, making certain that there is enough mobility to the fundus that the sutures are not under tension.

If a significant defect is present in the diaphragmatic hiatus, crural repair should be accomplished by a series of 2-0 silk sutures placed posteriorly to the esophagus. This should be done before the fundoplication is accomplished.

The laparotomy wound is then closed without drainage.

THE USE OF THE COLLIS GASTROPLASTY WITH FUNDOPLICATION

Some surgeons have advocated performing a fundoplication in the mediastinum in patients with shortening of the esophagus following esophagitis. Leaving the fundoplication above the diaphragm may be unavoidable unless some other procedure is done. Resection and esophagogastrostomy have invariably resulted in secondary stricture. Major procedures such as jejunal or colonic interposition have their advocates but carry greater risk than would normally seem necessary. Resection with any form of reconstruction is rarely required and must be reserved for strictures that are unmanageable by any form of dilatation. Almost every stricture can be dilated by the experienced surgeon with patient, careful effort. In many cases of "short esophagus," the shortening is more apparent than real, and in these patients fundoplication can be performed and the area of the cardia placed beneath the diaphragm without difficulty.

The Collis gastroplasty may be useful when esophageal shortening will not permit placing the cardia beneath the diaphragm. It can be associated with either a Nissen or a Belsey fundoplication because following gastroplasty alone reflux is not likely to be controlled.

The Collis-Nissen procedure will be described here.

Position

Left lateral.

Incision

Left posterolateral thoracotomy.

Procedure (Fig. 12–15)

The pleural space is entered through the sixth or seventh intercostal space. Following routine exploration, the esophagus is mobilized and encircled with a Penrose drain. The cardioesophageal junction and adjacent stomach are mobilized. It will be necessary to ligate and transect several short gastric vessels. A counterincision may be made in the diaphragm, but usually is not necessary. Fat-containing tissue is excised from the stomach in the surgical field, leaving the stomach and lower esophagus essentially bare.

The esophagus is progressively dilated using Hurst-Maloney dilators until a size No. 52 to No. 54 French has been reached. The last dilator is left in place. The fundus of the stomach is grasped with a Babcock clamp and countertraction applied.

A G.I.A. stapling instrument is then positioned with the instrument parallel to the esophagus. The stapler is applied to the stomach, taking care to stay lateral enough from the side of the in situ dilator so that the tissue will not be stapled under tension. The staples are fired and the tissue severed, after which the instrument is removed. This creates a tube the size of the esophagus 5 cm in length. This length is usually adequate, but if necessary, an additional staple application for 2 to 3 cm may be used. The staple line of the stomach

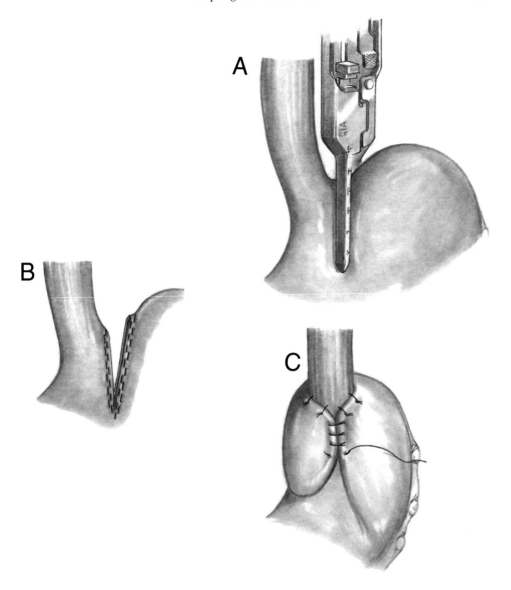

Figure 12–15. Collis-Nissen procedure (transthoracic).

A, The cardia, distal esophagus, and fundus of the stomach have been mobilized. A G.I.A. Stapling instrument has been placed on the stomach parallel to the esophagus. A Hurst-Maloney dilator (No. 44 to No. 52) should be present in the esophagus to prevent narrowing.

B, Note the result of stapling, which lengthens the esophagus by 5 cm. An additional cut may be made if necessary.

C, The fundus has been wrapped about the lengthened gastric esophagus and is being sutured to itself.

and esophagus may be oversewn with a 4-0 continuous or interrupted suture or the stapled suture line may be left free.

Fundoplication is then accomplished. Several of the short gastric vessels have already been severed. The fundus is wrapped about the terminal esophageal tube just created. Additional mobilization of the greater curvature may be required so that a wrap of 2–3 cm in length may be sutured without tension. Nonabsorbable material (4-0) is used to suture the wrapped fundus to the anterior wall of the stomach. Each suture includes a portion of the esophageal musculature as well as the gastric wall.

The completed fundoplication is then reduced through the hiatus. The sutures placed in the crura previously or placed at this time are tied, narrowing the hiatus to prevent herniation of the fundoplication. I prefer to place several 4-0 sutures at this point, suturing the musculature of the esophagus to the margin of the hiatus. The Hurst-Maloney dilator is removed.

A single drainage tube is placed in the pleural space, and the wound is closed.

Notes

1. **Severe transmural esophagitis may make dissection difficult and leave the esophagus more bulky than normal.**
2. **Previous attempts at hiatal hernia repair or fundoplication also make the procedure technically difficult or occasionally impossible; this will make resection mandatory.**

BELSEY MARK IV ANTIREFLUX PROCEDURE

Indications

This and other operative procedures are reserved for patients with proved ulcerative esophagitis, esophageal stricture, repetitive bleeding, demonstrated recurrent aspiration, and lesser degrees of esophagitis that have not been managed successfully by a good medical regimen.

The choice of the Nissen or the Belsey procedure depends on two considerations.

1. The Nissen can be performed by either laparotomy or left thoracotomy. If there is no other consideration, laparotomy is probably preferable. The Collis-Nissen modification requires thoracotomy.

2. The Belsey procedure is a thoracic operation. Therefore, the choice is a matter of preference, but in addition the surgeon must decide whether thoracotomy or laparotomy is preferable. Results of the two procedures are comparable with the thoracic procedures, carrying a slightly higher morbidity rate, probably unnecessarily so.

There is no indication for the repair of esophageal hiatal hernia in the absence of proved, symptomatic reflux.

Position

Left lateral.

Procedure (Fig. 12–16)

A posterolateral thoracotomy incision is made and the pleural space entered through the sixth or seventh intercostal space. The lung is retracted. The pulmonary ligament may be divided, but this is not usually necessary for exposure. The mediastinal pleura is incised from the diaphragm to the posterior pulmonary hilum, and the esophagus is mobilized over this distance, which is about 12 to 15 cm. All of the pleural and peritoneal tissue and attachments to the area of the cardia are dissected free, and the adipose tissue is excised. A Penrose drain is passed about the esophagus to facilitate exposure. The vagus nerves are noted and carefully protected. The margins of the hiatus are dissected until only muscle tissue is present.

The cardia is elevated, and the diaphragmatic crura are identified and dissected until only muscle and fascia are apparent. Then several sutures are placed through the crura, including generous amounts of tissue. These should be 0 or 2-0 nonabsorbable suture. The purpose of these sutures is to reduce the size of the hiatus. Usually, three to five stitches are sufficient. Making the hiatus tight about the esophagus serves no purpose except to increase the risk of dysphagia postoperatively. These sutures are left untied at this time.

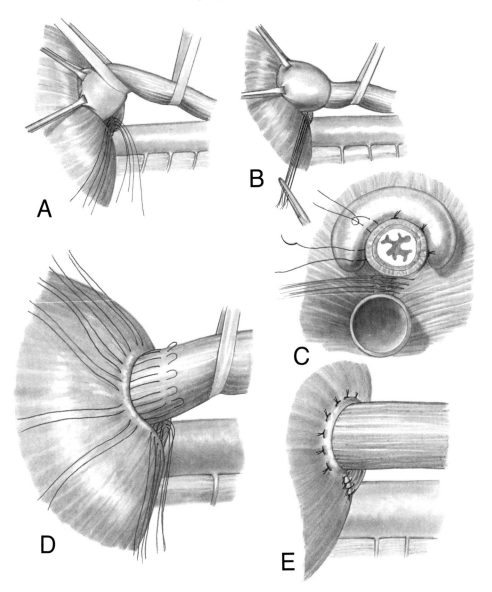

Figure 12–16. Belsey fundoplication (modified) (transthoracic).

A, The esophagus, cardia, and adjacent fundus of the stomach have been mobilized. Crural sutures of 2-0 or 0 silk have been placed to reduce the size of the hiatus. They are not tied at this time.

B, The completed dissection.

C, The first row of plication sutures is being placed. These include 3 cm of stomach; Belsey used only three. The plication involved about 280 degrees of the circumference of the esophagus.

D, The second row of plication sutures has been placed, plicating an additional 3 cm of stomach and then passing through the diaphragm. A total of 6 cm of stomach is now plicated over the cardia and held beneath the diaphragm.

E, Crural sutures are tied. The procedure is completed.

Two rows of three to five stitches each are then utilized to imbricate the stomach over the terminal esophagus. The first row are three sutures of 3-0 or 4-0 nonabsorbable material placed as horizontal mattress sutures encompassing about 5 to 6 mm of tissue with the esophageal suture 2 cm above the gastric suture area. These are tied and 2 cm of stomach becomes imbricated. The sutures are placed to involve about 270 degrees of the circumference of the esophagus.

A second row of sutures is then placed, again imbricating an additional 2 cm of stomach over and above the first suture line. The suture differs in that it includes the diaphragm about 1 cm lateral to the hiatus. Actually, the stitching begins with the diaphragm, picks up layers of the stomach wall, then ends with esophagus tissue. It passes again through the stomach wall and back through the diaphragm about 1 cm lateral or medial to the first strand.

These sutures are tied and effectively imbricate an additional 2 cm of stomach over the terminal esophagus, at the same time replacing the cardia and about 4 cm of the esophagus below the diaphragmatic hiatus.

The crural sutures are then tied, beginning with the most posterior suture and ending with the one at the hiatus. The tightness of the hiatal ring about the esophagus is evaluated after each suture is tied and the number of stitches is modified accordingly.

Modifications

1. Some surgeons prefer to use more than three stitches in each of the two layers.
2. Some surgeons have preferred to incise the hiatus to gain exposure to the fundus and close this incision at the completion of the repair.
3. Acute dilatation of a pre-existing stricture may be necessary before beginning the imbrication. Hurst-Maloney dilators may be used progressing up to No. 44 to No. 52 French size. An occasional situation may occur in which this method of dilatation is ineffective. A variant is to make a small gastrotomy and dilate the stricture retrogradely with progressive sizes of Hegar cervical dilators. Any form of acute dilatation of a fibrous stricture may rupture the esophageal wall; therefore, careful inspection is necessary to avoid leaving an unrepaired injury behind. I prefer to dilate strictures over 2 to 3 weeks preoperatively with Hurst-Maloney dilators to avoid acute dilatation, which is more likely to result in injury.
4. The surgeon must be absolutely certain that a stricture is a stricture and not a narrowed lumen produced by neoplasm.

THE HILL REPAIR (FIG. 12–17)

Indications

Gastroesophageal reflux is the primary indication, although Hill recommends it for several other situations.

Position

Supine

Anesthesia

General

Figure 12–17. *A,* Diagram of the operative field as seen in the Hill repair. Three mattress sutures have been placed in the diaphragmatic crura. Tying these will reduce the size of the esophageal hiatus. *B,* The crural sutures are now tied. The second five sutures are suturing the phrenoesophageal ligaments to the preaortic fascia and the median arcuate ligament. It is preferable to place small teflon pledgets on both ends of each suture to prevent sutures from cutting through the tissues. No sutures are placed in the esophagus.

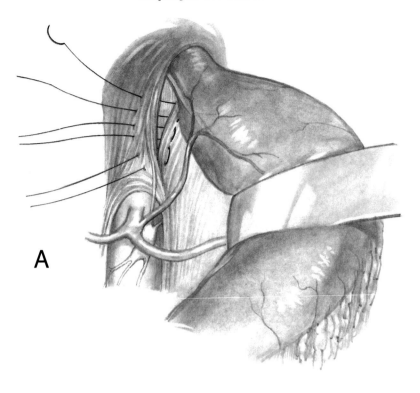

A

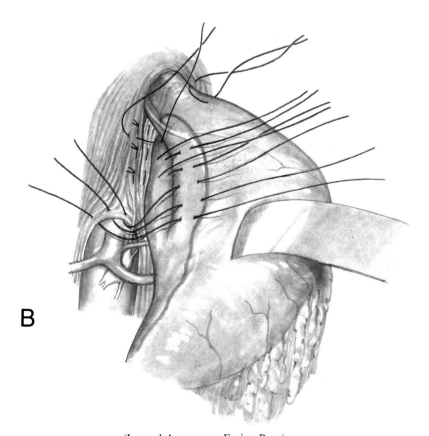

B

(Legend Appears on Facing Page)

Incision

Upper midline abdominal

Procedure

A lengthy upper midline incision is made, beginning at the xiphoid level, preferably with excision of the xiphoid process. Adequate exposure to this area is difficult to obtain and requires a mechanical table-mounted retractor. It is necessary to divide the triangular ligament so that the left lobe of the liver may be exposed. The phrenoesophageal membrane is divided, exposing the terminal esophagus. The gastrohepatic ligament is divided, with care not to injure the phrenoesophageal bundles or bronchus of the left gastric artery to the liver. The esophagus is further dissected and encircled with a Penrose drain for exposure posteriorly. About 6 to 8 cm of intra-abdominal esophagus is mobilized. The vagus nerves are protected carefully. The gastric fundus is then partially mobilized by dividing its attachments to the diaphragm and the upper portion of the gastrosplenic ligament including one or two short gastric arteries.

The esophagus and stomach are retracted laterally and the pancreas inferiorly, exposing the pre-aortic area. The celiac axis is identified by palpation so that injury is avoided. The median arcuate ligament is then identified and dissected free. A finger may be introduced superiorly between the diaphragmatic crura and gently advanced to the level of the arcuate ligament in the preaortic plane. The ligament is usually well defined. Dissection should be cautious to avoid vascular injury of aorta or celiac branches.

The crura of the diaphragm is then approximated with heavy nonabsorbable sutures buttressed by Dacron or Teflon pledgets. Two to four sutures are sufficient. Either an esophageal bougie should be indwelling or the final opening should admit the finger easily.

The two phrenoesophageal bundles are then visualized by the surgeon passing the right hand around the greater curvature of the stomach. Each bundle is grasped with a Babcock clamp. Sutures with pledgets are then placed. The first passes through the seromuscular gastric wall. The anterior bundle and the posterior bundle are then brought through the preaortic fascia just superior to the median arcuate ligament. This suture is left untied until at least four additional sutures are placed, each one more inferiorly on the stomach, the last being at approximately the gastroesophageal junction and in the median arcuate ligament. The vagus nerves should lie within the approximated bundles but not injured or involved by any suture. The proximal two sutures are then tied. Hill recommends measuring the lower esophageal sphincter pressure with an intraluminal catheter manometer. A desirable pressure between 35 and 45 mm Hg is advised. Additional sutures may be placed to achieve this level of pressure.

The laparotomy incision is then closed. Probably, if the manometric instrumentation is not available to the surgeon, it would be wise not to perform this procedure rather than do an inadequate procedure.

13
Diaphragm

REPAIR OF PARAESOPHAGEAL DIAPHRAGMATIC HERNIA

The paraesophageal or parahiatal hernia is produced by a defect in the phrenoesophageal membrane or ligament. There are several variations, sometimes categorized as types II, III, and IV. A hiatal hernia frequently coexists and may be symptomatic in terms of reflux esophagitis.

These hernias may be large and may contain most of the stomach. A sequence of volvulus, obstruction, necrosis, and perforation may be a fatal complication. Transient mechanical obstruction may result in severe pain, and ulceration and bleeding are also common. Herniation of other viscera into the mediastinum is not rare.

The presence of a paraesophageal hernia is an indication for repair because of the seriousness of the complications just mentioned.

Position

Left lateral.

Procedure (Fig. 13–1)

A left posterolateral thoracotomy incision is made, and the pleural space is entered through the sixth or seventh interspace. The lung is retracted, the inferior pulmonary ligament is divided, and hemostasis is produced. The mediastinal pleura is opened widely by a vertical incision, after which the esophagus is mobilized and encircled with a Penrose drain. The vagus nerves are identified and protected. There is always a hernia sac present. It should be entered at its lateral side 4 to 5 cm away from the cardia. After the extent of the herniation has been evaluated, the hernial sac is excised. This may require some time and patient ligating of numerous vessels. The excision should be terminated without entering the vasculature of the lesser curvature. Hemostasis must be perfect at this point. The fundus, cardia, and all other structures should be free of peritoneal, mediastinal, and pleural attachments. Patients who have large incarcerated hernias, of long duration, may have extensive adhesions to mediastinal structures and may require prolonged, meticulous dissection before the hernia can be reduced.

The hernia is reduced and retained by sponges or a sponge holder. The defect in the diaphragm is then delineated, and all adipose and peritoneal tissue is removed. The defect is evaluated and the extent of repair necessary is determined. Most often the defect can be converted to a single large hiatus, which can be repaired by simple sutures through the crura.

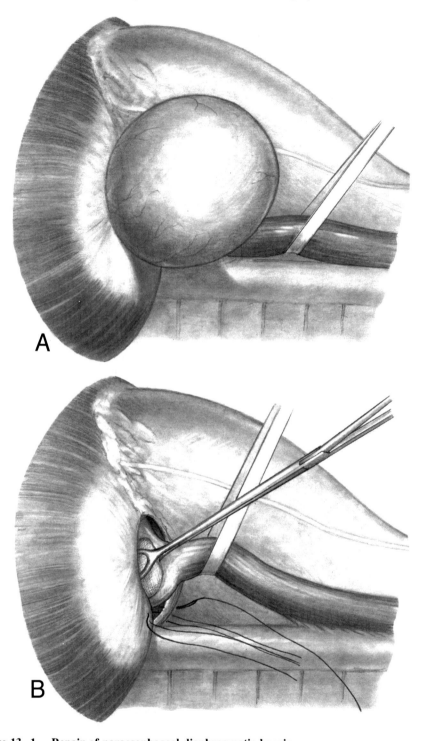

Figure 13–1.   Repair of paraesophageal diaphragmatic hernia.

   A, View of the herniated stomach through a left posterolateral thoracotomy. The esophagus is partially mobilized. *B,* The stomach has been dissected free from the diaphragm and reduced, and the hiatal margin and crura are completely freed. Crural sutures are being placed using 0 or 2-0 nonabsorbable material.   *Illustration continued on following page*

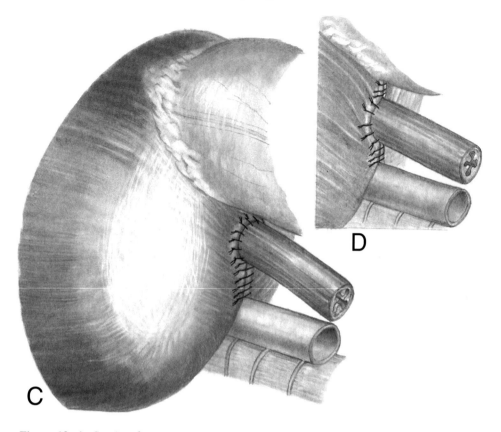

Figure 13–1. *Continued.*

C, Suturing has been completed. Additional sutures of 4-0 nonabsorbable material have been placed in the esophageal musculature and the margin of the hiatus to minimize sliding motion and recurrence.

D, A very large defect may be reduced in size by sutures placed anterior to the esophagus; this will prevent excessive displacement of the esophagus anteriorly.

If an antireflux procedure is indicated, it should be done at this time. The crural sutures are placed beginning posteriorly and inferiorly. Sutures should include a considerable amount of tissue and be placed about 1 cm apart. Suture material should be nonabsorbable of 0 or 2-0 size. These sutures should be left untied until all are placed and then tied, again beginning posteriorly. The area of the hiatus is checked after each suture is tied to judge the adequacy of closure.

After completing this suture line, a single chest tube is placed and the chest is closed.

Modifications

1. **I prefer to suture the esophagus with a series of four or five 4-0 sutures to the inferior surface of the diaphragm before beginning the crural repair. At the completion of the crural repair, a second row of 4-0 sutures is used to secure the esophagus to the superior margin of the hiatus. It is hoped that this will reduce the sliding ability of the esophagus and seal the hiatus.**
2. **Occasionally the defect is so large (8 to 10 cm) that, if all sutures are placed posteriorly, the hiatus is shifted anteriorly to a nonanatomic position. In this instance, it is preferable to place some sutures anteriorly, creating a new hiatus**

in its approximately normal position. The surgeon must be wary of making the hiatus too small by this technique, however.

3. **The diaphragmatic muscle may be attenuated or atrophied so that secure suture closure of a large defect is not possible. Marlex mesh may be used, preferably sutured superiorly over the repair, to give added strength. I would not use Marlex mesh to close the defect primarily if there is any alternative choice.**

REPAIR OF EVENTRATION OF THE DIAPHRAGM

Eventration of the diaphragm is most often an incidental finding rather than a symptomatic entity. In elderly patients for whom no previous x-ray films are available, a problem may arise in differentiating phrenic nerve paralysis related to malignancy from eventration. Also, an eventration discovered following major trauma must be differentiated from traumatic rupture of the diaphragm, particularly on the right side.

Only those patients with eventration of the diaphragm who have severe respiratory insufficiency on the basis of the diaphragmatic lesion should be considered for operation. Most of these are children or young adults.

Position

Lateral. (The description given here assumes a right-sided eventration.)

Incision

Posterolateral thoracotomy.

Procedure (Fig. 13–2)

A posterolateral thoracotomy incision is made. The contents of the pleural space are examined and the diagnosis is confirmed. The diaphragm is evaluated carefully. In some patients, it appears to be normal except for redundancy and elevation. In others, it contains a lesser amount of muscle than normal, and in still others the diaphragm consists only of pleura and peritoneum. As a variant, muscle may be limited to the lateral portions of the diaphragm.

Two or three Allyce clamps are used to grasp the diaphragm in an anteroposterior plane, and the diaphragm is elevated while the viscera are displaced inferiorly. Sutures of 2-0 or 0 nonabsorbable material are used to create a line of 6 to 10 horizontal mattress sutures at the base of the tented-up portion of the diaphragm (Fig. 13–2B). Sutures buttressed with pledgets of Teflon may be helpful if the muscle is thin and attenuated. After this suture line has been completed, the diaphragm should assume a lower, flattened contour with a fold of redundant tissue 5 to 10 cm in width. This layer of muscle is reflected laterally and sutured to the diaphragm near the chest wall or actually to the chest wall itself.

A circular piece of Marlex mesh is then fashioned to conform to the diaphragmatic surface and sutured to the diaphragm with a series of sutures about its periphery; additional sutures are placed in the central portion to obliterate any space between the mesh and the diaphragm. The purpose of this mesh is to prevent further attenuation or stretching of the noninnervated diaphragm and thereby a recurrence of its elevated position. This mesh also minimizes, to some degree, paradoxic diaphragmatic motion.

This procedure is essentially one of my devising, and several other approaches may serve as well. To reiterate, repair of eventration is rarely indicated and should not be done indiscriminately.

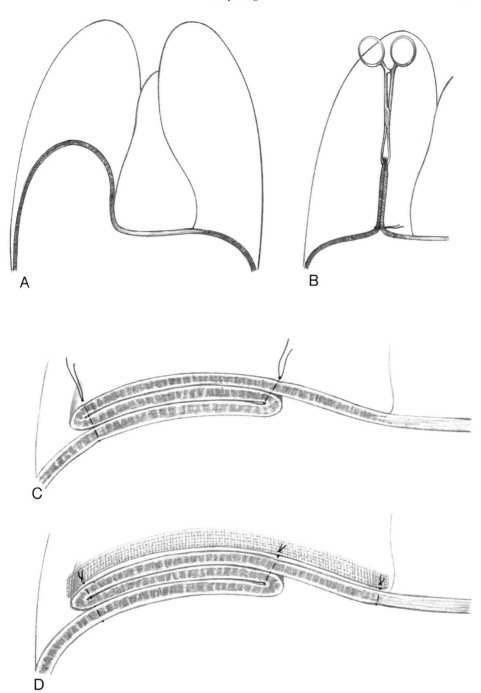

Figure 13–2. Eventration of the diaphragm.

A, Diagrammatic illustration of the defect.

B, The excess diaphragmatic tissue is grasped with Allyce clamps and a series of mattress sutures is used to suture the diaphragm to itself, restoring it to its normal position.

C, The redundant layer of diaphragm is sutured to the periphral area of the diaphragm near the chest wall.

D, Marlex mesh may be sutured over the completed repair to prevent further elevation of the denervated tissue.

REPAIR OF FORAMEN OF MORGAGNI HERNIA

Hernia of the foramen of Morgagni is a congenital defect that lies at the site of passage of the internal mammary artery through the diaphragm, where it becomes the superior epigastric artery of the abdominal wall. It is an uncommon lesion. The most common variety represents herniation of the preperitoneal fat to produce a circumscribed mass noted on x-ray films, which may be confused with a pericardial fat pad or a pericardial cyst. Occasionally the omentum and transverse colon herniate. A sac may or may not be present. Few patients require operation except to establish diagnosis or unless there is intestinal herniation.

This defect can be repaired either transthoracically or by laparotomy, the latter being technically more easily accomplished. The description given here will use the laparotomy approach.

Position

Supine.

Incision

Subcostal.

Procedure (Fig. 13-3)

The rectus muscle is transected, and the peritoneum is opened. Hemostasis is produced, after which the hernia is inspected and reduced. If a sac is present, it is excised. It is necessary to carry repair sutures through the full thickness of the chest wall because there is no remnant of diaphragmatic muscle anteriorly, and merely suturing the defect leaves an anterior defect still present. A row of interrupted nonabsorbable sutures is placed through the anterior edge of the defect with the stitches about 1 cm apart. Then a second row of mattress sutures is placed about 2 to 3 cm away from the margin on the left. This last row of sutures is passed through the chest wall using fairly large Fergueson or Mayo needles. After all sutures have been placed, the anterior sutures are then made through the chest wall in a similar fashion but through the next lower interspace. All of these sutures are tied, and the abdominal wall incision is closed. A single chest tube is introduced and left in place for 24 hours.

In the event that there is incarcerated bowel or bowel fixed in the thorax by adhesions, a separate thoracotomy incision in the anterior sixth or seventh interspace may be required to free the bowel safely and remove it from the thorax.

REPAIR OF FORAMEN OF BOCHDALEK HERNIA

Preoperative Management

Early diagnosis, before profound hypoxemia and acidosis occur, is probably the major factor influencing survival in patients with foramen of Bochdalek hernia. Early placement of a nasogastric tube will minimize gastrointestinal distention and any further respiratory distress. Early intubation and respiratory support may stabilize the condition of the patient temporarily. Correction of severe acidosis is mandatory, but operative intervention should not be delayed.

Position

Supine.

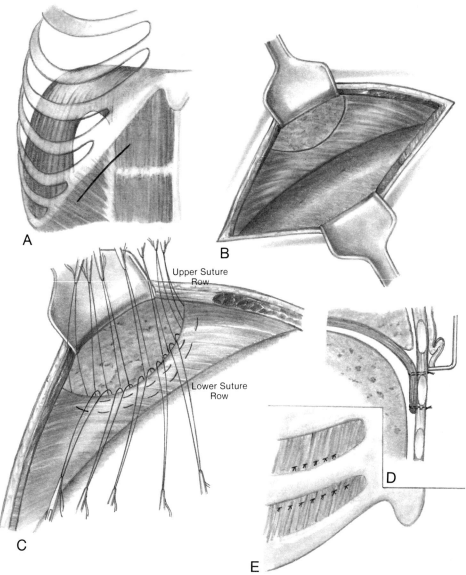

A

B

Upper Suture
Row

Lower Suture
Row

C

D

E

Figure 13–3. Repair of foramen of Morgagni hernia. *A,* The location of the defect. *B,* The defect as it would appear from the abdominal exposure. *C,* Two rows of sutures are usually used. The mattress sutures in the diaphragm are carried through the full thickness of the chest wall except for the skin and subcutaneous tissue. *D,* These two rows are tied and should obliterate the space produced by the congenital defect.

Incision

Left subcostal.

Procedure

The peritoneum is opened and the abdominal viscera are gently extracted from the thorax. Passage of a No. 10 or No. 12 catheter into the thorax, allowing air to enter, may facilitate removal of the intestine. It is preferable to extract first the small bowel, then the colon, and finally the stomach. Much care must be taken not to injure the spleen and left lobe of the liver.

The child's respiratory status should improve following removal of herniated viscera from the chest. A sac composed of pleura and peritoneum may be present, or the defect in the diaphragm may communicate freely with both cavities. A wide variety of defects may be seen, from a relatively small posterolateral defect to absence of a major part of the diaphragm (Fig. 13–4) or complete absence of the entire structure.

Most often the defect can be repaired by direct suture using interrupted nonabsorbable 3-0 sutures in two layers (Fig. 13–5). Absence of a segment of the diaphragm on the costal aspect will require that the sutures pass around the ribs to provide sufficient stability for closure. Complete absence of the diaphragm or even a very large defect may require a piece of Marlex mesh or Dacron cloth to effect closure. The area near the pericardium is a point where careful placement of sutures is necessary to avoid injury to the vena cava or aorta.

The abdominal wall is then closed. Closure may be difficult because the peritoneal cavity has not previously contained all the viscera and therefore is too small. Forcefully stretching the abdominal wall may be helpful. Using undue tension to close the wound may produce sufficient intraperitoneal pressure to make adequate ventilation impossible, however. Therefore, fascial closure can be abandoned and the skin merely closed over the viscera. Forceful efforts to reduce bowel and liver may damage viscera.

A single No. 12 catheter is placed in the left pleural space and left with either water seal drainage and no suction, or suction not exceeding 5 to 6 cm of water. Miniaturized tubing and bottle are desirable.

No effort should be made to forcefully expand the atelectic immature left lung. Attempts to do so will be unsuccessful and may result in pneumothorax on the right side.

Despite the great advances in neonatal care and anesthesia technique in infants, the overall mortality rate still remains near 50%. This is probably caused partly by the immaturity of both the contralateral and epsilateral lung and partly by the poor respiratory status of the patient before operation.

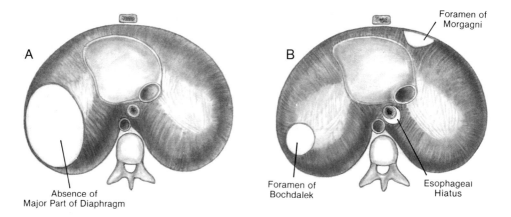

Figure 13–4.   Congenital defects of the diaphragm. *A,* Congenital absence of a major portion of the left leaf of the diaphragm, a relatively uncommon defect. *B,* Three defects, the foramen of Morgagni hernia anteriorly, the foramen of Bochdalek hernia in the posterolateral aspect of the left leaf of the diaphragm, and congenital enlargement of the esophageal hiatus.

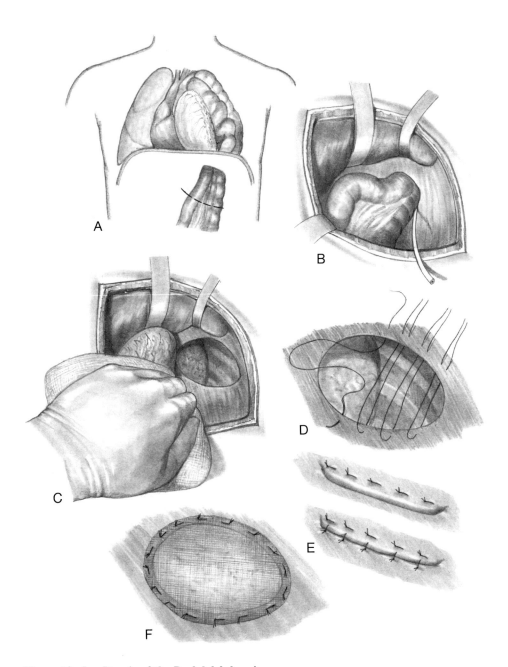

Figure 13–5.   Repair of the Bochdalek hernia.

   A, The structures herniating through the foramen and location of the incision in the subcostal region of the left upper quadrant.

   B, The technique of introducing a catheter into the pleural space, permitting air to enter and dissipating the vacuum, which makes reduction of the viscera easier.

   C, The defect as it appears after all viscera are reduced into the abdominal cavity.

   D, E, The placement of mattress sutures, resulting in a two-layer closure of the defect. This is applicable if there is adequate tissue for direct closure.

   F, The technique using prosthetic materials such as Marlex mesh when the defect is too large for a direct approximation of the diaphragmatic edges.

Selected Reading List

The object of this textbook has been to give a didactic approach to preoperative and postoperative care and to describe surgical procedures. There has been no attempt to place references in the text because of this approach. This reading list is intended to be a primary source reference; it is not meant to be complete or even comprehensive on any subject, but instead attempts to introduce the reader to other published material as a starting point. The reader is advised to make a comprehensive literature search of his or her own and not rely only on these references.

Some of the references are to publications that are out of print but usually available in medical libraries.

Standard Text Material

1. Blades B (ed): Surgical Diseases of the Chest. 3rd Ed. St Louis, CV Mosby, 1974.
2. Frazer RF, Pare JAP: Diagnosis of Diseases of the Chest. 2nd Ed. Philadelphia, WB Saunders Company, 1977.
3. Glenn WWL (ed): Thoracic and Cardiovascular Surgery. 4th Ed. Norwalk, Conn, Appleton-Century-Crofts, 1983.
4. Hinshaw HC, Murray JF: Diseases of the Chest. 4th Ed. Philadelphia, WB Saunders Company, 1980.
5. Hood RM, Boyd AD, Culliford AT: Thoracic Trauma. Philadelphia, WB Saunders Company, 1989.
6. Moore EE, Mattox KL, Feliciano DV: Trauma. 2nd Ed. Norwalk, Appleton-Lange, 1991.
7. Sabiston DC Jr, Spencer FC (eds): Gibbon's Surgery of the Chest. 5th Ed. Philadelphia, WB Saunders Company, 1990.
8. Shields TW (Ed): Mediastinal Surgery. Philadelphia, Lea & Febiger, 1991.
9. Shields TW (ed): General Thoracic Surgery. 4th Ed. Philadelphia, Lea & Febiger, 1993.
10. Spencer H: Pathology of the Lung. 3rd Ed. Philadelphia, WB Saunders Company, 1977.

Preoperative Evaluation

1. Bates DV, Madden PT, Christie RV: Respiratory Function in Disease. 2nd Ed. Philadelphia, WB Saunders Company, 1971.
2. Comroe JH Jr, et al: The Lung. 2nd Ed. Chicago, Year Book Medical Publishers, 1962.

3. Comroe JH Jr: Physiology of Respiration. 2nd Ed. Chicago, Year Book Medical Publishers, 1974.
4. Felson B: Fundamentals of Chest Roentgenology. Philadelphia, WB Saunders Company, 1960.
5. Nunn JF: Applied Respiratory Physiology. 2nd Ed. London, Butterworths, 1977.
6. West JB: Ventilation—Blood Flow and Gas Exchange. 3rd Ed. Philadelphia, JB Lippincott,
7. West JB: Respiratory Physiology: The Essentials. 2nd Ed. Baltimore, Williams & Wilkins, 1979.
8. West JB: Pulmonary Pathophysiology. Baltimore, Williams & Wilkins, 1977.

Postoperative Care

1. Altemeier WA, Burke JF, Pruitt BA, et al: Manual on Control of Infections in Surgical Patients. Philadelphia, JB Lippincott, 1976.
2. Artz CP, Hardy JD (eds): Management of Surgical Complications. 3rd Ed. Philadelphia, WB Saunders Company, 1975.
3. Ashbough EC, Bigelow DB, Petty TH: Acute respiratory distress in adults. Lancet 2:319, 1967.
4. Blaisdell FW, Lewis FR Jr: Respiratory Distress Syndrome of Shock and Trauma. Philadelphia, WB Saunders Company, 1977.
5. Bane RC: Treatment of severe hypoxemia due to the adult respiratory distress syndrome. Arch Intern Med 140:851, 1980.
6. Collins RD: Illustrated Manual of Fluid and Electrolyte Disorders. Philadelphia, JB Lippincott, 1976.
7. Cordell AR, Ellison RG: Complications of Intrathoracic Surgery. Boston, Little, Brown & Co, 1979.
8. Eklind J, Jarnberg PO, Narlander O, et al: Opsscula Medica 1981, Supplementum LIII, Intensive Care IV. New Aspects of Artificial Ventilation. Stockholm, Sweden, 1981.
9. Hardy JD: Critical Surgical Illness. Philadelphia, WB Saunders Company, 1971.
10. Kinney JM, Bendixon HH, Powers SR: Manual of Surgical Intensive Care. Philadelphia, WB Saunders Company, 1977.
11. Kinney JM, Egdahl RH, Zuidema GD: Manual of Preoperative and Postoperative Care. 2nd Ed. Philadelphia, WB Saunders Company, 1971.
12. Kirby RR, Graybar GB: Intermittent mandatory ventilation. Anesthesiol Clin 18:1, 1980.
13. Langston HT, Pantane AM, Melamed M: The Postoperative Chest, Springfield, Ill, Charles C Thomas, 1958.
14. Moore TD, et al: Posttraumatic Pulmonary Insufficiency. Philadelphia, WB Saunders Company, 1969.
15. Murray JE: Mechanisms of acute respiratory failure. Amer Rev Resp Dis 107:115, 1977.
16. Neville WE (ed): Care of the Surgical Cardiopulmonary Patient. Chicago, Year Book Medical Publishers, 1971.
17. Petty TL (ed): Intensive and Rehabilitative Respiratory Care. 3rd Ed. Philadelphia, Lea & Febiger, 1982.

Trauma

1. Arom KV, Richardson JD, Webb G, et al: Subxyphoid pericardial window in patients with suspected pericardial tamponade. Ann Thorac Surg 23:545, 1977.
2. Akins CW, Buckley MJ, Daggett W, et al: Acute traumatic disruption of the thoracic aorta: a ten year experience. Ann Thorac Surg 31:305, 1981.

3. Borrie J: The Management of Emergencies in Thoracic Surgery. New York, Appleton-Century-Crofts, 1958.

4. Brawley RK, Murray GF, Crisler C, et al: Management of wounds of the innominate, subclavian and axillary blood vessels. Surg Gynecol Obstet 131:1130, 1970.

5. Crawford ES, Walaker HSJ III, Saleh SA, et al: Graft replacement of aneurysms in the descending thoracic aorta: results without bypass or shunting. Surgery 89:73, 1981.

6. Daughtry DC (ed): Thoracic Trauma. Boston, Little, Brown & Co, 1980.

7. Grillo HC: Congenital lesions, neoplasms and injuries of the trachea. *In* Sabiston DC Jr, Spencer FC (eds): Gibbon's Surgery of the Chest. 4th Ed. Philadelphia, WB Saunders Company, 1983.

8. Grillo HC: Surgical treatment of post intubation injuries. J Thorac Cardiovasc Surg 78:860, 1979.

9. Hood RM (ed): Management of Thoracic Injuries. Springfield, Ill, Charles C Thomas, 1969.

10. Hood RM, Sloan H: Injuries of the trachea and major bronchi. J Thorac Cardiovasc Surg 38:458, 1959.

11. Kirsch MM, Sloan H: Blunt Chest Trauma. Boston, Little, Brown & Co, 1977.

12. Naclario EA: Chest Injuries: Physiologic Principles and Emergency Management. New York, Grune & Stratton, 1971.

13. Pillay SP, Ward M, et al: Oesophageal ruptures and perforations — a review. Med J Aust 150:246, 1989.

14. Rich NM, Spencer FC: Vascular Trauma. Philadelphia, WB Saunders Company, 1978.

15. Samson PC, Buford TH: Total pulmonary decortication: its evaluation and present concepts of indications and operative technique. J Thorac Cardiovasc Surg 16:127, 1947.

16. Schaff HV, Brawley RR: Operative management of penetrating vascular injuries of the thoracic outlet. Surgery 82:182, 1977.

17. Shires GT, Carrico CJ, Canigaro PC: Shock. Major Problems in Surgery. Philadelphia, WB Saunders Company, 1973.

18. Sugg WL, Rea WJ, Ecker RR, et al: Penetrating wounds of the heart: an analysis of 159 cases. J Thorac Cardiovasc Surg 56:531, 1968.

19. Symbas PN: Traumatic Injuries of the Heart and Great Vessels. Springfield, Ill, Charles C Thomas, 1972.

20. Trinkle JK, Richardson JD, Franz JL, et al: Management of flail chest without mechanical ventilation. Ann Thorac Surg 19:355, 1975.

21. Trinkle JK, Marcus J, Glover FL, et al: Management of the wounded heart. Ann Thorac Surg 17:230, 1974.

22. Urschel HC Jr, Razzuk MA, Wood RE, et al: Esophageal perforation, exclusion and diversion in continuity. Ann Surg 179:587, 1974.

23. Walt AJ (ed): Early Care of the Injured Patient. Philadelphia, WB Saunders Company, 1982.

24. Young CP, Large Sr, et al: Blunt traumatic rupture of the thoracic oesophagus. Thorax 43:794, 1988.

Thoracic Incisions

1. Alley RO: Thoracic incisions and postoperative drainage. *In* Cooper P (ed): Craft of Surgery. London, J&A Churchill, 1964.

2. Becker RM, Munro DD: Transaxillary minithoracotomy: the optimal approach for certain pulmonary and mediastinal lesions. Ann Thorac Surg 22:259, 1976.

3. Overholt RH: Technique of Pulmonary Resection. Springfield, Ill, Charles C Thomas, 1954.

4. Sweet RH: Thoracic Surgery. 2nd Ed. Philadelphia, WB Saunders Company, 1954.
5. Williams VL, Hanlon GL: Transverse median sternotomy incision. Am J Surg 100:799, 1960.

Pulmonary Anatomy

1. Birnbaum GL: Anatomy of the Bronchovascular System: Its Application. Chicago, Year Book Medical Publishers, 1954.
2. Bloomer WC, Liebow AA, and Hales MR: Surgical Anatomy of the Bronchovascular Segments. Springfield, Charles C Thomas, 1960.
3. Boyden EA: Segmental Anatomy of the Lungs. New York, McGraw-Hill, 1955.
4. Jackson CL, Huber JF: Correlated applied anatomy of the bronchial tree and lungs with system nomenclature. Dis Chest 9:319, 1943.

Pulmonary Surgery

1. Adebo OA: Post-operative complications in pulmonary resections. West Afr J Med 8:270, 1989.
2. Allison PR: Intrapericardial approach to the lung root in the treatment of bronchogenic carcinoma by dissection pneumonectomy. J Thorac Cardiovasc Surg 15:99, 1946.
3. Baldwin JC, Mark JP: Treatment of bronchopleural fistula after pneumonectomy. J Thorac Cardiovasc Surg 90:813, 1985.
4. Bayes AJ, Wilson JA, et al: Claggett open-window thoracostomy in patients with empyema who had not undergone pneumonectomy. Can J Surg 30:329, 1987.
5. Beltrami V: Surgical transsternal treatment of bronchopleural fistula postpneumonectomy. Chest 95:379, 1989.
6. Braun J, Allica E, et al: Omental pedicle flap used to treat a bronchopleural fistula after diaphragma-pericardio-pleuropneumonectomy. Thorac Cardiovasc Surg 38:318, 1990.
7. Breyer RH, Jensik RJ: Lung-sparing operations in elderly patients. Ann Thorac Surg 40:636, 1985.
8. Brock R, Whytehead LL: Radical pneumonectomy for bronchial carcinoma. Br J Surg 43:8, 1955–1956.
9. Burch BH, Miller AC: Atlas of Pulmonary Resection. Springfield, Ill, Charles C Thomas, 1954.
10. Carlens C: Mediastinoscopy: a method for inspection and tissue biopsy in the superior mediastinum. Dis Chest 36:343, 1959.
11. Crabbe MM, Patrissi GA, et al: Minimal resection for bronchogenic carcinoma. An update. Chest 99:1421, 1991.
12. Daniels A: A method of biopsy in diagnosing certain intrathoracic diseases. Dis Chest 16:36, 1949.
13. Dartevelle PG, Khalife J, et al: Tracheal sleeve pneumonectomy for bronchogenic carcinoma: report of 55 cases. Ann Thorac Surg 46:68, 1988.
14. Eckersberger F, Moritz E, et al: Treatment of postpneumonectomy empyema. Thorac Cardiovasc Surg 38, 352, 1990.
15. Faber LP: Individual ligation technique for lower lobe lobectomy. Ann Thorac Surg 49:1016, 1990.
16. Frist WH, Mathisen DJ, et al: Bronchial sleeve resection with and without pulmonary resection. J Thorac Cardiovasc Surg 93:350, 1987.
17. Ginsberg RJ, Pearson FG, et al: Closure of chronic postpneumonectomy bronchopleural fistula using the transsternal transpericardial approach. Ann Thorac Surg 47:231, 1989.

18. Gregoire R, Deslauriers J, et al: Thoracoplasty: its forgotten role in the management of nontuberculous postpneumonectomy empyema. Can J Surg 30:343, 1987.

19. Hasse J: Patch-closure of tracheal defects with pericardium/PIFE. A new technique in extended pneumonectomy with carinal resection. Eur J Cardiothorac Surg 4:412, 1990.

20. Hood RM, et al: The use of automatic stapling devices in pulmonary resection. Ann Thorac Surg 16:85, 1973.

21. Jensik RJ, Faber LP, et al: Sleeve lobectomy for bronchogenic carcinoma: the Rush-Presbyterian-St. Luke's Medical Center experience. Int Surg 71:207, 1985.

22. Jensik RJ, Faber LP, Milloy FJ, et al: Segmental resection for lung cancer: a fifteen year experience. J Thorac Cardiovasc Surg 66:563, 1973.

23. Johnson J, Kirby CK: Surgery of the Chest. 3rd Ed. Chicago, Year Book Medical Publishers, 1964.

24. Kaplan DK, Whyte RI, et al: Pulmonary resection using automatic stapling devices. Eur J Cardiothorac Surg 1:152, 1987.

25. Keszler P: Sleeve resection and other bronchoplasties in the surgery of bronchogenic tumors. Int Surg 71:229, 1986.

26. Kirksey JD, et al: Techniques of pulmonary resection. Ann Thorac Surg 9:525, 1970.

27. Mathisen OJ, Grillo HC: Carinal resection for bronchogenic carcinoma. J Thorac Cardiovasc Surg 102:16, 1991.

28. McNeil TM, Chamberlain JM: Diagnostic anterior mediastinoscopy. Ann Thorac Surg 2:533, 1966.

29. Morice RC, Peters EJ. et al: Exercise testing in the evaluation of patients at high risk for complications from lung resection. Chest 101:356, 1992.

30. Mud HJ, VanHouten H, et al: A modified pectoralis muscle flap for closure of postpneumonectomy esophagopleural fistula: technique and results. Ann Thorac Surg 43:359, 1987.

31. Overholt RH: Technique of Pulmonary Resection. Springfield, Ill, Charles C Thomas, 1954.

32. Rusch VW, Piantadosi S, et al: The role of extrapleural pneumonectomy in malignant pleural mesothelioma. A lung cancer study group trial. J Thorac Cardiovasc Surg 102:1, 1991.

33. Sarot TRW, Gilbert L: Extrapleural pneumonectomy and pleurectomy in pulmonary tuberculosis. Thorax 4:173, 1949.

34. Sarsam MA, Moussali H: Technique of bronchial closure after pneumonectomy. J Thorac Cardiovasc Surg 98:220, 1989.

35. Sellman M, Henze A, et al: Extended intrathoracic resection for lung cancer. Follow-up of 49 cases. Scand J Thorac Cardiovasc Surg 21:69, 1987.

36. Shields TW: Pulmonary resections. *In* Shields TW: General Thoracic Surgery. 2nd Ed. Philadelphia, Lea & Febiger, 1983.

37. Shirai T, Amano J, et al: Thoracoscopic diagnosis and treatment of chylothorax after pneumonectomy. Ann Thorac Surg 52:306, 1991.

38. Slinger PD: Anaesthesia for lung resection. Can J Anaesth 37:15, 1990.

39. Sugarbaker DJ, Mentzer SJ: Improved technique for hilar vascular stapling. Ann Thorac Surg 53:165, 1992.

40. Sugarbaker DJ, Heher EC, et al: Extrapleural pneumonectomy, chemotherapy, and radiotherapy in the treatment of diffuse malignant pleural mesothelioma. J Thorac Cardiovasc Surg 102:10, 1991.

41. Sweet RH: Thoracic Surgery. 2nd Ed. Philadelphia, WB Saunders Company, 1954.

42. Toledo J, Roca R, et al: Conservative and bronchoplastic resection for bronchial carcinoid tumors. Eur J Cardiothorac Surg 3:288, 1989.

43. Van-Schil PE, Brutel-de-la-Rivière A, et al: TNM staging and long-term follow-up after sleeve resection for bronchogenic tumors. Ann Thorac Surg 52:1096, 1991.

44. Watanabe Y, Murakami S., et al: The clinical value of high-frequency jet ventilation in major airway reconstructive surgery. Scand J Thorac Cardiovasc Surg 22:227, 1988.
45. Weber J, Grabner D., et al: Empyema after pneumonectomy—empyema window or thoracoplasty? Thorac Cardiovasc Surg 38:355, 1990.
46. Yaman M, Goklen AN, et al: Endoscopic treatment of bronchus stump fistula with fibrin sealant following pneumonectomy. Chest 100:288, 1991.
47. Zollinger RM, Zollinger RM Jr: Atlas of Surgical Operations. Vol II. New York, Macmillan, 1967.

Endoscopy

1. Jackson C, Jackson CL: Bronchoesophagology. Philadelphia, WB Saunders Company, 1950.
2. Stradling P: Diagnostic Bronchoscopy. 4th Ed. Edinburgh, Churchill Livingstone, 1981.

Single Lung Transplantation

1. Cooper JD, Pearson FG, Patterson GA, et al: Technique of successful lung transplantation in humans. J Thorac Cardiovasc Surg 93:173, 1987.
2. Cooper JD: The evolution of techniques and indications for lung transplantation. Ann Surg 212:3, 1990.
3. Dark JH, Patterson GA, Al-Jilaihawi AN, Hsu H, Egan T, Cooper JD: Experimental en bloc double-lung transplantation. Ann Thorac Surg 42:394, 1986.
4. Grossman RF, Frost A, Zamel N, et al: Results of single-lung transplantation for bilateral pulmonary fibrosis. N Engl J Med 322:727, 1990.
5. Hardy JD, Webb WR, Dalton ML, Walker GR: Lung homotransplantation in man. JAMA 186:1065, 1963.
6. International Lung Transplant Registry, Suite 3107 Queeny Tower, One Barnes Hospital Plaza, St. Louis, MO 63110.
7. Todd TR: Lung transplantation. The experience of the Toronto group. Critical Care Report 2:202, 1991.
8. Truloc EP, Egan TM, Kouchoukos NT, et al. Single lung transplantation for severe chronic obstructive pulmonary disease. Chest 96:738, 1989.
9. Veith FJ, Kamholz SL, Mollenkopf FP, Montefusco CM: Lung transplantation 1983. Transplantation 35:271, 1983.

Thoracoscopy

1. Coltharp WH, et al: Videothoracoscopy: Improved technique and expanded indications. Ann Thorac Surg 53:776, 1992.
2. Landreneau RJ: Thorascopic removal of an anterior mediastinal tumor. Ann Thorac Surg 54:142, 1992.
3. Lewis RJ, et al: Imaged thoracic lobectomy: should it be done? Ann Thorac Surg 54:80, 1992.
4. Lewis RJ, et al: Imaged thoracoscopic lung biopsy. Chest 102:60, 1992.
5. LoCicero J: Minimally invasive thoracic surgery, video-assisted surgery and thoracoscopy. Chest 102:330, 1992.
6. Mathisen OJ: Don't get run over by the bandwagon. Editorial, Chest 102:2, 1992.
7. McKneally MT, et al: Statement of the AATS/STS joint committee on thorascopy and video-assisted thoracic surgery. Ann Thorac Surg 54:1, 1992.

8. Wakabayashi, Akio: Expanded applications of diagnostic and therapeutic thoracoscopy. J Thorac Cardiovasc Surg 102:721, 1991.

Mediastinum

1. Grasfield JL, et al: Primary mediastinal neoplasm in infants and children. Ann Thorac Surg 12:179, 1971.
2. Payne WS, Bernatz PE: Surgery of the thymus gland. *In* Shields TW (ed): General Thoracic Surgery. 2nd Ed. Philadelphia, Lea & Febiger, 1983.
3. Sabiston DC Jr: The mediastinum. *In* Sabiston DC Jr, Spencer FC (eds): Gibbon's Surgery of the Chest. 4th Ed. Philadelphia, WB Saunders Company, 1983.
4. Shields TW: General Thoracic Surgery. 2nd Ed. Philadelphia, Lea & Febiger, 1983.
5. Silverman NA, Sabiston DC Jr: Primary tumors and cysts of the mediastinum. Curr Probl Cancer 2:1, 1977.
6. Wychallis AR, Payne WS, Claggett OJ, et al: Surgical treatment of mediastinal tumors: a 40 year experience. J Thorac Cardiovasc Surg 62:379, 1971.

Pleura and Chest Wall

1. Alexander J: The Collapse Therapy of Tuberculosis. Springfield, Ill, Charles C Thomas, 1937.
2. Anderson CV, Philpott GW, Ferguson TB: The treatment of malignant pleural effusions. Cancer 33:916, 1974.
3. Andrews NC: The surgical treatment of chronic empyema. Dis Chest 47:533, 1965.
4. Borrie J: Emergency thoracotomy for massive spontaneous hemopneumothorax. Br Med J 2:16, 1953.
5. Brooks JW: Open thoracotomy in the management of spontaneous hemothorax. Ann Surg 77:798, 1973.
6. Burford TH, Parker EF, Sampson PC: Early pulmonary decortication in the treatment of posttraumatic empyema. Ann Surg 112:163, 1945.
7. Claggett OT, Gelaci JE: A procedure for the management of postpneumonectomy empyema. J Thorac Cardiovasc Surg 45:141, 1963.
8. DeMeester TR: The pleura. *In* Sabiston DC Jr, Spencer FC (eds): Gibbon's Surgery of the Chest. 4th Ed. Philadelphia, WB Saunders Company, 1983.
9. Eloesser L: An operation for tuberculosis empyema. Surg Gynecol Obstet 60:1096, 1935.
10. Findlay CW Jr: The management of the pleural space following partial resection of the lung (especially for tuberculosis). J Thorac Cardiovasc Surg 31:601, 1956.
11. Gregoire R, Deslauriers J, et al: Thoracoplasty: its forgotten role in the management of nontuberculous postpneumonectomy empyema. Can J Surg 30:343, 1987.
12. Horrigan TP, Snow NJ: Thoracoplasty: current application to the infected pleural space. Ann Thorac Surg 50:695, 1990.
13. Jaretzki A III: Role of thoracoplasty in the treatment of chronic empyema. Ann Thorac Surg 52:584, 1991.
14. Konvolinka CW, Olearczyk A: Subphrenic abscess. Curr Probl Surg, Jan 1972, p 1.
15. Langston HT: Thoracoplasty: the how and the why. Ann Thorac Surg 52:1351, 1991.
16. Pate JW: One-stage operation for chronic empyema. Ann Thorac Surg 49:342, 1990.
17. Ravitch MM: Congenital Deformities of the Chest Wall and Their Operative Correction. Philadelphia, WB Saunders Company, 1977.
18. Ravitch MM: Disorders of the sternum and chest wall. *In* Sabiston DC Jr, Spencer FC (eds): Gibbon's Surgery of the Chest. 4th Ed. Philadelphia, WB Saunders Company, 1983.
19. Ravitch MM, Fein R: The changing picture of pneumonia and empyema in infants and children. JAMA 175:1039, 1961.

20. Roos DB: Transaxillary approach for first rib resection to relieve thoracic outlet syndrome. Ann Surg 163:354, 1966.
21. Samson PC: Empyema thoracis. Essentials of present-day management. Ann Thorac Surg 11:210, 1971.
22. Sarot IN: Extrapleural pneumonectomy and pleurectomy in pulmonary tuberculosis. Thorax 4:173, 1949.
23. Schede M: Die behandlung der empyema. Verh Congr Ann Med 9:41, 1890.
24. Takaro T, Scott SM, Bridgman AH, et al: Suppurative disease of the lungs, pleurae and pericardium. Curr Probl Surg 24:1, 1977.
25. Tschopp JM, Evequoz D, et al: Successful closure of chronic BPF by thoracoscopy after failure of endoscopic fibrin glue application and thoracoplasty. Chest 97:745, 1990.
26. Youmans CR Jr, Williams RDM, McMinn MR, et al: Surgical management of spontaneous pneumothorax by bleb ligation and pleural dry sponge abrasion. Ann Surg 120:644, 1970.

Anatomy of the Esophagus

1. DeMeester TR: Surgical anatomy of the esophagus. *In* Shields TW (ed): General Thoracic Surgery. Philadelphia, Lea & Febiger, 1983.

Esophagus

1. Anderson KD: Gastric tube esophagoplasty. Prog Pediatr Surg 19:55, 1986.
2. Bar-Maor JA, Shoshany G, et al: Wide gap esophageal atresia: a new method to elongate the upper pouch. J Pediatr Surg 24:882, 1989.
3. Beasley SW, Auldist AW, et al: Current surgical management of oesophageal atresia and/or tracheo-oesophageal fistula. Aust NZ J Surg 59:707, 1989.
4. Beasley SW, Shann FA, et al: Developments in the management of oesophageal atresia and tracheo-oesophageal fistulas. Med J Aust 150:501, 1989.
5. Belsey R: Mark IV repair of hiatal hernia by transthoracic approach. *In* Glenn WWL, Baue AE, Geha AS, Hammond GL, Laks H (eds): Thoracic and Cardiovascular Surgery. Norwalk, Conn, Appleton-Century-Crofts, 1983.
6. Bishop PJ, Klein MD, et al: Transpleural repair of esophageal atresia without a primary gastrostomy: 240 patients treated between 1951 and 1983. J Pediatr Surg 20:823, 1985.
7. Donnelly RJ, Sastry MR, et al: Oesophagogastrectomy using the end to end anastomotic stapler: results of the first 100 patients. Thorax 40:958, 1985.
8. Ellis FH: Esophagomyotomy by the thoracic approach for esophageal achalasia. Hepatogastroenterology 38:498, 1991.
9. Ellis FH Jr, Olsen AM: Achalasia of the esophagus. Philadelphia, WB Saunders Company, 1969.
10. Ellis FH Jr: Disorders of the esophagus in the adult. *In* Sabiston DC Jr, Spencer (eds): Gibbon's Surgery of the Chest. 4th Ed. Philadelphia, WB Saunders Company, 1983.
11. Fok M, Cheng SW, et al: Pyloroplasty versus no drainage in gastric replacement of the esophagus. Amer J Surg 162:447, 1991.
12. Freeman NV: Colonic interposition. Prog Pediatr Surg 19:73, 1986.
13. Gossot D, Sarfati E, et al: Early blunt esophagectomy in severe caustic burns of the upper digestive tract. Report of 29 cases. J Thorac Cardiovasc Surg 94:188, 1987.
14. Gross R: The Surgery of Infancy and Childhood. Philadelphia, WB Saunders Company, 1953.
15. Gurkan N, Terzioglu T, et al: Transhiatal oesophagectomy for oesophageal carcinoma. Br J Surg 78:1348, 1991.

16. Hagberg S, Rubenson A, et al: Management of long-gap esophagus: experience with end-to-end anastomosis under maximal tension. Prog Pediatr Surg 19:88, 1986.
17. Haight C, Towsley HA: Congenital atresia of the esophagus with tracheoesophageal fistula. Extrapleural ligation of fistula and end-to-end anastomosis of esophageal segments. Surg Gynecol Obstet 76:612, 1943.
18. Halsband H: Esophagus replacement by free, autologous jejunal mucosa transplantation in long-gap esophageal atresia. Prog Pediatr Surg 19:22, 1986.
19. Hankins JR, Attar S, et al: Carcinoma of the esophagus: a comparison of the results of transhiatal versus transthoracic resection. Ann Thorac Surg 47:700, 1989.
20. Hendren WH, Hendren WG: Colon interposition for esophagus in children. J Ped Surg 20:829, 1985.
21. Hill LD, Gelfand M, Bauermeister D: Simplified management of reflux esophagitis with stricture. Ann Surg 172:638, 1970.
22. Holder TM, Ashcroft KW: Esophageal atresia and tracheoesophageal fistula. Curr Probl Surg 1:68, 1966.
23. Howell CG, Davis JB Jr, et al: Primary repair of esophageal atresia: how long a gap? J Pediatr Surg 22:42, 1987.
24. Hyduke JF, Pineda JJ, et al: Severe intraoperative myocardial ischemia following manipulation of the heart in a patient undergoing esophagogastrectomy. Anesthesiology 71:154, 1989.
25. Kaplan DK, Whyte RI, et al: Oesophagogastrectomy using stapling instruments. Eur J Cardiothorac Surg 2:95, 1988.
26. King RM, Pairolero PC, et al: Ivor Lewis esophagogastrectomy for carcinoma of the esophagus: early and late functional results. Ann Thorac Surg 44:119, 1987.
27. Klingman RR, DeMeester TR: Surgery for carcinoma of the thoracic esophagus: Adams and Phemister in perspective. Ann Thorac Surg 46:699, 1988.
28. Little AG, Soriano A, et al: Surgical treatment of achalasia: results with esophagomyotomy and Belsey repair. Ann Thorac Surg 45:489, 1988.
29. MacGillivray DC, Etienne HB, et al: Transhiatal esophagectomy in the management of perforated esophageal cancer. J Milit Med 156:634, 1991.
30. Mannell A, Becker PJ: Evaluation of the results of oesophagectomy for oesophageal cancer. Brit J Surg 78:36, 1991.
31. Mathisen DJ, Grillo HC, et al: Transthoracic esophagectomy: a safe approach to carcinoma of the esophagus. Ann Thorac Surg 45:137, 1988.
32. Mitchell RL: Abdominal and right thoracotomy approach as standard procedure for esophagogastrectomy with low morbidity. J Thorac Cardiovasc Surg 93:205, 1987.
33. Muehrcke DD, Kaplan DK, et al: Anastomotic narrowing after esophagogastrectomy with the EEA stapling device. J Thorac Cardiovasc Surg 97:434, 1989.
34. Myers NA, Beasley SW, et al: Secondary esophageal surgery following repair of esophageal atresia with distal tracheoesophageal fistula. J Pediatr Surg 25:773, 1990.
35. Najem AZ, Neville WE, et al: Unified approach for nonmalignant esophageal lesions using right colon and terminal ileum. A 30-year experience. Am Surg 53:10, 1987.
36. Nissen R, Rosetti J, Stewart R: Twenty years in the management of reflux disease using fundoplication. Chirurgie 48:634, 1977.
37. Page RD, Khalil JF, et al: Esophagogastrectomy via left thoracophrenatomy. Ann Thorac Surg 49:763, 1990.
38. Papachristou DN, Skandalakis P, et al: Total esophagectomy without thoracotomy for cancer. Am Surg 53:587, 1987.
39. Parker EF, Gregory HB: Carcinoma of the esophagus. Current Problems in Surgery. Vol 4. Chicago, Year Book Medical Publishers, 1967.
40. Parrilla-Paricio P, Martinez-deHaro L, et al: Achalasia of the cardia: long-term results of oesophagomyotomy and posterior partial fundoplication. Brit J Surg 77:1371, 1990.
41. Payne WS, Olsen AM: The esophagus. Philadelphia, Lea & Febiger, 1974.

42. Poenaru D, Laberge JM, et al: A more than 25-year experience with end-to-end versus end-to-side repair for esophageal atresia. J Pediatr Surg 26:472, 1991.
43. Postlewait RW: Surgery of the Esophagus. New York, Appleton-Century-Crofts, 1979.
44. Randolf JG: Surgical problems of the esophagus in infants and children. *In* Sabiston DC Jr, Spencer FC (eds): Gibbon's Surgery of the Chest. 4th Ed. Philadelphia, WB Saunders Company, 1983.
45. Scott HW Jr, DeLozier JB III, et al: Surgical management of esophageal achalasia. South Med J 78:1309, 1985.
46. Shaul DB, Schwartz MZ, et al: Primary repair without routine gastrostomy is the treatment of choice for neonates with esophageal atresia and tracheoesophageal fistula. Arch Surg 124:1188, 1989.
47. Sillen U, Hagberg S, et al: Management of esophageal atresia: review of 16 years' experience. J Pediatr Surg 23:805, 1988.
48. Spitz L, Kiely E, et al: Esophageal atresia: five year experience with 148 cases. J Pediatr Surg 22:103, 1987.
49. Stipa S, Fegiz G, et al: Heller-Belsey and Heller-Nissen operations for achalasia of the esophagus. Surg Gynecol Obstet 170:212, 1990.
50. Stone MM, Fonkalsrud EW, et al: Esophageal replacement with colon interposition in children. Ann Surg 203:346, 1986.
51. Templeton JM Jr, Templeton JJ, et al: Management of esophageal atresia and tracheoesophageal fistula in the neonate with severe respiratory distress syndrome. J Pediatr Surg 20:394, 1985.
52. Valente A, Brereton RJ, et al: Esophageal replacement with whole stomach in infants and children. J Pediatr Surg 22:913, 1987.

Diaphragm

1. Garver L: Congenital diaphragmatic hernia. South Med J 67:59, 1974.
2. Gross R: The Surgery of Infancy and Childhood. Philadelphia, WB Saunders Company, 1953.
3. Hill LD: Paraesophageal hernia. *In* Sabiston DC Jr, Spencer FC (eds): Gibbon's Surgery of the Chest. 4th Ed. Philadelphia, WB Saunders Company, 1983.
4. Hood RM: Traumatic diaphragmatic hernia. Ann Thorac Surg 12:311, 1971.
5. Shochal SJ, Naeye RR, et al: Congenital diaphragmatic hernia—new concept in management. Ann Surg 190:332, 1979.
6. Skinner DB: Esophageal hiatal hernia. *In* Sabiston DC Jr, Spencer FC (eds): Gibbon's Surgery of the Chest. 4th Ed. Philadelphia, WB Saunders Company, 1983.
7. Tharnas TV: Congenital eventration of the diaphragm. Ann Thorac Surg 10:180, 1970.

Index

Page numbers in *italics* indicate illustrations; pages followed by "t" indicate tables.